The Platelet
and its
Disorders

To A. E. McGuinness and C. R. B. Blackburn,
who introduced me to
clinical medicine and platelets.

The Platelet and its Disorders

Barry G. Firkin

Chairman of Medicine
Monash University, Alfred Hospital
Victoria, Australia

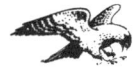 SPRINGER-SCIENCE+BUSINESS MEDIA, B.V.

British Library Cataloguing in Publication Data

Firkin, Barry G.
  The platelet and its disorders.
  1. Blood platelets
  I. Title
    612'.117   QP97

ISBN 978-94-011-8119-8   ISBN 978-94-011-8117-4 (eBook)
DOI 10.1007/978-94-011-8117-4

Library of Congress Cataloging in Publication Data

Firkin, Barry G., 1930–
  The platelet and its disorders.
  Includes bibliographies and index.
  1. Blood platelet disorders. I. Title.
[DNLM: 1. Blood platelets—Physiology. 2. Blood
platelet disorders. WH 300 F523p]
RC647.B5F57 1984   616.1'5   84–891
  ISBN 978-94-011-8119-8

Copyright © 1984 Springer Science+Business Media Dordrecht
Originally published by MTP Press Limited in 1984
Softcover reprint of the hardcover 1st edition 1984

Typesetting by Georgia Origination, Liverpool

Contents

Preface

The aim of this book is to introduce the medical student, recent medical graduates involved in postgraduate training and physicians in practice to the role of the platelet in physiology and disease. It is not intended to be an encyclopaedic review of all the literature over the past few decades, but largely represents a personal account, and although resultant prejudices occur, an attempt has been made to emphasize to the reader areas of doubt, and point the way to other sources which may explore these questions more fully in selected references at the end of each chapter. I acknowledge the help of my secretaries, Ms Carolyn Harvey and Mrs Marjorie Brown without whom the book would never have been started, let alone completed. Some illustrations and figures were made by Mr W. Shepherd of Monash University and Ms A. Leaman of the Alfred Hospital. I am indebted to Mrs E. Hagon who read and corrected a number of the chapters, and for the constant help through discussion and debate with my two close collaborators in research, Dr Margaret Howard and Dr Sharron Pfueller. Dr Siew Choong, Mrs Maureen Broadway and Ms Ilona Lakatos documented the methods used in our laboratory to study platelets as outlined in the Appendix. I acknowledge research funding from the National Health and Medical Research Fund of Australia, the Life Assurance Fund of Australia, The Victorian Anti Cancer Council, The National Heart Foundation of Australia and the Alfred Hospital and Monash University Research Funds for support for my investigations over the past twelve years.

In conclusion I must thank my wife Ruth with whom I corrected the proofs.

Barry G. Firkin

1
Introduction

As multicellular organisms developed from their unicellular forebears in the seas and/or ponds on earth, an evolutionary train of events occurred to aid survival. This revolved around essential mechanisms of repair, nutrition and ultimately defence against foreign predators. Initial life forms consisted of a colony of similar cells bathed in their surrounding water milieu, from which they absorbed their nutrients. With time specialization occurred, so that some cells became capable of movement to sites where trauma had resulted in a fracture or tear of the multicellular colony, and these cells affected a reunion to reconstitute the integrity of the organism. Such cells probably developed humoral components in their cytoplasm, which on release following secretion or the cells' rupture could aid in such repairs. These cells were the forebears of the platelets and the fibroblasts. Increase in the size of multicellular organisms rapidly produced problems of nutrition which became difficult to sustain by the simple process of diffusion from the organism's gaseous and/or liquid environs. Specialized systems had to be developed to ingest and digest food, to enable movement to capture food, an internal circulation to distribute the gaseous and nutritional elements to all parts of the organism, and ultimately to ensure defence against physical injury or attack by other invading organisms.

The mammalian circulation is a system consisting of structural elements which not only act as conduits for blood, which contains the body's cellular and humoral elements concerned with nutrition, repair and defence, but is also specialized in some areas to enable gaseous exchange (the lungs) to eliminate waste products (the kidney) and to maintain circulatory flow (the heart). Socratic argument could reason that these vessels would not merely be passive, but would be able to actively contribute to these basic functions of the circulation, and this has been amply supported by work over the past years which has shown vessels to play an important role, both from a structural and metabolic view, to the maintenance of the integrity of the circulation to all parts of the body. The two major areas which have so far been identified in this regard are firstly, the ability of the vasculature to set up collateral systems to bypass areas of block and to establish new supplies to endangered tissue, and secondly the properties of the endothelial cells lining the wall and their metabolic role in prevention of blockages occurring in the system which would result in the death of tissue supplied by the vessel.

The platelet is a cell evolved to maintain the integrity of the vascular compartment and, as would be expected, has an intimate association with other humoral and cellular elements in the blood concerned with repair, defence and nutrition, although its functional attributes and properties are more important for some aspects compared to others. Nonetheless, it should not be thought of as a cell in isolation, it has a particular affinity and integration with cellular elements of the vessel wall and humoral elements concerned with the maintenance, surveillance and repair of vascular integrity and more peripherally with the inflammatory response and the body's defence systems.

Three fluid phase systems have been identified in blood which appear intimately interrelated, and which have some striking similarities. One is that of blood coagulation wherein the platelet has a most important role and intimate connection, whilst the others concern inflammatory response and body defence mechanisms, namely the complement and kinin systems. All three systems rely on complicated interactions of enzyme precursors which are interlocked and perhaps interdependent for optimal efficiency. These fluid and cellular body defence mechanisms have been identified in most species studied. The degree to which they contribute to the body's defence seems to vary, but in all submammalian species there is a cell, which has a similar role to the platelet, called the thrombocyte. This cell is morphologically strikingly different to the platelet since it is nucleated, often has only a thin rim of cytoplasm, and is difficult to distinguish from a small lymphocyte, although in some species, e.g. the chick, it possesses a characteristic inclusion body. The basic properties of this cell and the platelets are similar, and since they exist from teleost to reptilia and aves, would seem to be fundamentally essential for this cell's function. These properties are:

(1) The ability to stick to foreign surfaces and traumatized vessels,
(2) The ability to stick to one another, i.e. aggregate,
(3) Their ability to take up certain foreign particles, e.g. virus or latex particles.

While the importance of the first two properties can be readily understood from current theories of haemostasis (v. infra), the role of the third in the function of the thrombocyte or platelet is still a mystery. In view of its universal presence in thrombocytes in all species so far examined, including mammalian platelets, it would seem likely that it has some major import or may be related in some inseparable way with one of the other two functions of the cell (see Glanzmann disease).

2

ORIGIN OF THE PLATELET

In man the platelet is produced in the cytoplasm of a cell called the megakaryocyte, which is a large cell most commonly located in the haematopoietic tissue in the bone marrow. This cell may also be seen in capillaries in lung and in other sites where haematopoiesis occurs embryologically, such as the liver and spleen. In the latter instances, such a location is usually associated with some disease state such as myelofibrosis.

The megakaryocyte is an unusual cell because it is polyploid, and to achieve this undergoes a number of nuclear divisions without the cytoplasm of the cell dividing — termed *endomitosis*. Morphologically megakaryocytes are divided into three types which reflect the degree of polyploidy and maturity of the cell. Type I megakaryocyte or megakaryoblast is a cell $15\,\mu m$ in diameter, and is largely constituted of a nucleus and a small rim of deep blue cytoplasm. The ploidy of the nucleus is usually between $4n$ and $8n$. The Type II megakaryocyte or basophilic megakaryocyte is a larger cell, 20–$30\,\mu m$ in diameter, with a relatively higher cytoplasm to nuclear ratio (1:1), whose cytoplasm is usually blue with Romanowsky stains and whose nuclear ploidy ranges up to $64n$. Type III megakaryocyte or granular megakaryocyte is the classical mature megakaryocyte whose cytoplasm to nuclear ratio is approximately 3:1, and which has an overall size of somewhere between 30 and $50\,\mu m$. The cytoplasm is pinker in colour, and in it can be seen the granules and inclusions which are characteristic of platelets. The nucleus has a ploidy which again ranges up to $64n$. Both Type II and III megakaryocytes have a similar range of ploidy and both produce platelets (see Table 1.1). Morphological studies suggest that these platelets are produced by a cleaving of the cytoplasm of the cell, rather as one would tear a postage stamp from a stamp booklet, and arise from protuberances of the cell cytoplasm projecting into the venous sinuses of the bone marrow. One proposal is that this occurs along a membrane system which is found in the megakaryocytes' cytoplasm termed the demarcation membrane system, and this would account for the doubling or trebling of the surface membrane needed to produce the numbers of platelets from a single megakaryocyte. An alternative proposal is that the

Table 1.1 (After Penington). Approximate distribution of ploidy of megakaryocytes *Type I, II and III in human bone marrow*

Ploidy	Percentage	Platelets produced
$4n$	1%	*Dense*
$8n$	16%	Large platelet with high granule count and little intracellular
$16n$	66%	membrane.
$32n$	16%	*Light*
$64n$	1%	Small platelets with few granules and plentiful intracellular membrane synthesized during endomitosis.

3

demarcation membrane system is in fact an invaginated membrane system, which in response to the appropriate stimuli becomes evaginated to form the long thin megakaryocyte cytoplasmic processes, these may protrude into the intravascular spaces by a mechanism similar in principle to platelet shape change (Figure 2.2). The open canalicular system in the platelet is perhaps a residue of the so-called demarcation membrane system. In some instances a larger portion of cytoplasm containing many unseparated platelets may be detached into the vascular stream, and the individual cells separated at distal sites, either in the bloodstream itself or in capillaries, lungs or spleen. In other instances the megakaryocyte may enter the circulation and lodge in the lungs where its cytoplasm may fragment to produce platelets. Some authorities estimate that between 20 and 50% of the circulatory platelet mass may be derived in this fashion. Following the platelets' entry into the circulation they remain there, like the red cell, until their death when they are thought to be removed by tissue macrophages in the reticulo-endothelial system. Since most studies put the average lifespan of a platelet in man as being between 8 and 10 days, each individual cell would be expected to traverse the circulatory system on many occasions, but how long cells spend in secluded areas of the circulation such as the sinusoidal system of the spleen, is not known. Microscopic observations in animals show that in blood flowing in the arterial vessels, platelets occupy a position between the centrally placed stream of red cells and the more peripheral white cells. The latter roll along the vessel wall like a number of cartwheels. Artificial model systems would suggest that vigorous jet streams, with or without eddy currents, around narrowings in vessels could result in the formation of platelet aggregates thereby precipitating thrombus formation in the arteries. Similarly, the arterial jet streaming could account for some of the dramatic clinical thrombotic problems which occur on the arterial side of the system, namely cerebral thrombosis and coronary occlusion.

Two major functions have been identified for the platelet – one is to support the normal integrity and physiology of the vessel wall; the other is to act as a police force to patrol the vasculature, and should any interruption or damage be located to pinpoint it by sticking to it and forming an aggregate around which coagulation occurs and repair is aided by such cells as the fibroblasts. In man the platelet count is maintained somewhere between 150 and $350 \times 10^9/l$. Taking the platelet lifespan as 10 days, and the platelet count to be $250 \times 10^9/l$ with a blood volume of 5 litres, approximately 125×10^9 platelets are produced per day. The mechanisms by which the numbers of platelets produced by megakaryocytes are controlled remain uncertain. A postulated hormone thrombopoietin, is a poorly defined plasma protein which stimulates platelet production, and which is increased in activity when the platelet count is lowered by such methods as plateletpheresis or the injection of platelet antibodies. Artificially increasing the platelet count by platelet transfusion has also been shown to reduce the numbers of platelets produced, but again the mechanism by which this is achieved is unknown. Although it has been felt for some time that platelets contribute to vascular integrity it has only been recently that apparently convincing evidence has been offered in support of this. This is based on animal studies in which the animal has been rendered thrombocytopenic either by irradiation or the use of platelet antibodies. Subsequent electron microscopic examination of the vasculature following exposure to agents such as thorotrast has shown that the thrombocytopenic animal's vessels are readily penetrated by thorotrast, and that the tight junctions between the endothelial cells become less evident. Such changes may be lessened by the exhibition of drugs such as prednisolone. Other workers have not been able to reproduce this work. The idea that platelets might in some way be continuously contributing to vascular integrity gave rise to the suggestion that platelets might be removed from the circulation in a random fashion rather than by senescence. Analysis of platelet survival data in the late 1950s and early 1960s led to a consensus view that the most important factor in the platelet's lifespan was age, and that random intravascular destruction of platelets was unlikely in physiological states. This is supported today by the lack of evidence of a free specific-platelet-protein in plasma such as β-thromboglobulin or platelet factor 4 (*v. infra*) which can be readily identified in situations where intravascular destruction of platelets has occurred, such as disseminated intravascular coagulation. In addition, there is no prolongation of platelet lifespan in people with normal platelet survival who are fully anti-coagulated. The interpretation of lifespan data has usually been based on there being only one type of platelet population. In 1965 Webber and Firkin examined the effects of osmotic shocks on platelets, and found that two morphological types could be distinguished by electron microscopy following either hypo-osmotic or hyper-osmotic shock. One type was highly crenated in appearance, had a very well developed surface connecting system, and was darker than the second type which appeared blown up and light but still contained some granules. Serial section showed that these appearances were consistent in an individual cell, and it was therefore suggested that there might be two different types of platelets in the circulation which could be due to either:

(1) Ageing, or
(2) Different types of platelets with possibly different functional attributes.

When platelet sizing techniques became available it was appreciated that there could be considerable differences in platelet sizes, and that there were some genetic characteristics, i.e. people from the Mediterranean area usually seemed to have bigger platelets than Caucasians. The introduction of density gradient techniques by Karpatkin (1969) demonstrated differing populations of platelets which he believed to result primarily from an ageing process, the lighter platelets being the younger and the cells becoming more dense as they grew older. He supported this contention by pulse labelling experiments using [75]Se (selenomethionine). This was supported by another group employing radioactive ^{51}Cr and another with ^{35}S. It was pointed out that density is related to the presence of dense granules, and after the release reaction (*v. infra*) platelets become lighter and their density may reflect previous platelet activation, perhaps, therefore, one might expect old platelets to be less dense, i.e. the reverse of the above. Penington *et al.* (1976) believes a more likely explanation of the differing subsets of platelets is that populations of platelets are derived from megakaryocytes of varying ploidy, those with the lower ploidy producing the larger dense platelets containing the most granules and the higher ploidy producing the smaller and lighter platelets (see Table 1.1). This would envisage a whole family of circulating platelets of differing size with similar lifespans. The megakaryocyte does not divide, but the membrane produced during nuclear division is increased intracellularly to produce an extensive and highly ramified surface connecting system. The less dense platelets contain fewer granules, have a much higher content of membrane and a more extensive surface connecting system. They, therefore, may be more important for adhesion or in providing fibrillar bayonet type platelets important in the interaction with other cells and fibrin (*v. infra*). These platelets are derived from megakaryocytes with higher ploidy, 32 n–64 n (Table 1.1). It would be interesting to know whether the distribution of ploidy in megakaryocytes was different in the Mediterranean races who produce larger platelets, but so far this information is not available.

The role of the spleen in the physiology of the platelet has been much debated over the years. At one stage it was proposed that it might secrete hormones which were important in the stimulation or inhibition of platelet production. The present view is that the spleen acts as a filter, perhaps retaining the stickier and larger of the platelets to form a 'pool' of between 10 and 20% of the total platelet population in the vascular system. The presence of this pool was postulated because it was noted that there was a difference in the percentage of labelled platelets recovered after infusion in patients with splenomegaly secondary to portal hypertension compared to normal people. It was further found that such patients with splenomegaly had a yield following infusion of radioactive platelets of only 4% which following splenectomy rose to 50% (Firkin, 1963). This was confirmed by more definitive studies showing that the platelets in the spleen were available to the circulation (Aster, 1966) and that platelets could be recovered from spleens removed following splenectomy by direct perfusion (Penny *et al.*, 1966). Under pathological conditions of splenic enlargement, the pool may be dramatically increased, so that in some instances the spleen may contain seven times the number of platelets circulating in the blood. This is most classically seen in congestive splenomegaly secondary to portal hypertension, the peripheral blood platelet count will appear to be reduced to approximately $\frac{1}{2}$ to $\frac{1}{3}$ normal but the overall mass of platelets in the body, because of the accumulation in the spleen, remains the same.

The spleen in some instances may act as a safety mechanism to prevent

6

active or sticky platelets entering the circulation; there is an increased incidence of thromboses reported after splenectomies in numerous clinical situations, especially in patients who have had splenectomy for hereditary haemolytic situations which are not completely remedied. In these circumstances it may be as much a result of an overall increase in platelet count rather than a circulation of platelets which are 'stickier than normal'.

References

ASTER, R. H. (1966). Pooling of platelets in the spleen: role in pathogenesis of 'hypersplenic' thrombocytopenia. *J. Clin. Invest.*, **45**, 645

FIRKIN, B. G. (1963). The platelet. *Aust. Ann. Med.*, **12**, 3

KARPATKIN, S. (1969). Heterogeneity of human platelets. I. Metabolic and kinetic evidence suggestive of young and old platelets. *J. Clin. Invest.*, **48**, 1073

PENINGTON, D. G., STREATFIELD, K. and ROXBURGH, A. E. (1976). Megakaryocytes and the heterogeneity of circulating platelets. *Br. J. Haematol.*, **34**, 639

PENNY, R., ROZENBERG, M. C. and FIRKIN, B. G. (1966). The splenic platelet pool. *Blood*, **27**, 1

RADLEY, J. M. and HALLER, C. J. (1982). The demarcation membrane system of the megakaryocyte: A misnomer. *Blood*, **60**, 213

WEBBER, A. J. and FIRKIN, B. G. (1965). Two populations of platelets. *Nature*, **205**, 1332

2
Morphology of the platelet

When examining peripheral blood, either with phase-contrast illumination or a fixed film and a Romanowsky stain, the smallest elements seen are platelets. These cells usually range from 1 to 3 μm in diameter, although an occasional larger cell up to 5 μm may be seen. With higher magnification a central area is seen, termed the granulomere because it contains granules, and a peripheral clearer area called the hyalomere. When wet preparations are examined by phase-contrast the granules move within the cell. If a fixed film has been obtained from a finger prick, rather than from venous anticoagulated blood, clumps of platelets are observed due to the triggering of platelet aggregation following the tissue trauma and glass contact. Artifacts may occur in the platelets' appearance if the blood is collected into anticoagulants and allowed to stand for any length of time. This is particularly so when the anticoagulant used is ethylene diamine tetra-acetic acid (EDTA) in which the platelets swell on incubation. Studies of recalcification of platelet-rich plasma using phase-contrast microscopy showed a rapid change in shape from disc to a spiny sphere and the early appearance of long thin filaments with aggregation into masses of cells which coalesce and lose the granules, and from these radiate strands of fibrin. This phenomenon was called viscous metamorphosis, but examination by electron microscopy shows that each individual cell retains its integrity, and that the changes observed by the light microscope reflect both the release reaction (*v. infra*) and the redistribution of the cells' organelles during platelet aggregation as well as changes in the platelets' shape.

Figure 2.1 is a diagrammatic representation of the platelet viewed in coronal and longitudinal section by transmission electron microscopy. The cell is bound by a typical unit membrane consisting of a phospholipid bilayer, on the external surface of which is glycoprotein and protein components with the internal surface lined by protein components alone. In this trilaminar structure the glycoprotein surface is quite dense when it is viewed with stains such as

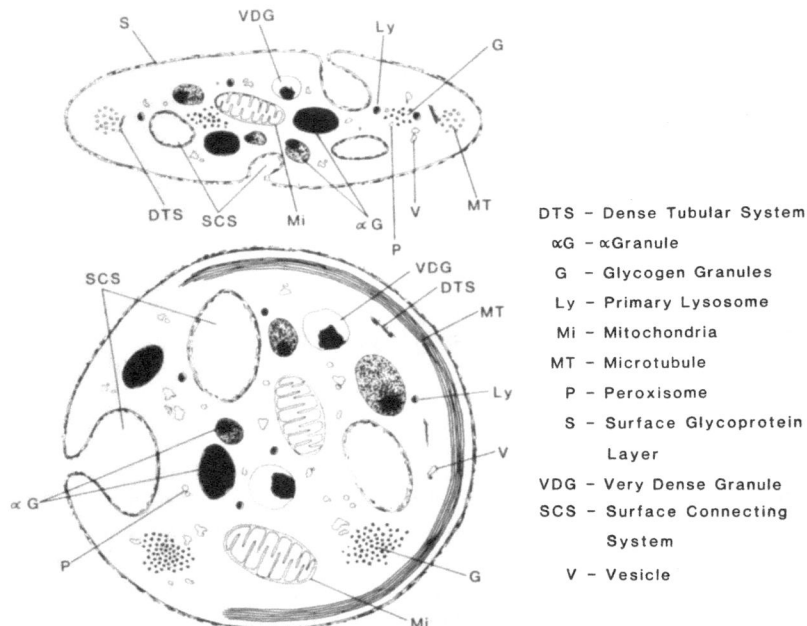

Figure 2.1 Diagrammatic representation of longitudinal (above) and coronal (below) section of the platelet seen by transmission electron microscopy

ruthenium red, giving the platelet an atmosphere of some 20–40 nm. There are lake-like areas in the cell's interior which are also lined by glycoprotein, and which are believed to connect to the surface through a continuous canalicular system called the surface connecting system (see Figure 2.1). The electron micrographs of cells which have been either incubated in EDTA or with a proteolytic enzyme such as trypsin demonstrate a complex canalicular system which interlinks the lakes of the cell with each other and with other sectors of the surface connecting system (SCS), and in some instances platelet granules (*v. infra*) are contained within this system. How much of the SCS is freely connected to plasma and therefore part of the cell's surface is conjectural, but inert particles such as thorotrast are able to pass along it to finally lodge in the α-granules (*v. infra*) of the cell. Immediately subjacent to the unit membrane fibrillar components of the cell can be recognized, which range from 5 to 6 nm in width. In disrupted platelets two types of filaments have been distinguished, one 6 nm in width and resembling actin filaments varying in length up to 1–2 μm. These were found to react with high molecular weight myosin to form arrow head complexes, supporting the contention that these were actin filaments. The other filaments have a width which varies in the central part from 8 to 18 nm and these correspond to myosin. These filaments were often closely associated in disrupted platelets. Actin comprises 10% of the platelet protein, whereas only 1% is myosin. It is likely that the filamentous structures seen in the intact cell are important from the viewpoint of the cell's contractability. The polymerization of these filamentous actin and myosin components is thought to be induced when the cell is activated, and to result in the extended filaments which have been termed filopodia when the platelet changes from disc to spiny sphere (Figure 2.2). These filopodia are composed largely of actin and attach to fibrin. Although the cell is relatively small the extensive ramifications of the SCS give it a potentially very large surface area. On stimulation individual platelets can project fine filaments up to 10 μm in length, termed sword or bayonet forms by earlier workers, and it has been postulated that this is accompanied by a deepening and opening up of the SCS; others conclude that activation of the platelet's contractile protein causes an increased pressure which propels long pseudopodia, composed largely of actin, which join with fibrin strands and on retraction cause clot retraction (Figure 2.2).

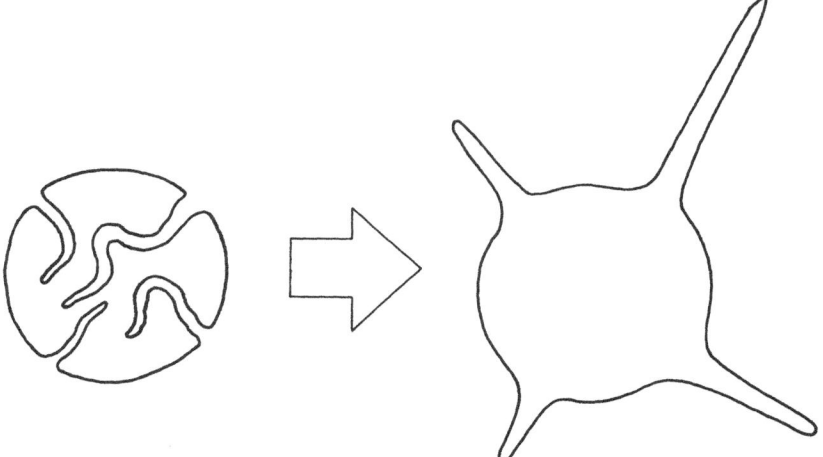

Figure 2.2 Platelet activation changes the cell from a disc to 'spiny' sphere in a few seconds after a stimulus perhaps by eversion of the SCS as illustrated here

Also situated in the peripheral area of the cell are the microtubules which consist of 5–20 bundles placed in parallel circumferentially around the cell, and appearing in longitudinal section as circular structures at the apices of the disc some 20–25 nm in diameter (*see* Figure 2.1). Some believe that the microtubules are a continuous single structure which is wound in a spiral fashion around the platelet's circumference. Microtubules are made of protein dimer subunits with a molecular weight of approximately 110 000. Both subunits contain guanosine triphosphate (GTP) on a specific binding site, i.e. 2 moles of GTP per dimer, these nucleotides are thought to stabilize the protein's configuration. This protein is termed tubulin and when denatured produces a monomer of 55 000–60 000 daltons. It is postulated that *in vivo* an equilibrium exists between the monomeric units and the fully polymerized microtubules, and that *colchicine* binds to a specific site and prevents polymerization, shifting the balance towards solubilization of the micro-tubules. One colchicine molecule binds to one dimer. *Vinblastine* on the other hand binds to a different site and aggregates the microtubule protein, breaking down the microtubules into subunits and causing inclusions of hexagonally packed crystals. Studies by Behnke (1970) and White (1973) have shown that microtubules are important in the retention of the platelets' disc shape and that colchicine causes sphering of the cell by disrupting the microtubules. Cooling of the cell results in a loss of these structures and is concomitantly associated with a sphering effect and pseudopod formation; this can be corrected by re-warming the cell when the microtubular systems reappear, initially in a random fashion but in time the cell resumes its disc shape and with it the radial arrangement of the microtubules becomes evident. The effect of cold on the cell shape can be prevented by raising the platelet's cyclic AMP (cAMP) levels either using prostaglandin, e.g. PGE_1, or by adding cAMP. Incubation of normal platelets for 60 minutes, with either PGE_1 or cAMP, increases the number of marginal microtubules. Glycolysis is important in the retention of the cell shape, since the exhibition of the inhibitor sodium fluoride does not disrupt the microtubules but results in alterations in the cell's shape. Microtubules may also be important in the release reaction since it has been shown that the exposure of cells to colchicine is associated with a loss of second wave platelet aggregation which is dependent on the release reaction. This corresponds with microtubular function in other cells where it is related to ordered movement of material within the cells and sometimes release, e.g. insulin release from the cells in the Islets of Langerhans.

A pharmacological agent cytochalasin B has been shown to inhibit a number of contractile events in other cells, and was found to abolish clot retraction when added to platelet-rich plasma. When its effects on platelet aggregation were examined it was seen that shape change was inhibited and the first wave of aggregation was greatly inhibited (*v. infra*), but after delay the release reaction occurred normally and normal second phase aggregation ensued. Curiously, platelets pre-exposed to cytochalasin B and then cooled to 4 °C preserved their shape, and even after 60 min incubation the microtubular systems remained intact in 25% of the cells, suggesting that inhibition of the microfilaments had inhibited the effect of cooling in disrupting microtubules and that microfilaments may play a role in microtubule assembly and disruption.

Another tubular system which has been called the dense tubular system (DTS) contains an amorphous relatively electron dense substance in a narrow organelle, varying from 40 to 60 nm in diameter. Its location in the cell varies, but one is usually seen close to the marginal microtubules (Figure 2.1). This structure is believed by White and others to be analogous to the sarcomere in muscle; it contains a high concentration of calcium which can be readily mobilized when required by the cell and may be central to the interaction of the release reaction and aggregation (*v. infra*). Scattered throughout the cell are groups of vesicles and vacuoles which may represent highly ramified conduits connecting the cell's membranous systems or may simply be individual organelles. Recently one group of such vesicles which are 17.5–25 nm in diameter have been shown to contain acid phosphatase and could be primary lysosomes. Another organelle which also appears as a vesicle, unless special stains are employed, is the peroxisome which contains catalase.

There are at least three types of 'granules' present in the granulomere, *viz.* the α-granule, the very dense granule, as well as mitochondria and possibly others. The most frequently observed characteristic of the mammalian platelet is the α-granule. They usually measure 30–50 nm in diameter, and on occasions may be seen to lie within another membranous system. They are commonly oval or rod-shaped granules which are finely granular on transmission electron microscopy, and which sometimes possess an eccentrically placed darker nucleoid structure. Some reside in the surface connecting system. α-granules contain fibrinogen, factor VIII antigen, fibronectin, β thromboglobulin, platelet factor 4, thrombospondin and the platelet growth factor (mitogenic factor). Whether all these components are in each individual granule or whether there are subtypes of granules awaits further investigation.

Another very typical structure in the platelet is the so called very dense granule or δ-granule. This is smaller in size than the α-granule (25–30 nm in diameter) and consists, as its name implies, of a very electron dense area which usually is an eccentrically placed black sphere set in a circular membranous structure with occasional streaks of homogeneous material radiating out towards the periphery from this central dense core. This contains heavy concentrations of calcium, 5-hydroxytryptamine (serotonin), adenosine triphosphate (ATP), adenosine diphosphate (ADP) and other catecholamines. The numbers of these structures vary in mammalian species. There is, for example, a very high concentration in rabbits and this relates to the high serotonin content of this animal's platelets. The serotonin is thought to be held in a micellar complex with Ca^{2+} and ATP. The ADP which is concentrated in these structures is relatively metabolically inert, being stored in the dense granules until the cell is excited and undergoes the release reaction.

The mitochondria have their characteristic structure, but are somewhat smaller than in other cells. Another striking feature are clumps of glycogen granules (*see* Figure 2.1).

When the endothelial surface of an arterial vessel is damaged in a living animal, the platelets are seen to adhere to the surface denuded of endothelial cells, initially retaining their disc shapes and remaining as a lining of a single layer of cells. This is thought to result from an interaction between the platelet surface, von Willebrand factor in plasma and the underlying exposed microfibrils or collagen. If the surface is redamaged, the initial layer of platelets is followed by the formation of a clump of platelets and coagulation may or may not ensue. Studies with the scanning electron microscope show platelet aggregates and red cells enmeshed in fibrin threads much like a disordered spider's web with tendrils from platelets adhering to individual fibrin strands.

The phenomenon of platelet aggregation has been repeatedly studied morphologically in *in vitro* systems with platelet-rich plasma where aggregation is initiated by the addition of calcium, collagen, adrenalin and thrombin to name a few of the more commonly used reagents. Of these, adrenalin is unusual in that shape change is not induced, but the platelets aggregate retaining their oval to disc like shapes. With the remaining substances the first change that is observed is that of shape change, in which the cell becomes rounded with small spiky protuberances (Figure 2.2), although some cells also develop long thin pseudopodia which may be several μm in length (sword forms). Following this shape change, the platelets become closely associated with apparent movement of their contained granules towards the centre of the cell with a resultant wider hyalomere. White (1973) initially proposed that this was due to a contraction of the microtubules, since these circumferentially arranged bundles follow the granular structures towards the centre of the cell, leaving a wider hyalomere. However, Behnke (1970) has shown that this central movement of the granules occurs even when the microtubules have been disrupted, e.g. by exposure to cold, and that this movement is resultant upon activation of the contractile actin and myosin elements of the cell.

Next there is a closer approximation of a number of the cells which are linked by bridges between their outer glycoprotein surfaces. Probably coinciding with the release reaction, the adjacent cell membranes of the platelets become very closely aligned and many platelets appear to lose their δ-granules. Alpha granules may still be seen, but they are less in number. If the aggregate is examined some 30 minutes later, the appearance is of closely intertwined cells of various sizes and shapes and often the only remaining granules are mitochondria. The margin of the cells in these *in vitro* platelet aggregates is retained, but *in vivo* the individual cell membranes are probably eventually broken down by enzymes released intracellularly by lysosomes, and the agregate attaches to the vessel wall and is covered by endothelial cells growing in from the margin. It is thought by some that this is one mechanism by which early lipid deposits occur in the vessel wall as the platelets are broken down by their lysosomal enzymes.

References

BEHNKE, O. (1970). Effects of some chemicals on blood platelet microtubules, platelet shape and some platelet functions *in vitro*. *Scand. J. Haematol.*, **7**, 123

BEHNKE, O. (1968). Electron microscopical observations on the surface coating of human blood platelets. *J. Ultrastr. Res.*, **24**, 51

WHITE, J.G. (1973). Identification of platelet secretion in the electron microscope. *Ser. Haematol.* VI, **3**, 429

3
Biochemistry and metabolism of the platelet

THE PLATELET MEMBRANE

The cell's membrane is its window to the outside world and determines its affinity for other cells, tissues and fluids. Through it must be transmitted the signals which set in train the appropriate physiological responses. Currently there is widespread interest on the nature of the substances or chemicals which may stimulate a cell (the best studied being the hormones), the nature of the receptor on the cell surface, the mechanism of the transmission of the signal and the train of events leading to the cell's response. It may be anticipated that each family of cells will have an individual and specialized cell surface, even though the overall structural pattern may be similar. The individuality of a cell's surface is largely determined by the glycoproteins and/or other carbo-hydrate moieties and their arrangement on the surface of the individual cells. This is strikingly shown by the wide variety of blood groups which may be expressed on the surface of a human erythrocyte, and even more so by the HLA antigens which are present on the surface of most other cells and are responsible for problems in the transplantation of human tissues. Most of our early understanding and many of the techniques developed in the study of membranes' structure and function have been derived from work on red cell membranes. Erythrocytes are readily separated from other blood elements and their membrane can be isolated in uncontaminated form, since the mature red cell is anucleate and lacks the nuclear membranes as well as organelles in the cytoplasm, such as mitochondria, endoplasmic reticulum, Golgi apparatus, etc. Application of these techniques to other cells has already led to much valuable information, but in the case of the platelet the peculiar anatomy of this cell's membrane, together with the difficulty in isolating it without other cytoplasmic structural membranes, must be remembered.

The morphological studies of Behnke (1968) were the first to establish the

15

protein elements on the surface of the platelet membrane. These and subsequent studies emphasized that glycoproteins were also located in the cell's interior due to the extremely complex ramification of the surface connecting systems of the cell (*see* Figure 2.1). As a result, techniques employed in the red cell to label elements concentrated on the outer surface of the cell must be interpreted cautiously in the platelet since there is as yet little information as to how much of the internally placed surface membrane is labelled by these techniques. Studies which have used external labels of glycoproteins and which show a loss of these components during the circulation of the cell may be interpreted as meaning that this is due to cell–cell contact or adhesion during such circulation, but it could also result from internalization of cell glycoprotein, metabolism and excretion rather than any loss from cell surface to the exterior. Analysis of the platelet membrane's glycoproteins has been undertaken by disrupting the cell and using gradient diffusion techniques and ultracentrifugation to isolate the cell's membrane then solubilizing it with sodium dodecyl sulphate (SDS). These preparations are electrophoresed in appropriate gel support media and then analysed by staining with glycoprotein (periodic acid Schiff - PAS) or protein stains. Using these techniques initially only three or four glycoprotein bands were identified. The introduction of bidirectional techniques, whereby the solubilized membrane is initially electrophoresed in one direction in a non-reduced form and then in another after reduction with agents such as mercaptoethanol – which breaks disulphide bonds – has enabled the identification of many more individual glycoproteins. The terminology relating to the identification of the glycoproteins is still confused, and in this book, the convention will be adopted of allocating Roman numerals to the individually recognized glycoprotein, so that Roman number I represents the largest of these proteins by molecular weight, Roman number II would be the next in order and so on (Phillips, 1980). Since it has been recognized that there may be several discrete molecular types at the same molecular weight, Arabic lettering has been used to indicate where this has been recognized, e.g. glycoprotein Ia and glycoprotein Ib, and subscripts using the Greek alphabet have been applied where glycoproteins are made up of separate polypeptide chains. Thus glycoprotein Ia and Ib are different molecular species which have the same molecular weight, glycoprotein Ib has two polypeptide chains linked by disulphide bonds, the larger chain is called glycoprotein Ib_α and the smaller glycoprotein Ib_β.

Surface glycoproteins in the platelets play a similar role to those in other cells providing receptor sites for various molecules and enabling cell–cell recognition and adhesion. The platelet is negatively charged due to a large proportion of its surface glycoproteins having sialic acid as the terminal sugar. As with other cells it has been shown that removal of sialic acid by neuraminidase digestion results in the exposure of the next sugar in the glycoprotein chain which is generally galactose, and cells so treated have a reduced survival *in vivo*.

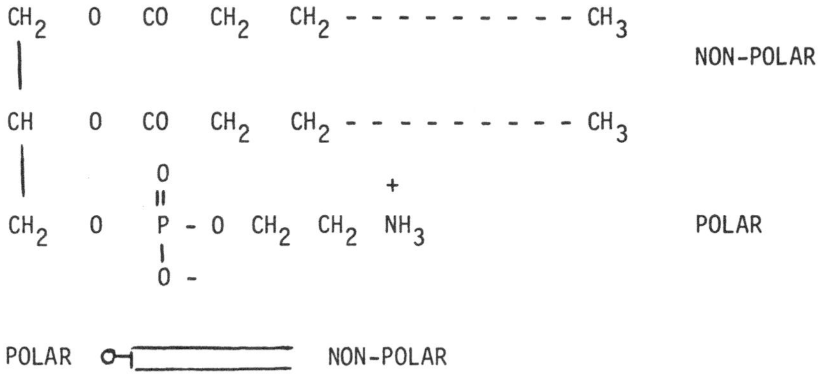

$$CH_2 \quad O \quad CO \quad CH_2 \quad CH_2 - - - - - - - - - CH_3$$

NON-POLAR

$$CH \quad O \quad CO \quad CH_2 \quad CH_2 - - - - - - - - CH_3$$

$$CH_2 \quad O \quad \overset{\overset{O}{\parallel}}{P} - O \quad CH_2 \quad CH_2 \quad \overset{+}{NH_3}$$

POLAR

$$O -$$

POLAR o—[＿＿＿＿＿] NON-POLAR

Figure 3.1 Phospholipids have polar and non-polar regions as illustrated here by phosphatidyl ethanolamine and may be represented diagrammatically as a clothespeg. (Adapted from *Progr. Haematol.*, **V**, 26 (1966), reproduced by permission of the Editor)

There is $280 \mu g$ of lipid per mg of platelet protein in human platelets. Figure 3.1 is the clothes peg diagrammatical illustration of a phospholipid, illustrating the glycerol backbone with two non-polar fatty acid chains linked by acyl bonds and a phosphate radical joined to a base. The major classes of phospholipid found in the platelet are phosphatidyl choline – 37%; phosphatidyl ethanolamine – 27%; sphingomyelin – 17%; phosphatidyl serine – 10%; and phosphatidyl inositol – 5%. There are also small amounts of phosphatidic acid and other sphingolipids and proteolipids.

The glycolipids consist of a fatty acid, a carbohydrate and sphingosine. The carbohydrate is usually glucosamine, glucose or galactose; the sphingosine fatty acid part of the structure is called a ceramide which is the non-polar group embedded in the lipid of the membrane. Free ceramide, i.e. sphingosine and the fatty acid, has also been isolated from platelets and is present in higher concentrations than has been reported in other cells, being 1.5% of the platelet lipid. The gangliosides are another minor but important component of membrane differing from other glycolipids in that they contain sialic acid, they have been shown to bind serotonin and to be the cell's receptor for this metabolite.

Figure 3.2 is a representation of the conventional view of the platelet surface membrane, which is based on the classical Davson–Danielli model of a bilayer of phospholipids with polar groups directed outwardly from a central core or hydrophobic region of the membrane. Polar groups of molecules are situated at the external and internal surface of the membrane, but only the external surface has glycoproteins. In addition to the phospholipids and glycoproteins there are other glycolipids and proteolipids, the carbohydrate portion of which is probably externally orientated. Interpolated between the phospholipids, and not shown in Figure 3.2, are cholesterol molecules which play an important role in the fluidity of the membrane in conjunction with the

17

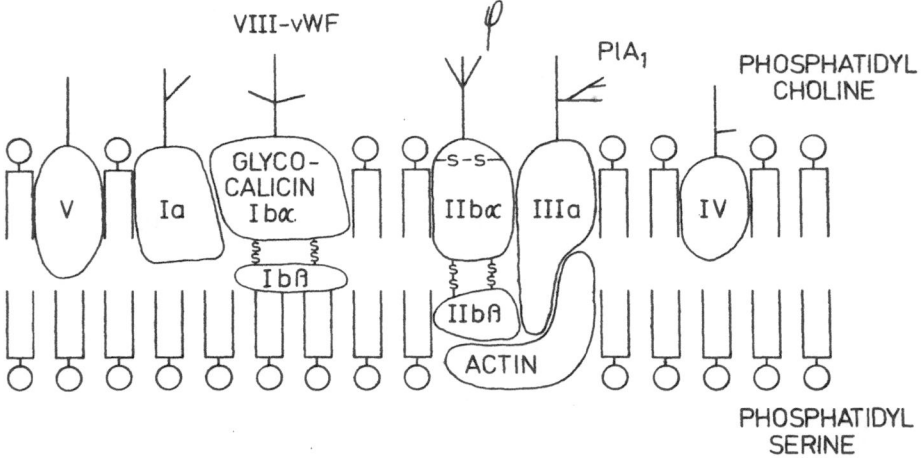

Figure 3.2 Modified Davson-Danielli model of platelet plasma membrane. Glycoprotein components are represented as branches on the outer surface of the membrane. Phosphatidyl choline is predominantly on the outer surface and phosphatidyl serine on the inner when the platelet is unactivated. Note that some membrane proteins may traverse the membrane and be in contact with proteins on the inner surface e.g. actin

saturation of the fatty acids of the phospholipids. The more cholesterol the greater the membrane viscosity and the more saturated the fatty acids the greater the stability. Membranes with low cholesterol content and a high concentration of unsaturated fatty acids are more fluid. The cell's membrane is a very dynamic structure which is in a constant state of flux and perturbation with alterations in the conformation of the fatty acid side chains, as well as a constant exchange of fatty acids and cholesterol with the surrounding plasma. The proteins in the membrane and phospholipid components are in many, if not all, instances capable of lateral movement, although those proteins which are transmembrane and stretch from the external to the internal surface may be less mobile or indeed be anchored *in situ* due to their interactions with other structures on the internal surface of the cell such as the microfibrils (actin), or microtubular elements. Some of these glycoproteins exist on the cell surface as microclusters (glycoprotein Ib), whereas others are randomly distributed but may cluster after being exposed to an appropriate stimulus, e.g. glycoprotein IIb and glycoprotein IIIa (*v. infra*). The modern fluid membrane mosaic model envisages a lipid bilayer – which imposes a viscosity resembling high grade machine oil – on the surface of which float globular proteins with antennae of sugar side chains often branched and frequently terminating with sialic acid. When the proteins traverse the lipid bilayer the hydrophilic portions of the molecule locate themselves on the external and internal surface of the membrane while its hydrophobic component is central in the membrane. Such proteins may be anchored like buoys to cytoplasmic structures, and in many cells including the platelet a membrane protein resembling actin has also been identified. Using appropriate fluorescent probes, lateral movement of both lipid and protein moieties has been established, the mobility of the lipid being much more rapid than that of protein and in some instances, e.g. where the protein is anchored, no movement may occur at all. It seems highly likely that the mobility may vary from place to place in the membrane, depending on the properties of viscosity. This in turn is dependent on temperature, cholesterol concentration, calcium content, and methylation or unsaturation of the fatty acids. Just as there is a mosaic of proteins there may be a mosaic of lipids. Apart from the lateral movement, lipids are capable of changing their orientation so that their polar groups which were initially outwardly placed may 'flip-flop' to face the interior or *vice versa*. Phosphatidyl ethanolamine and phosphatidyl serine are predominantly placed on the interior of the lipid bilayer, whilst phosphatidyl choline is predominantly on the exterior surface of the platelet although activation of the cell may result in the exposure of phosphatidyl ethanolamine and serine, the former being particularly involved in one of the procoagulant activities (*v. infra*). Actinomyosin may be located on the cell's surface following its exposure to activating agents such as thrombin, but is not normally detected there.

The mosaic pattern of the membrane is probably maintained by three constraints:

(1) The external glycoprotein branches with sialic acid repelling other glycoproteins and lectin-like effects of plasma proteins drawing some surface glycoproteins towards each other,

(2) The integral composition of the membrane proteins with certain hydrophobic components of the surface glycoproteins, having a preference for certain hydrophobic environs of the lipids and hence a congregation in a mosaic of lipid soil, and

(3) The effects of cytoplasmic metabolism exerted through contractile proteins on protein molecules which penetrate the lipid bilayer and which may thereby secure some of the membrane proteins at particular points. Perhaps in turn these may influence the surrounding lipids in the membrane and via their carbohydrate side chains also influence neighbouring untethered glycoproteins.

Some surface proteins may be covalently bound to cytoplasmic protein components such as adenyl cyclase.

It can be seen from this discussion that metabolic events in the cell's cytoplasm may affect membrane composition. For example, changes in membrane lipid may change membrane fluidity, the protein contractile elements may be altered and thus tether or untether certain glycoproteins which express themselves on the surface and enhance, or otherwise, opportunities for lateral movement perhaps also increasing 'flip-flop' of the lipid components by causing changes in the polar groups of lipids and/or fatty acid side chains. Similar changes may be exerted by alterations of the external plasma lipid content, hence external forces or cytoplasmic metabolism may modify the fluidity and perhaps stability of the membrane. Such changes may have considerable importance in human pathology. Recent work in diabetes has shown that the increased cholesterol content of the plasma may reflect itself by changes in the platelet membrane, which in turn result in the platelet being hyperaggregable (*see* Chapter 9).

RECEPTORS

Conceptually receptors are sites which bind specific compounds (agonists), and may be situated either on the surface of the cell or anywhere within it. The combination of an agonist with its receptor is thought of in much the same way as an antigen–antibody lock and key situation; just as in antibody–antigen reactions there may be differing affinities, so a receptor site may have low, intermediate or high avidity for a certain compound. A receptor on the external surface of the cell is either a glycoprotein or glycolipid which when bound to its agonist, and perhaps secondary to a resultant allosteric conformational change, undergoes lateral movement in the membrane mosaic. Perhaps propelled by an induced aversion to its lipid environs it moves to other areas containing the effector molecule to which the receptor becomes attached causing its activation. This effector is usually a protein which is genetically distinct from the receptor molecule, and which is often separately placed in the membrane but sometimes covalently linked to the receptor, e.g. adenosine and adenylate cyclase in the turkey erythrocyte.

The activation of adenylate cyclase to produce the hormone cAMP within the cell is one of the most frequently implicated mechanisms of inducing a cell's response to a hormone, and cAMP has been called a second messenger hormone. How cAMP exerts such differing actions in the cell remains unclear, but it may be inherent in the target cell, the receptor or in the compartmentalization of the particular adenylate cyclase which is activated by the receptor stimulus complex. Another mechanism by which receptor agonist complexes may activate intracellular action is by inducing clustering of such complexes on the cell surface, endocytosis then carrying the complex within the cell where it is transported to lysosomes and digested, or to endoplasmic reticulum where it may activate protein synthesis, or to the cell's nucleus where it may induce various metabolic effects including mitosis. The latter is proposed as the mechanism whereby lymphocyte mitosis is induced. The antibody complexes with the antigen on the lymphocyte surface, is clustered and capped then ingested into the cell where it is transported to the nucleus, subsequently lymphocyte proliferation induces a clone of cells producing the required antibody. In this type of process the receptor may be lost from the cell's surface, explaining the so-called *down* regulation where there is a decreased

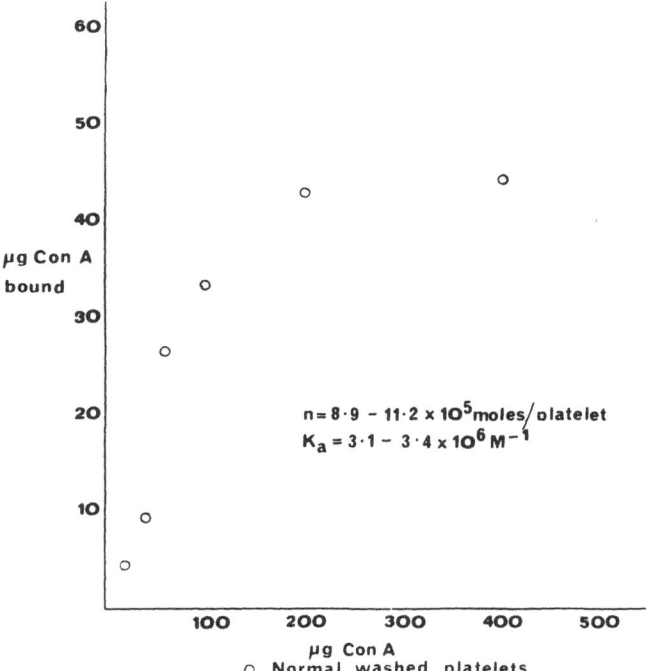

$$n = 8 \cdot 9 - 11 \cdot 2 \times 10^5 \text{moles/platelet}$$
$$K_a = 3 \cdot 1 - 3 \cdot 4 \times 10^6 \text{ M}^{-1}$$

Figure 3.3 Con A binding to washed human platelets. (Adapted from *Thromb. Res.,* **13**, 337 (1978)

number of receptors on the cell's surface when the cell is subjected to elevated levels of hormones or chemical agonists.

Surface or membrane receptor sites are usually determined by incubating whole cells or isolated cell membranes with a radiolabelled agonist or a specific antagonist, e.g. α-bungarotoxin for acetylcholinesterase receptors, or using ^{125}I-labelled yohimbine for α_2-adrenergic receptors. The specificity is determined by ensuring that the binding is reversible, and the amount of non-specific binding calculated by determining the percentage of binding of the radiolabelled ligand in the presence of cold ligand or in an excess of its specific antagonist. This is well illustrated by the binding of the lectin concanavalin A (con A) which binds to mannose sugars, and whose binding is therefore inhibited by an excess of α-mannopyranoside. Figure 3.3 shows the binding of ^{125}I-labelled con A to a constant number of platelets incubated with increasing concentrations of con A. In the presence of an excess of α-mannopyranoside, the non-specific binding was less than 5%, and it is seen that at a concentration of con A greater than 10^{-4} mol/l, a plateau has occurred, in other words all the binding sites for this lectin have been saturated. This should always be the case unless there is a turnover of the receptor sites by a mechanism such as endocytosis where the receptor site is internalized. By knowing the amount of labelled con A bound to the platelet and that remaining free at varying concentrations, a Scatchard plot may be constructed where the bound/free con A is plotted on the ordinate and bound on the abscissa. If such a plot is linear, the number of binding sites (n) will be given by its interception with the abscissa and the slope of the curve will give an affinity constant K. The steeper the slope the greater the affinity and the higher the constant. If the plot is not linear it will imply that there is more than one binding site, and from its shape this may be resolved into two or more receptors with differing numbers of affinity and binding sites.

In general, it seems that high affinity binding sites are the important ones physiologically, and usually only a proportion of these need to be occupied to produce a maximal effect (the remaining receptors are termed spare receptors). In some instances curvilinear plots may result from the property of negative co-operativity which implies that the binding of an agonist to a receptor may decrease the affinity for neighbouring receptors. This concept once widely held is in disfavour, and such a circumstance is now thought to reflect differing populations of receptors. There are also instances where cross-linking of surface receptors by lectins or antibodies may cause an enhancement of the receptor binding to its specific agonist. Patching of surface receptors is associated with localized changes of contractile proteins, such as actin or tubulin, and so cAMP and cGMP (cyclic guanosine monophosphate) through their effects on microtubular function may be of importance in determining the external arrangement of receptor molecules and their affinity and response to an agonist.

Another way cAMP may function is to dissociate an inhibitor subunit from a protein kinase, which in turn may phosphorylate specific seryl and threonyl units of structural or regulatory enzymes within a cell and thereby cause the characteristic hormonal response. In addition, the agonist receptor interaction may result in a number of basic changes in the cell membrane altering either physical, electrical or biological properties. For example, following the platelet's exposure to ADP or thrombin there is a change in its electrophoretic mobility and in the neuroreceptor response to acetylcholine, there follows a rapid influx of sodium through channels opened in the cell membrane which changes the membrane potential to establish the action potential of neuro-humoral responses. This may occur by its inducing phosphorylation of an endogenous membrane protein kinase. Guanosine triphosphate (GTP) has been shown to reduce binding affinities of certain membrane receptors such as β-adrenergic receptors, but has also been shown in some circumstances to be a requirement for hormone induced coupling of a receptor to adenylate cyclase. Thus there are clearly many points in the cell's metabolism, both externally and internally, which may modify its receptor sites and thereby its responses.

In the case of the platelet these involve the properties of adhesion, aggregation and to a lesser degree the release reaction. The importance of intra-

22

cellular events is also emphasized by studies showing that cap formation in peripheral polymorphonuclear leukocytes and lymphocytes is markedly increased when the cells are exposed to colchicine, and this effect is inhibited by exposing the cells to cGMP or by using agents such as carbamylcholine and phorbolmyristate which increase intracellular cGMP levels. The role of cAMP *vis à vis* cGMP in the stabilization of microtubules is still to be clarified, and may vary from cell type to cell type.

PLATELET ANTIGENS

Platelet membranes contain ABO blood group antigens, but it seems likely that these antigens are expressed in a different way to those of the erythrocytes, since transfusions of platelets to patients with different red cell blood groups have shown similar survival times to those with the same blood type. Thus it is standard practice for blood banks to use pooled platelets in routine supply for hospital use. These antigens are perhaps differently orientated in the platelet membrane compared to the red cell, or located primarily in the surface connecting system within the cell and not as antigenically available as those on the surface of the red cell. More important from the point of view of platelet transfusion are the HLA components. The nearer the match of HLA typing of the blood platelets, the less likely the patient is to develop resistance or antibodies to the infused platelets with repeated usage. *In vitro* experiments have shown that platelets from blood group O individuals can take up Group A and B antigens from the plasma of people with these respective groups, and similarly platelets which are HLA-A1 or -A2 negative can absorb-A1 and -A2 + ve properties if incubated in serum from HLA-A1 or -A2 + ve individuals. How much serum blood group or transplant antigens contribute to *in vivo* platelet groups is uncertain, but it is of interest that HLA antigens B8, B13 and B14 are low in plasma and little expressed in platelets, whereas B5 and B7 are high in both serum and platelets. Whilst HLA antigens undoubtedly play a role in the development of refractoriness to platelet transfusion, selection of platelets with a low HLA content from HLA-B8, 13 and 14 individuals may reduce this problem. Rh blood groups on the other hand have not been shown to be present in platelet membranes.

Platelets do possess specific isoantigens which have been identified, usually following blood transfusion purpura or neonatal thrombocytopenia

Table 3.1 Compounds for which there are receptors in human platelets

α-Adrenergic	Insulin
Fibrinogen	Collagen
ADP	Thromboxane A_2
Thrombin	Xa
Ristocetin cofactor VIII:AG	Prostacyclin PGI_2
DNA	Quinine antibody
Fc	Serotonin

(*v. infra*). One of the best studied is called PlA1 which is present in 98% of platelets of unrelated humans, is related to glycoprotein IIIa and is missing from patients with thrombasthenia (Glanzmann disease), but individuals with PlA1 deficiency alone do not have the faulty platelet function associated with thrombasthenia. Other antigens which have been identified are the PlE system, the Ko, Duzo, Bak and Lek systems. Undoubtedly others await recognition. These antigens are expressed as autosomal dominants and the PlA, PlE and Ko systems are di-allelic, whereas Bak, Lek and Duzo are mono-allelic.

Table 3.1 lists the various receptors which have been so far identified in the platelet. The majority of these will be discussed in other sections of this book. Glycoprotein Ib is the platelet receptor for the ristocetin cofactor (VIII-RCoF) and may be the thrombin receptor, but other workers have implicated glycoprotein V. Glycoprotein Ib is often the receptor for the quinine antibody in man (*v. infra*). Glycoprotein IIIa not only carries the PlA1 antigen, but is also the receptor for fibrinogen (Figure 3.2). Since many of these receptors act as a trigger for platelet aggregation and the release reaction, they will be discussed in more detail in the section on platelet aggregation.

PLATELET METABOLISM

Lipid metabolism and the platelet prostaglandin pathways

Lipids

The platelet's ultrastructure illustrates its high membrane content. Lipids are not merely structurally important, but provide substrates for the prosta-

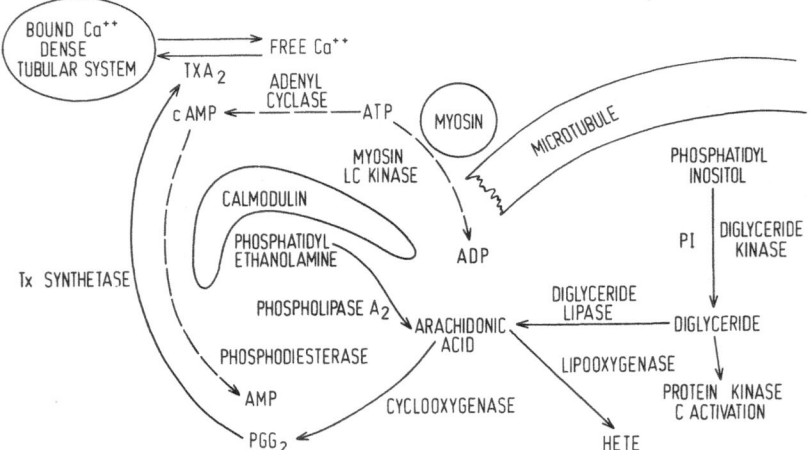

Figure 3.4 Thrombin (or another agonist) binds to a membrane receptor which releases bound Ca^{2+}. This interacts with calmodulin to orchestrate a series of biochemical events illustrated here. A second synergistic pathway results from the simultaneous release of diglycerol from phosphatidyl in ositol. This activates protein kinase C and constitutes an alternative pathway to that of increased sytosol Ca^{2+} (Michell 1983)

glandin pathways in the cell as well as providing its procoagulant activity. There is approximately 7.8 mg of membrane lipid per 10^{11} platelets.

In vitro studies with ^{32}P revealed that this isotope was actively incorporated into platelet phospholipids, with phosphatidyl inositol and phosphatidic acid being the most heavily labelled, although there was a significant incorporation into all classes of phospholipid. This labelling pattern was in contrast to that found when platelets were examined in patients with myeloproliferative disorders or leukaemia who had been given ^{32}P therapeutically and where platelet samples were obtained over the next few days. The most intensively labelled phospholipids were then found to be phosphatidyl choline, phosphatidyl ethanolamine and the sphingolipids which may represent the more stable structural lipids.

The platelet possesses the enzymes to synthesize phospholipids *de novo* and as in red cells the platelet's membrane lipid content is influenced by the plasma lipids and therefore by diet. Accordingly, the platelet's lipid content can be altered particularly with regard to its cholesterol concentrations and also the length and composition of fatty acid side chains in its phospholipid molecules. Eskimos who live on a diet of raw fish containing a high amount of unsaturated fatty acids show a high unsaturated fatty acid content in their platelets. It has also been found in volunteer human experiments that feeding

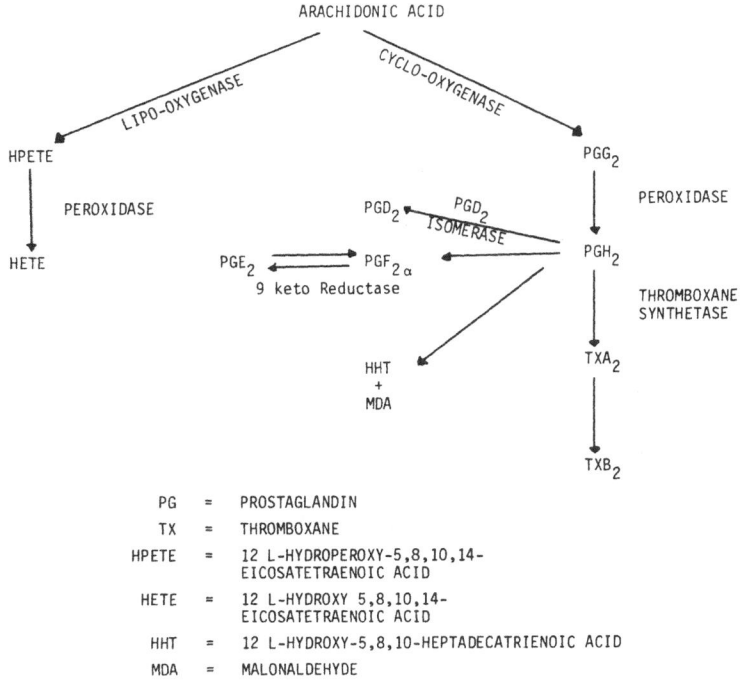

PG	=	PROSTAGLANDIN
TX	=	THROMBOXANE
HPETE	=	12 L-HYDROPEROXY-5,8,10,14-EICOSATETRAENOIC ACID
HETE	=	12 L-HYDROXY 5,8,10,14-EICOSATETRAENOIC ACID
HHT	=	12 L-HYDROXY-5,8,10-HEPTADECATRIENOIC ACID
MDA	=	MALONALDEHYDE

Figure 3.5 Arachidonic acid pathway in the platelet (see text)

various chain length fatty acids can alter the content of the fatty acid side chains of platelet phospholipids. This is of particular importance when examining the platelet prostaglandin pathway, the initiation of which is the release of free arachidonic acid, a 20 carbon unsaturated fatty acid, from its parent phospholipid molecule in the cell's membrane (Figure 3.4).

Arachidonic acid comprises 23% of the total fatty acids in platelet membranes from people on a standard Western diet. The proposed two major phospholipid sources of arachidonic acid are phosphatidyl ethanolamine and/or phosphatidyl inositol. Both these phospholipids contain a high percentage of arachidonic acid as their fatty acid side chains on position 2. In the case of phosphatidyl ethanolamine it is believed that the calmodulin modulated enzyme, phospholipase A_2 may liberate arachidonic acid. Arachidonic acid may also be released from phosphatidyl inositol in two steps, diglyceride kinase releases the diglyceride which is then attacked by diglyceride lipase to produce free arachidonic acid (Figure 3.4).

Prostaglandin pathway

Arachidonic acid (Figures 3.4 and 3.5) is converted by cyclo-oxygenase to PGG_2 which is acted upon by a peroxidase to become PGH_2 which in turn may be converted to a number of other derivatives including HHT, which is a chemotactic substance for polymorphonuclear leukocytes, and malonaldehyde, which is often used as a marker of this metabolic pathway. PGF_2 and PGE_2 have little effect on platelet aggregation, but PGD_2 has been found to be a potent inhibitor, and when added exogenously is twice as effective as the classical prostaglandin PGE_1. PGD_2 stimulates adenylate cyclase to increase cAMP as does PGE_1 but the effect may be mediated by two individual receptors on the membrane. The amount of PGD_2 produced during platelet aggregation is sufficient to block platelet aggregation to a standard stimulus added exogenously, and therefore it may be an important inbuilt modulatory control of platelet aggregation and a limit to its extent. The major product of the prostaglandin pathway in the platelet is thromboxane A_2 (TXA_2). Although PGH_2 is thought by some to promote platelet aggregation directly, TXA_2 is much more potent and it seems probable that PGH_2 has to be converted to TXA_2 for this effect. The early burst of oxygen consumption in platelets, which was first described following exposure to thrombin and lasts only 10–20 seconds, is largely due to the oxidative steps in this pathway (Figures 3.4 and 3.5) and can be inhibited by cyclo-oxygenase inhibitors such as aspirin or indomethacin. The oxygen burst then does not occur even when higher concentrations of thrombin produce aggregation.

TXA_2 is one of the most potent aggregating agents of platelets weight for weight known, and is also a very potent vasoconstrictor. TXA_2 is released from the platelet and interacts with a receptor on the cell surface. Thromboxane A_2 inhibits the cAMP increases stimulated by substances such as PGE_1

or PGI_2 (prostacyclin) by inhibiting their effect on adenylate cyclase, but it has no effect on the basal cAMP levels. Since calcium ions (Ca^{2+}) can also inhibit PGI_2-stimulated cAMP increases in the platelet, it has been suggested that TXA_2 acts by releasing calcium from its bound state thus inhibiting adenylate cyclase. This has been examined by looking at the effects of substances which are known to inhibit calcium release from membrane, such as TMB-8 which has been shown to cause similar effects in platelets to prostacyclin. TXA_2 is a very unstable substance and is rapidly converted in 10–30 seconds to thromboxane B_2 (TXB_2). Alternatively, the free arachidonic acid may be acted upon by the enzyme lipo-oxygenase (Figure 3.5) to form the product 12-hydroperoxyeicosatetraenoic acid (HPETE), and this is subsequently converted to 12-hydroxyeicosatetraenoic acid (HETE). This metabolite is a potent chemotactic substance for eosinophils, and HETE and HHT may explain the accumulation of granulocytes around platelet aggregates seen in thrombosis.

The enzyme cyclo-oxygenase may be blocked by substances such as aspirin and indomethacin which do not affect lipo-oxygenase. However, glucocorticoids affect lipo-oxygenase activity possibly by blocking the release of arachidonic acid, drug ibuprofren, and compounds, e.g. imidazole, are now available which specifically inhibit other individual enzymes such as thromboxane synthetase (Figure 3.5). There is still some dispute as to whether or not thromboxane A_2 can cause platelet aggregation in its own right or whether there is always a requirement for the presence or release of ADP as a prerequisite for thromboxane aggregation. Marcus' group (1978) has shown that when platelets are subjected to arachidonic acid in the presence of ADP removing enzymes, such as creatinine phosphokinase or apyrase, the normal platelet oxygen burst follows implying that the cyclo-oxygenase reaction has proceeded, but the platelet aggregation does not occur supporting the concept that ADP release or presence is required for thromboxane to cause aggregation, although other evidence opposes this view (Meyers *et al.*, 1979).

The major end product of the prostaglandin pathway via cyclo-oxygenase is thromboxane A_2 in the platelet, but the end product in the endothelial cells lining blood vessels is a potent inhibitor of platelet aggregation and a vasodilator, *viz.* prostacyclin (PGI_2). The pathway in the endothelial cell is similar to the platelet except that PGH_2 is converted by prostacyclin synthetase to PGI_2. PGI_2 is the most potent inhibitor of platelet aggregation yet discovered, but like thromboxane it is unstable with a half life of 3 minutes, and is rapidly converted by spontaneous hydrolysis to 6-keto $PGF_{1\alpha}$ which is inactive. Prostacyclin induces a marked increase in cAMP in the platelet and this effect may persist for up to one hour *in vitro*. PGI_2 is effective *in vivo* in inhibiting platelet thrombus formation for 30 minutes, despite the short half life of PGI_2. The endothelial cells may be stimulated to produce PGI_2 by exposure to thrombin, arachidonic acid, the ionophore AT 3187 or trypsin. The most potent stimulus is ionophore, next arachidonic acid and then thrombin, whereas ADP and adrenalin have no effect. Aspirin inhibits prostacyclin production in endothelial cells by blocking the enzyme cyclo-oxgyenase as it inhibits thromboxane production in platelets. It has been shown that endothelial cells so blocked are still capable of producing prostacyclin if arachidonic acid metabolites beyond the cyclo-oxygenase steps are exhibited to them. Thus PGH_2 added to aspirin treated endothelial cells results in a production of prostacyclin. Similarly, it has been shown that stimulation of platelets by an ionophore which will bring about the release reaction with release of endoperoxides as well as thromboxane A_2 results in aspirin treated endothelial cells producing prostacyclin. Thus the beneficial effects of aspirin in thrombotic situations may relate to the endothelial cells' capacity to re-synthesize cyclo-oxygenase unlike the platelet, and that regardless, should platelet aggregation occur, the release of endoperoxides (PGH_2) from the platelets would result in the endothelial cells producing PGI_2.

Protein metabolism

Amino acids are actively transported into the platelet, valine, proline and glutamic acid being less rapidly taken up than leucine, serine, cysteine or lysine. This may in part depend on the pools of amino acids found in the

Table 3.2 Platelet protein

1. *Shape and contractility*	Tubulin Actin Myosin
2. *Coagulation proteins*	*Agonist* Fibrinogen VIII:Ag Factor V Factor XIII
	Antagonist Platelet factor 4 α_1 Antitrypsin α_2 Macroglobulin α_2 Antiplasmin
3. *Metabolic regulation*	Enzymes in the cells' metabolic pathway Lysosomal enzymes Calmodulin
4. *Miscellaneous*	Mitogenic factor Fibronectin γ-Globulin β-Thromboglobulin Platelet factor 4 Complement activating factor β-Lysin Permeability factor Thrombospondin Albumin

platelet since glutamic acid, proline and in particular taurine are present in very high amounts compared with lysine, leucine and cysteine. The taurine may be derived from the metabolism of cysteine. Studies employing ^{14}C-labelled amino acids have not only shown the transport, but have shown some incorporation into the soluble protein of the cell obtained by precipitation with trichloracetic acid, and also the platelets' fibrinogen obtained by precipitating it with thrombin. The amounts incorporated are tiny and of questionable significance and are possibly derived from mitochondrial activity since this incorporation could be abolished by previous incubation of the cell with chloramphenicol; no ribosomes have been observed in the platelet by electron microscopy. Therefore, the platelet has little capacity, if any, for *de novo* synthesis of protein, and thus drugs which irreversibly inactivate enzymes will be effective throughout the cell's lifespan and can only be overcome by the arrival of freshly synthesized cells from the megakaryocytes. The best known example of this is aspirin which irreversibly acetylates and inactivates cyclo-oxygenase, whereas drugs such as indomethacin are effective for 6–8 hours only.

The total protein content of one platelet is 2.1 ± 1.0 pg of protein, and some of the individually important ones are listed in Table 3.2. The micro-tubules and their major building block, tubulin, together with contractile proteins of the cell initially called 'thrombasthenin', and now identified as actin and myosin, play a major role in the release reaction of the cell. Platelet actin comprises 10% of the total platelet protein and has a molecular weight of 43 000. It polymerizes into long filaments which can form arrow heads when reacted with skeletal muscle myosin, and is capable of activating ATPase activity in muscle heavy myosin in the same way as muscle actin. Platelet actin more closely resembles actin which has now been isolated from other cells in the body, e.g. the erythrocyte, and has minor amino acid sequence differences to muscle actin. Platelet myosin comprises only 1% of the platelet's total protein (far less than myosin in muscle), has a molecular weight which is similar to the muscle myosin being 460 000, and is composed of heavy chains of 200 000 molecular weight and light chains of platelet myosin which differ from that found in skeletal or cardiac tissue. Platelets also contain a myosin light chain kinase which phosphorylates one of the platelet myosin's light chains and greatly enhances its actin activated ATPase activity. It is thought that this effect is a major factor in platelet actin–myosin interaction, and this step may precede the onset of contraction in the cell which results in the release reaction.

Calmodulin is a recently identified calcium binding protein which regulates a large number of enzyme systems by means of its 'presentation' of calcium to them or perhaps by conformational shape changes induced in the calmodulin by allosteric reactions following calcium binding. It is a widely distributed protein which has been found in most mammalian cells including the platelet. It has a molecular weight of 16 790 and its amino acid sequence has been established. It has four binding sites for calcium, and on binding to calcium undergoes different conformational changes depending on the number and combination of sites to which calcium has been bound. It is believed to play an important part in microtubule association, and its control of protein kinase activity has been established as having a role in cyclic nucleotide phosphodiesterase activity, e.g. cAMP phosphodiesterase, as well as activating myosin light chain kinase; and it is important in the calcium pump in erythrocytes. It has now been established that platelet myosin light chain kinase requires calmodulin for its activity, and that calmodulin also regulates stimulation of phospholipase A2. As is seen in Figure 3.4, this regulating protein may be one of the most important elements in the instigation of the release reaction since it is intimately involved in several key enzyme steps, namely the phosphorylation of myosin to enable contraction, its production of thromboxane A2 through the initiation of this pathway via phospholipase A2 and its regulation of cAMP levels which is so important in the response of the platelet to various agonists.

The platelet mitogenic factor or platelet derived growth factor is a very cationic protein with a molecular weight between 10 000 and 30 000, and which has the remarkable property of inducing mitogenesis in a variety of cells such as smooth muscle, fibroblasts and glial cells. It has been shown to have strikingly similar amino acid sequences to some oncogenes. It has no effect on the proliferation of endothelial cells. It is extremely potent and has effects on cells in culture at levels of 100 ng/ml. Since one of the first changes in the initiation of an atherosclerotic lesion is the proliferation of smooth muscle in the intima of the blood vessels, this protein has attracted a lot of attention since it is released from platelets when they are stimulated by thrombin. It has, therefore, been postulated that atherosclerosis is the result of endothelial cell damage resulting in the deposition of platelets which release the mitogenic factor and cause intimal smooth muscle proliferation, which if the insult continues or is reinstituted will eventually result in the development of a full blown atheromatous lesion. Other cationic proteins have also been described in the platelet. One is a permeability factor which induces histamine release from mast cells, and another is a chemotactic factor which activates the fifth component of complement releasing a chemotactic factor for segmented neutrophils. A bactericidal factor has also been described and called β-lysin, but other work has not revealed any antibacterial factor in platelets.

Thrombospondin is a glycoprotein with a molecular weight of 450 000, and is released from platelets after they are treated with thrombin. This protein contains three polypeptide chains and binds to heparin. Thrombospondin may be the endogenous platelet lectin activity which appears following platelet activation by thrombin or ionophore, and may be important in stabilizing platelet aggregation. It was previously called the thrombin sensitive protein, and is believed to be located in the α-granules.

Beta thromboglobulin (β-TG) and platelet factor (PF4) are proteins which are believed to be uniquely derived from platelets, and are released during the release reaction; they may be useful markers following situations where platelet activation has occurred, such as thrombosis. β-TG has a molecular weight of 35 400 daltons, and is a tetramer of four identical subunits. When released from the platelets *in vivo* it is thought to have a half-life ($T_{\frac{1}{2}}$) of approximately 100 minutes. β-TG is believed to be a cleavage product of the precursor protein called low affinity platelet factor 4. The latter is unrelated to PF4 which is also a tetramer of four identical subunits with an overall molecular weight of 30 800 daltons. PF4 has a very short lifespan in plasma being < 10 minutes, following its release from platelets, PF4 binds to endothelial cells and this may account for its rapid clearance. It can be mobilized back into the plasma by heparin so that heparin infusions cause quite dramatic elevation of plasma PF4 levels. Whereas β-TG is metabolized by the kidney and its level is raised in patients whose renal function is reduced, PF4 is normal. Therefore, elevated plasma β-TG can be equated with platelet activation *in vivo* provided renal function is normal and provided it is considerably in excess of PF4. Should both β-TG and PF4 be varied equally the most likely explanation is that of platelet activation during blood collection.

The lysosomal enzymes include acid phosphatase, β-glucuronidase, aryl sulphatase, etc. and are secreted to varying degrees following stimuli such as collagen, the ionophore A23187 and thrombin. It has been said that acid P-nitrophenyl phosphatase is the exception, and if this is the case the falsely raised serum acid phosphatase seen in the sera of patients with very high platelet counts is presumably derived from β-glycerol phosphatase which is also present in the platelet. Gammaglobulin represents 0.3% of the total protein in platelets, and its significance is not known. The platelet has been shown to contain fibronectin which is released and which may play a role in platelet aggregation. As well it contains a number of coagulation factors (Chapter 4).

Carbohydrate and nucleotide metabolism in platelets

A frequent analogy has been drawn between the platelet and the muscle cell. However, the platelet does not undertake the repetitive contractile efforts of such a cell, but rather can be envisaged as circulating in a resting state, which on activation by appropriate stimuli, results in an orgastic contraction of the cell with release of specific components and the initiation of platelet aggregation and support of clot retraction. Until recently it was felt that the platelet once activated automatically self-destructed and like the bee defending its hive, died. Work from Mustard's group (1973) has refuted this concept by showing that platelets which have been activated to bring about the release reaction can circulate in animals for a relatively normal lifespan, and an acquired storage pool disease has been described in man which results from *in vivo* platelet activation with the release and circulation of cells with reduced or

31

absent granules. Such cells are capable of replenishing their serotonin stores, but cannot restore their secreted α-granule constituents. As in other cells the major energy source is believed to be adenosine triphosphate (ATP) which is generated by glycolysis. It has been estimated that 55% of the ATP generated in the platelet comes from the classical Embden–Meyerhof pathway, 35% by oxidative phosphorylation in mitochondria and the remaining 10% by the pentose–phosphate or hexose–monophosphate shunt. The normal level of glycogen in the platelet is very similar to that of muscle, and a decrease in glycogen may be an explanation for some of the inhibitory effects of agents such as PGE_1, adenosine and cAMP which are all well known in inhibiting platelet function. It has been shown that all of these agents can activate cAMP dependent protein kinase which causes activation of phosphorylase with a subsequent decrease in glycogen content. During platelet aggregation by substances such as ADP, there is a similar fall in glycogen level, but the mechanism is different and is due to a calcium activated phosphorylase activity which directly stimulates phosphorylase kinase activity. The release of calcium initiates both the platelet contractile activities through its effect on calmodulin activating the myosin light chain kinase, and by activating the phosphorylase to initiate glycogen breakdown which provides the necessary energy and explains the accompanying stimulation of glycolysis with the production of lactic acid. Cyclic AMP, apart from increasing glycogen breakdown, also reduces glycogen synthetase activity and inhibits glucose uptake by the platelet. The reverse applies during aggregation induced by ADP where there is an increased uptake of glucose by the cell and glycogen synthetase activity is, if anything, increased.

When the profile of nucleic acids in the platelet in a resting state is examined the three present in the highest concentration are ATP, ADP and GTP. Following stimulation of the platelets, either by thrombin or some other agonist, there is relatively little change over the first few minutes in this constitution, but studies by Holmsen (1969) and others have shown this is because of a burst in ATP synthesis which largely occurs through the conversion of glucose and glycogen to lactic acid. There is a recovery of the ATP broken down to ADP by salvage pathways so that the end product of ATP metabolism in the platelet, inosine monophosphate (IMP), is only slightly increased in the first few minutes. This initial burst of energy consumption is thought to be related to the initiation of the platelet's release reaction, and subsequently ATP is consumed in the more prolonged exercise of clot retraction. GTP which is intimately concerned with microtubular function is also diminished. It is important to remember that there are basically two pools of nucleic acid in the platelet. One is the stable or storage pool which is concentrated in the very dense granule consisting of ATP, ADP, calcium and α_2 antiplasmin which is secreted when the release reaction is initiated. The other nucleotide pool is constantly being turned over and is employed as an energy source within the cell unlike the storage pool nucleotide. All the enzymes required for *de*

32

novo synthesis of purines have been identified in the platelet, but most of the experiments undertaken have employed labelled adenosine which readily enters the metabolic pool after it crosses the platelet membrane, and under the action of adenosine kinase is converted to AMP which in turn is converted to ADP and ATP by adenylate kinase. The other label commonly employed is ^{14}C-labelled adenine which together with 5-phosphoribosyl-1-pyrophosphate may be converted to AMP by nucleotide-1-pyrophosphorylase. In interpreting various experimental results obtained by these techniques it is important to appreciate that only one subset of a metabolic pool may be labelled during the period of incubation of the cell with a radioactive label, and similarly measurement of total amounts of nucleotides may be very misleading since they may remain constant even in situations where there is a very high turnover. This point is especially important when considering the roles of cAMP and cGMP in the platelet. A simplistic view at present would be that these compounds have opposing effects from the point of view of release reaction and platelet aggregation, in that high levels of cAMP are associated with an inhibition of release and aggregation and the reverse occurring with cGMP. A popular thesis at present is that cAMP levels determine the activity of the calcium pump and may exert their effect by controlling calcium fluxes (Figure 3.6),

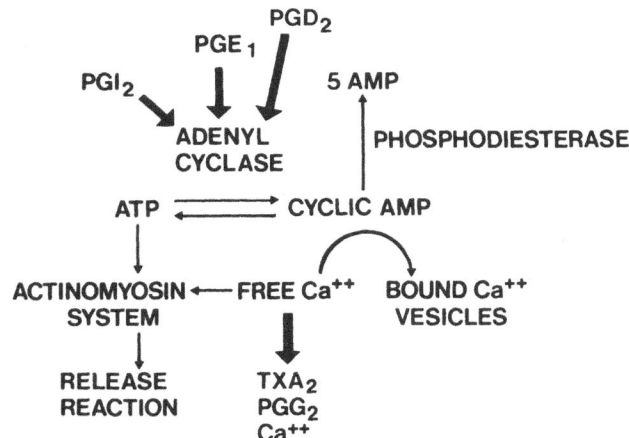

Figure 3.6 Role of cAMP in control of cytosal Ca^{2+} levels

thereby influencing calmodulin regulated enzyme systems. However, platelet agonists such as ADP and adrenalin, show no change in ^{14}C-adenine labelled cAMP levels or unlabelled cAMP levels, although there is dispute concerning this in the literature, and interpretation of the studies must take into account that labelled adenosine can also increase cAMP in the platelet of its own accord. PGE_1 increases cAMP in the platelet by activating adenylate kinase and this is greatly increased if cyclic AMP phosphodiesterase is inhibited, and the breakdown of cAMP is, therefore, decreased. ADP is found to markedly reduce the increase in cAMP caused by PGE_1 whether or not the cAMP phosphodiesterase is inhibited. ADP appears to affect its action as a non-competitive inhibitor of adenylate cyclase. Adrenalin on the other hand stimulates adenylate cyclase activity in the presence of phosphodiesterase inhibitors, and other agonists such as vasopressin or 5-hydroxytryptamine (serotonin) have no effect. Whereas overall cAMP is not altered by the addition of agonists, cGMP has been shown to have a 2–4 fold increase when platelets are stimulated with ADP or collagen.

Serotonin (5-hydroxytryptamine)

The platelet has a striking ability to accumulate serotonin by an active transport mechanism against a negative gradient. Platelets contain between 150 and 600 ng/10^9 cells of serotonin, and there is usually less than 30 ng/ml circulating in plasma. It is believed that the 5-hydroxytryptamine (5HT, serotonin) is released from the enterochromaffin cells in the intestine, and that this is accumulated in platelets in the circulation, explaining the higher serotonin content of platelets in portal blood to those in the systemic circulation. Once accumulated the platelet retains the serotonin unless its release reaction occurs. This is supported by the *in vivo* labelling studies of human platelets conducted by Heyssel (1961), wherein platelets labelled with ^{14}C-5HT had a slightly longer lifespan than platelets labelled with chromium. The physiological significance of the platelets' capacity to take up serotonin and of its release during the release reaction is still unknown. Serotonin produces a small, but variable aggregation of human platelets *in vitro* and is also a vasoconstrictor, but in none of these effects is it anywhere as potent as other agonists of human platelets (*see* Chapter 4).

RELEASE REACTION

This is a term which describes the specific release of platelet components found in the very dense granules and in the α-granules of the cell. It must be distinguished from cell lysis which follows an immune attack with destruction of the cell's membrane, since here the cellular contents, including cytosol enzymes such as lactic acid dehydrogenase (a frequently used marker), and enzymes present in mitochondria are freed. The physiological importance of release can be debated since drugs which can inhibit it do not usually result in bleeding problems, and patients with disorders in which this reaction is either ineffective or absent are usually little troubled by haemorrhages. However, activation of this release may be of prime importance in the instigation of platelet aggregation, and have a role in clinical situations such as the initiation of thrombotic events, migraine and even asthma (*v. infra*). Holmsen and Day (1969) have divided the mechanism of this phenomenon into:

(1) The receptor on the cell's surface,
(2) Transmission of the signal across the cell membrane, and
(3) Activation of release.

They have also divided the release reaction itself into release reaction 1, which they define as the release of substances in the very dense granules, and release reaction 2 which includes the substances found in the very dense granules and those in the α-granules. As markers for these events most laboratories use serotonin for release reaction 1, and platelet factor 4 and β-thromboglobulin for release reaction 2, and for cell lysis lactic acid dehydrogenase is used. Receptor sites for signal transmission have already been discussed in the section on the membrane of the cell.

It is important to emphasize that there are inhibitory receptor sites as well as excitatory receptor sites on the cell's surface. Most of the inhibitory sites appear to enhance the activity of adenylate cyclase and cause an increase in the levels of cAMP. Most excitatory stimuli have not been found to alter cAMP levels in the resting cell, but appear to prevent or lessen the effects of inhibitors on cAMP levels. The best identified and most studied biochemical pathway associated with the release reaction is that of thromboxane A_2 synthesis, but it is known that there must be other mechanisms of release since a complete blockade of this pathway can be overcome by thrombin and collagen in sufficient concentration without the activation of this pathway. It has been postulated that the effects of cAMP depend on a protein kinase which phosphorylates myosin kinase, and this decreases this protein's ability to bind calmodulin which regulates calcium mediated enzyme activity. The effects of the strongest inhibitors of platelet action such as PGI_2, PGE_1, PGD_2 can be blocked by calcium, and the mobilization of calcium by calcium ionophores induces platelet aggregation despite the presence of PGI_2, PGE_2 or PGD_2 (Figure 3.6). Increase in free calcium in the cell binds to calmodulin and this calmodulin-calcium complex in turn complexes with the inactive myosin kinase, activating it, this then interacts with actin causing contraction and the release reaction. The levels of cAMP in the cell are not only controlled by the activity of adenylate cyclase, but also by the enzyme phosphodiesterase which breaks cAMP down to AMP. Figure 3.6 sets out these events.

How this activation of the contractile system of the cell enables the release reaction is still unknown. The two favoured hypotheses are:

(1) That the granules are drawn close to the surface connecting system by the contractile process until they are bound, then the surface membrane of the granules fuses with that of the surface connecting system and breaks down the membrane by enzymatic attack allowing the release of the contents through the surface connecting system to the exterior of the cell.

(2) The so called 'hit and stick' hypothesis which envisages that the Brownian movement within the cell's granules usually does not have

sufficient energy for it to approach the surface connecting system, but that the activation of the contractile system results in the release of this energy which propels the granules with sufficient force to overcome any negative factors and to hit the membrane, stick on it, then fuse and release their contents.

It is important to emphasize that this release reaction refers to the release of platelet components into the liquid phase, but other alterations occur on the cell's membrane causing increased platelet factor 3 activity and providing the environs for coagulation. In normal circumstances these events occur simultaneously, but they may be independent of each other as illustrated by Glanzmann disease platelets in which the release reaction is normal, but platelet factor 3 activation is not. Similarly, some platelet contents such as factor VIII-Ag and Platelet factor 4 may be released from the cell but to a greater or lesser degree adhere to the cell's membrane, and respectively be of physiological significance in its adherence to collagen or microfibrils and to protect thrombin generation on the cell's surface (Chapter 4).

References

ADELSTEIN, R.S. and POLLARD, T.D. (1978). Platelet Contractile Proteins. In Spaet, T.H. (ed.). *Progress in Hemostasis and Thrombosis. Vol. 4*, p. 37. (New York: Grune and Stratton)

HEYSSEL, R.M. (1961). Determination of human platelet survival utilizing C14-labelled serotonin. *J. Clin. Invest.*, 40, 2134

HOLMSEN, H., DAY, H.J. and STORMORKEN, H. (1969). The blood platelet release reaction. *Scand. J. Haematol.*, (Suppl. 8)

LALEZARI, P. and DRISCOLL, A.M. (1982). Ability of thrombocytes to acquire HLA specificity from plasma. *Blood*, 59, 167

MARCUS, A.J. (1978). The role of lipids in platelet function: with particular reference to the arachidonic acid pathway. *J. Lipid Res.*, 19, 793

MARCUS, A.J. and ZUCKER, M.B. (1965). *The Physiology of Blood Platelets: Recent Biochemical, Morphologic and Clinical Research*. (New York: Grune & Stratton)

MEYERS, K.M., SEACHORD, C.L., HOLMSEN, H., SMITH, J.B. and PRIEUR, D.J. (1979). A dominant role of thromboxane formation in secondary aggregation of platelets. *Nature*, 282, 331

MICHELL, R.H. (1983). Ca2+ and protein kinase C: two synergistic cellular signals. *Trends Biochem. Sci. (TIBS)*, 8, 263

PHILLIPS, D.R. (1980). Surface labelling as a tool to determine structure–function relationships of platelet plasma membrane glycoproteins. *Thromb. Haemostas.*, 42, 1638

POLLET, R.J. and LEVEY, G.S. (1980). Principles of membrane receptor physiology and their application to clinical medicine. *Ann. Intern. Med.*, 92, 663

POLLEY, M.J., LEUNG, L.L.K., CLARK, F.Y. and NACHMAN, R.L. (1981). Thrombin-induced platelet membrane glycoprotein IIb and IIIa complex formation. An electron microscope study. *J. Exp. Med.*, 154, 1058

REIMERS, H.J., PACKHAM, M.A., KINLOUGH-RATHBONE, R.L. and MUSTARD, J.F. (1973). Effect of repeated treatment of rabbit platelets with low concentrations of thrombin on their function, metabolism and survival. *Br. J. Haematol.*, 25, 675

SHATTIL, S.J., ANAYA-GALINDO, R., BENNETT, J., COLMAN, R.W. and COOPER, R.A. (1975). Platelet hypersensitivity induced by cholesterol. *J. Clin. Invest.*, 55, 636

4
Platelet function

PLATELET ADHESIVENESS

One of the most basic and important biological phenomena is the property of a cell to adhere to one surface and not to another. Without such a property, sperms would not fertilize ova and morphogenesis would not occur, since changes in the properties of an individual cell's adhesiveness determine the company it keeps and may alter cell association and orientation to cause the configurational changes in embryogenesis which eventually produce an adult. This property is of importance in the defence mechanisms in the body such as phagocytosis, and the invasion of a cell by viruses or parasites is dependent on the ability of the foreign organism to adhere to the cell's surface prior to penetration. Its role in the spread of malignant cells is another example of why this property has attracted so much attention.

Platelet adhesiveness is the ability of platelets to adhere to other cells and/or surfaces, rather than to each other where the term aggregation or agglutination is used. Morphological studies have long emphasized the importance of platelet adhesion, but its mechanism is still poorly understood, largely resting on inference and circumstantial evidence provided by hereditary disorders of platelets in man, rather than on tight experimental evidence. In part this is due to the difficulty in measuring adhesiveness.

The lining cells of all blood vessels are endothelial cells which can now be isolated and grown in tissue culture. These cells have a glycoprotein layer covering their surface and exhibit properties of pinocytosis. *In vivo* they are joined to one another by tight junctions as well as desmosomes and have half demosome junctions with the basement membrane. Their surface also carries an antigen which is identical to factor VIII:related antigen (VIII:RAg) and probably has von Willebrand factor (VIII:vWf) activity but has no procoagulant VIII (VIII:CAg) or clotting activity (VIII:C). Tissue cultures of endothelial cells obtained from umbilical cords synthesize factor VIII:RAg, but not VIII:C. Unless endothelial cells are damaged, there is no evidence of other cells adhering to their surface, and cinemicrographs of intact vessels show white cells rolling along their surface with an axial stream of red cells and platelets. The endothelial cells exist as a single layer orientated to the longitudinal axis of the vessel and in parallel to flow. They are $50\,\mu$m in length and extend 2–$3\,\mu$m into the lumen of the vessel, occasionally displaying small projections which may be involved in phagocytosis. The number of mitotic figures and, therefore, the turnover rate of vascular endothelial cells is extremely small. However, there is an increased rate of turnover as judged by mitotic figures at vessel junctions which may be related to the increased trauma at these sites, and to the increased incidence of atheroma deposits. Human venous, but not arterial, endothelial cells elaborate a plasminogen activator. Arterial endothelial cells synthesize prostacyclin (PGI_2) and thereby may discourage platelet aggregation or initiation of clotting (*v. infra*). An ADPase has been found on the surface which could destroy ADP in the plasma, and thereby inhibit its platelet aggregating ability. The endothelial cells produce a heparin-like mucopolysaccharide which could act as a physiological anticoagulant. In culture they release a protein thrombomodulin which activates protein C, an enzyme which destroys the clotting factors V and VIII (*v. infra*).

Beneath the endothelial cells is the basement membrane which is composed of glycoprotein microfibrils having a high hydroxyproline content although their precise structure is unknown. When gaps appear between endothelial cells following injury, platelets adhere to the subendothelial surface and rapidly fill them. A simple *in vivo* experimental procedure which removes endothelial cells from medium sized vessels is to pass a catheter containing a balloon and then inflate the balloon and withdraw the catheter, which results in the stripping of the endothelium leaving the basement membrane intact. Within 10 minutes a single layer of disc shaped platelets which appear to act as a pseudo-endothelium has replaced the lost endothelial cells and thrombosis does not ensue. A repair process is established whereby the platelets are in turn replaced or covered by endothelial cells, and in many instances the platelets are incorporated into the subendothelium giving rise to early features of atheroma. If a vessel so damaged is repeatedly subjected to similar insults, there is not only a re-lining with a single layer of flattened platelets, but platelet clumps appear; in other words, the initiation of a thrombus. The requirement of repeated damage to the vessel wall to cause platelet aggregates and thrombus formation may relate to a necessity of damaging the endothelium sufficiently so that the cells are no longer capable of synthesizing prostacyclin as well as the other antithrombotic factors previously outlined. In any event, the damage to the vessel now predisposes to thrombus formation.

The layers surrounding the endothelium and basement membrane vary with the nature and type of the vessel. In the larger arteries there will be internal elastic lamina as well as smooth muscle cells, but the structure which appears to be the most significant from the haemostatic point of view is that of collagen. In vessels possessing an internal elastic lamina the collagen layer lies outside, i.e. peripheral to that layer. Collagen is believed to be of considerable importance in the response of an injured vessel, since its exposure results in activation of factor XII (Hageman factor) which commences the clotting cascade, as well as providing a surface to which platelets strongly adhere. Platelets also adhere to other elements in the basement membrane, namely the microfibrils, but to a lesser degree than to collagen, and microfibrillar adherence requires the presence of red cells and calcium ions whereas collagen platelet adherence occurs even in the presence of EDTA. Baumgartner (1972) has developed an experimental technique for examining platelet adhesiveness to damaged vessel walls *in vitro*. Using this technique he has shown that platelet adhesiveness is dependent on intrinsic properties of the cell which are lacking in Bernard–Soulier platelets, and which therefore may be dependent on glycoprotein Ib or one of the other minor components not yet completely identified as also lacking in this disorder (*v. infra*) – the plasma protein von Willebrand factor and the microfibrils or collagen beneath the endothelial layer. The specificity of this reaction is emphasized by the fact that Glanzmann platelets which lack glycoprotein IIb and IIIa adhere normally in this system.

There are as yet no widely adopted laboratory tests which specifically measure this function of the cell. Tests which in part depend on the properties of platelet adhesiveness are Borchgrevink's *in vivo* platelet adhesiveness test (1961) and a variety of tests for platelet retention to glass bead columns. The principle of the former test is to undertake platelet counts at fixed time intervals and compare these counts with a venous sample, after standard incisions with a template are made on the forearm and following the inflation of a blood pressure cuff to 40 mmHg. The difference between the venous sample and those obtained from the incisions from the forearm being regarded as representing the platelet's adherence and expressed as a difference, having a range of between 20 and 60%. Patients with Glanzmann disease show no difference between the venous and capillary samples, and clearly this test is dependent on the formation of a platelet plug as well as adhesion. Similarly the *in vitro* technique of glass bead adhesion depends on other plasma factors, von Willebrand factor and fibrinogen to coat the glass beads and also on platelet aggregation, so that patients with Glanzmann disease show a reduced glass bead adhesion. This is a time honoured test, and provided it is performed meticulously and is well standardized in the laboratory, has some diagnostic usefulness. The technique employed by most laboratories was developed from the original observations of Hellem (1960) that the percentage retention of platelets in a glass bead column was dependent on some factor that he found in red cells and which proved to be adenosine diphosphate. Confusing results were obtained in von Willebrand disease until it was realized that the rate of passage of the platelets through the glass beads was critical – should the rate be slow, ADP release from the platelets would cause aggregation and result in a high percentage of platelet retention on the glass beads, whereas rapid passage would cause a less than normal platelet retention. As a result Bowie (1971) developed a technique which employs a constant infusion with standardized glass beads contained in a tube of fixed diameter and size and passing platelet-rich plasma through the beads. The diameter of the glass beads, the surface of the containing tube as well as the volume of the column and the rate of infusion are all critical and must be standardized in each labora-

Table 4.1 Platelet retention on glass beads reduced or glass bead adhesiveness decreased

Congenital
Bernard–Soulier syndrome
Glanzmann disease
Storage pool deficiency
von Willebrand disease
Afibrinogenaemia

Acquired
Myeloproliferative disorders
Uraemia
Anaemia
? Aspirin defect
Disseminated intravascular coagulation
Acquired storage pool disease

Table 4.2 Platelet retention on glass beads increased or glass bead adhesiveness increased

Congenital
Homocystinuria

Acquired
Atherosclerosis
Hypertension
Hyperlipaemia
Diabetes
Post-operative period
Cancer
Multiple sclerosis
Oral contraceptives

tory. It is important that the glass bead columns are stored under constant atmospheric conditions, and that appropriate controls and standards are regularly undertaken. Even so, in our own laboratory we prefer to have three independent estimations on each individual patient, giving constant results before we are prepared to accept the result as definitely normal or abnormal. Table 4.1 shows the conditions, hereditary and acquired, which have been reported to have decreased platelet retention on glass beads or decreased glass bead adhesiveness. Table 4.2 shows disorders in which the reverse has been reported, i.e. increased glass bead adhesiveness or increased platelet retention. These tables represent reports from a number of laboratories, and in many instances there have been conflicting results. This is especially true with regard to coronary disease, atherosclerosis and diabetes. The diversity of these reports may reflect a number of factors which include patient selection and the methods employed.

ROLE OF PLATELETS IN BLOOD COAGULATION

Development of coagulation tests and concepts

Although the clotting of blood has been one of the most studied biological phenomena over the past 50 years, its precise nature still remains uncertain. It has been bedevilled by complicated terminology, and only in the past 5 years has a precise chemical structure for many of the components been established. Even now one of the most important, factor VIII (the factor which is abnormal in the disorder haemophilia), is poorly characterized and its role in coagulation is uncertain.

When blood is collected in a glass tube a clot is formed which after a varying time interval, usually between $\frac{1}{2}$ and 1 hour, retracts from the walls of the tube. Within 2 hours the process is complete, leaving a small deposit of free cells in the bottom of the tube, clear pale yellow serum and the fibrin clot, in which is enmeshed red cells, white cells and platelets. The property of clot retraction depends on a sufficient number of normally functioning platelets. Serum is the cell-free fluid in blood after clotting and differs from plasma since some of the plasma proteins are consumed whilst others are altered or activated. Some plasma proteins are not present in serum, e.g. fibrinogen which is totally converted to fibrin, whereas others remain either in a reduced amount and/or altered state, some being more active in the clotting process, e.g. IX, others being inactive, e.g. VIII (see Table 4.3).

Table 4.3 Coagulation factors

Serum	Aluminium hydroxide absorbed plasma
VII	Fibrinogen
IX	V
X	VIII
XI	XI
XII	XII

At the turn of the century the only tests available to investigate patients with haemostatic defects were the time it took for blood to clot in glass (whole blood coagulation time), the observation of clot retraction, the skin bleeding time and the platelet count. It was on the basis of such tests that haemophilia was distinguished from thrombocytopenia. In haemophilia the whole blood

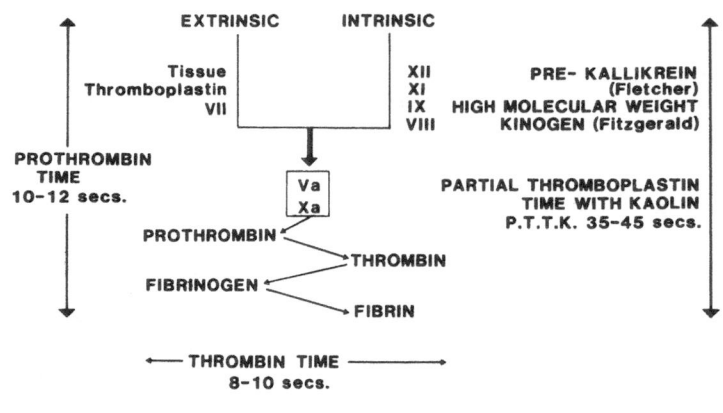

Figure 4.1 Simplified scheme of coagulation with commonly employed screening tests

clotting time was prolonged, clot retraction was normal after coagulation had occurred, the skin bleeding time was normal and the platelet count normal, whereas in thrombocytopenia the whole blood clotting time was normal, there was no clot retraction, the skin bleeding time was prolonged and the platelet count reduced. Haemophilia also had its striking inheritance pattern, being a sex-linked recessive disorder with expression of the disease in males but transmission by the otherwise normal females. It was this different hereditary pattern which enabled the first inherited haemostatic disorder to be distinguished from haemophilia; *viz.* von Willebrand disease (1911) where the disorder afflicted both male and female, and it was found that unlike haemophilia there was a prolonged skin bleeding time as well as a coagulation abnormality common to both disorders (Chapter 6).

The addition of calcium to plasma obtained by centrifuging blood collected into an anticoagulant such as citrate, resulted in a reproducible clotting time, and this was significantly shorter when platelet-rich plasma was compared with platelet-poor plasma. It was found that recalcification of plasma from patients with haemophilia, who had a strikingly longer clotting time than normal, was corrected by the addition of normal plasma. The prolonged clotting time of platelet-poor plasma required either the addition of platelets or phospholipids for its correction.

The introduction of the one stage prothrombin time by A. J. Quick represented a major advance. This test consists of adding tissue factor, sometimes called tissue thromboplastin (usually an acetone extract of brain), to platelet-poor plasma together with calcium. Fibrin formation occurs in 10–12 seconds in normal blood, but is found to be much longer in patients who have a vitamin

42

K deficiency or liver disease. Normal results depend on normal concentrations in plasma of the inactive enzyme precursor prothrombin, factor V (labile factor of Quick), factor VII (stable factor of Quick), factor X and fibrinogen (Figure 4.1). The clotting time of this test is far more rapid (10–12 seconds) than those seen on recalcification of platelet-rich plasma which depending on technique would be around 300–400 seconds, while the whole blood clotting time in glass would be 10–12 minutes. The prothrombin time was quite normal in patients with haemophilia, and eventually the concept was reached that there is an intrinsic coagulation system which is abnormal in haemophilia (VIII:C deficiency) and an extrinsic one involving tissue thromboplastin activation which is abnormal in liver disease and vitamin K deficiency. Both systems are haemostatically important in man, because isolated factor VII deficiency which is only involved in the extrinsic pathway may result in a severe haemorrhagic diathesis as does haemophilia (VIII:C deficiency) which only involves the intrinsic pathway.

The extrinsic blood coagulation system

Both the extrinsic and intrinsic systems lead to the activation of factor X (Xa) (Figure 4.1) and the subsequent conversion of prothrombin to the enzyme thrombin. The extrinsic system is unique in that it requires tissue factor and factor VII for the activation of factor X, neither of these factors are required in the intrinsic system. The tissue factor or tissue thromboplastin is not precisely characterized, but it is a combination of protein and lipid moieties, the protein having a peptidase activity which is separate from its clotting function, and a lipid phosphatidyl choline. This lipid is not active in the intrinsic pathway. Both lipid and protein are necessary for the extrinsic system activity. The extrinsic pathway is independent of platelets, and the composition of the tissue thromboplastin itself is critical and species specific so that tissue extracts from the animal under investigation are most efficient. This system appears early in evolution since species evolving in the Triassic period, such as the *Heterodontus portus Jacksoni* (The Port Jackson Shark), have an active extrinsic system. Studies of the distribution of tissue factor in mammals have shown high concentrations in organs such as lung, brain, placenta and in blood vessels where it is located on the surface of the endothelial cells lining these vessels. It is thought that tissue thromboplastin provides a binding site for factor VII and perhaps also X enabling the activation of the latter factor whose reaction is accelerated approximately 1000 times by the presence of factor V. A popular theory is that it is the activation of this system which provides small amounts of thrombin which in turn activate other clotting factors such as V and VIII involved in the intrinsic system, and hence these systems are biologically linked. Other proposals which have been advanced are that the two systems simply summate and support one another in the amounts of thrombin produced or there may be different physiological functions, perhaps related to anatomy, type of trauma or stress to which the tissue is subjected. Evidence has been presented to support an alternative extrinsic pathway which can be demonstrated *in vitro* by using dilute thromboplastin, Ca^{2+} and factor VII, and activates IX which together with VIII cofactor activates X, thus bypassing earlier steps in the intrinsic pathway. The importance, or otherwise, of this mechanism in physiological and pathological coagulation remains to be elucidated. The concept of extrinsic or intrinsic system is currently very helpful in the identification of a bleeding problem (Chapter 10).

The intrinsic system

The recalcification of platelet-rich plasma in a glass tube is normal in patients with isolated factor VII deficiency, and is dependent upon glass contact activation of clotting factors as well as lipids in the platelet, principally phosphatidyl ethanolamine. Quick introduced another test which he called the 'prothrombin consumption test' in which he allowed blood to clot in a glass tube, and at defined time intervals, e.g. at 0.5 hour, 1 hour and 2 hours after the blood had clotted, took aliquots of serum and added them to another tube containing fibrinogen, tissue thromboplastin and calcium and observed the clotting time (serum prothrombin time). The object of this test was to determine whether components which are required for the one stage prothrombin time remained in serum after coagulation. Using this approach Quick was able to show abnormalities in patients with haemophilia who had a normal whole blood clotting time in glass although their histories suggested a moderate to severe bleeding diathesis. In addition, patients with thrombocytopenia also failed to consume plasma components as completely as patients with normal platelet counts. In some severe haemophiliacs the serum prothrombin time was more rapid than the plasma prothrombin time, so that in severe factor VIII:C deficiency there was not only a reduced consumption or inactivation of clotting factors but also an increased activation resulting in a shortened clotting time. Although this test was helpful in diagnosing moderate to severe forms, it was unrewarding in all the mild forms of haemophilia where it was often normal. Some years later Bernard and Soulier showed that this test was abnormal in an hereditary platelet anomaly (the Bernard-Soulier syndrome). These data emphasize the collaborative role between the platelets and clotting factors in plasma when contacted with glass in the conversion of prothrombin to thrombin.

Another dramatic advance occurred when blood from two apparently identically severe haemophiliacs was mixed and mutual correction of the clotting time resulted. This observation led to the discovery of two coagulation factor deficiencies, both inherited in a sex-linked manner. One is termed true haemophilia and is the more common (haemophilia A), and is due to an abnormality of the factor VIII molecule. The other is haemophilia B or

Christmas Disease (after the name of one of the early patients described), and is due to an abnormality of the factor IX molecule. Some time later there was an even more puzzling finding when it was shown that if plasma from patients with factor VIII:C deficiency (true haemophilia) was infused into patients with von Willebrand disease who also had low factor VIII:C activity, the skin bleeding time was corrected and there was a restoration of the VIII:C levels to normal. This elevation in factor VIII:C lasted for a far longer period of time than would have been the case had normal plasma been infused into haemophiliacs. It was shown that serum which has no VIII:C activity had the same effect.

In 1953 Biggs and Douglas introduced the thromboplastin generation test. This is a two stage test in which appropriately diluted samples of serum and aluminium hydroxide-absorbed plasma are mixed together with platelets or a phospholipid substitute and calcium. At 1 minute intervals sub-samples are taken and added to a tube which contains either plasma or fibrinogen, calcium is then added and the clotting time is determined. Where the serum and plasma is obtained from a normal control the clotting time rapidly diminishes, particularly after the 3 minute sample to the order of 10–12 seconds. This test relies on the difference in clotting factor content in plasma absorbed with aluminium hydroxide and serum from which thrombin has been removed (Table 4.3). Since factor IX activity is present in serum, but absent in aluminium-absorbed plasma and factor VIII:C is absent in serum, but present in aluminium-absorbed plasma, IX and VIII deficiencies could readily be distinguished. It was a much more sensitive test to deficiencies in either factor VIII:C or IX than any previously established investigation, and it became possible to classify mild haemophiliacs in whom clotting examinations had been normal. From this approach there developed techniques for accurately assaying the clotting activities of factor IX and factor VIII:C. Table 4.4 sets out the various permutations and combinations when this test is employed in the diagnosis of haemostatic defects.

Table 4.4 Thromboplastin generation test

	Patient Deficiency					
	V	VIII	IX	X	XI	XII
CS + CP	N	N	N	N	N	N
CS + PP	A	A	N	N	N	N
PS + CP	N	N	A	A	N	N
PS + PP	A	A	A	A	A	A

CS = control serum; CP = control plasma; PS = patient serum; PP = patient plasma
N = normal: A = abnormal
VII is not required for the intrinsic system

Two stage tests such as the thromboplastin generation test have now been largely replaced by one stage techniques in most routine laboratories. The most commonly employed of these is called the 'activated partial thromboplastin time' (APTT) or the 'partial thromboplastin time with kaolin' (PTTK). In this test platelet-poor plasma is mixed with a phospholipid platelet substitute together with a potent surface activant such as kaolin, celite or ellagic acid, calcium is added and the clotting time determined. The normal range for the test varies with the reagents employed, and must be determined for the individual laboratory. It is a very useful screening test for all coagulant deficiencies with the exception of factors VII and XIII. This test has the added advantage of being readily automated, and by using the ability of the patient's plasma to correct plasma known to be deficient in individual clotting factors it can be used to diagnose precise coagulation defects as well as monitoring heparin therapy. It is the screening test par excellence at present for the intrinsic clotting pathway. Figure 4.2 is a schematic representation of the steps in this pathway. The general principles of this pathway were simultaneously

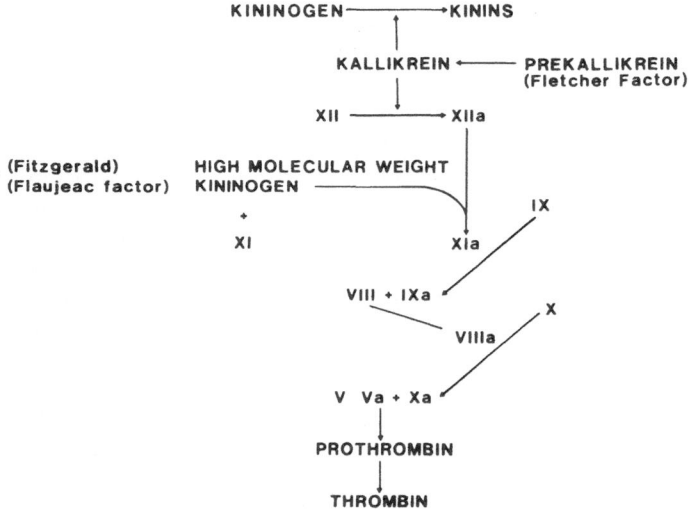

Figure 4.2 The intrinsic coagulation pathway

enunciated by R. G. McFarlane, and Davie and Ratnoff (1964), in which they proposed a scheme for intrinsic factor coagulation which was termed the cascade or amplification theory, stating that there was a progressive activation of clotting factors commencing with factor XII or contact factor and ending in the activation of factors X and V. All of these factors, with the exception of factor VIII, have been purified and their structure and amino acid sequence determined. These reactions consist of the activation of an inactive zymogen to produce a proteolytic enzyme (a serine protease) which splits off a peptide from its substrate in turn to convert another zymogen to a zymase. Some have proposed that factor VIII may have a similar function to factor V by enabling more efficient binding to a phospholipid micelle, thus enabling an acceleration of factor IX activation.

Following McFarlane's and Davie and Ratnoff's original proposals, it was appreciated that there were other plasma factors which were concerned in contact activation. These are prekallikrein (PK) or the Fletcher factor and the high molecular weight kininogen (HMWK) or the Fitzgerald, Flaujeac or Williams factor which together with factors XI and XII make up the 'contact factor system' (Figure 4.3). Apart from the surface activants already mentioned, which result in activation of Hageman factor (Factor XII), other negatively charged materials such as connective tissue or collagen, endotoxin and even sodium urate crystals have been shown to be able to initiate this intrinsic clotting system. Activated factor XII (XIIa) is capable of initiating the conversion of HMWK to bradykinin. Together with HMWK XIIa converts PK to kallikrein which activates both the complement and fibrinolytic pathways (Figure 4.3), and kallikrein in turn potentiates the further activation of factor XII. These reactions are closely related and interdependent. Thus this

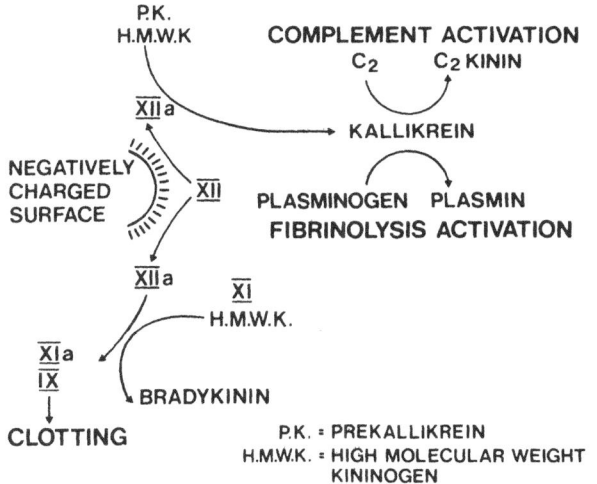

Figure 4.3 Contact factor activation

particular system serves as an interface with a number of other biologically important reactions which may be important for the body's response to a traumatic insult, and mount not just a clotting response but an inflammatory response as well. Walsh (1974) demonstrated that stimulation of human platelets could enhance activation of factor XII and factor XI and showed that there was a platelet pathway for activating factor XI which could bypass factor XII. Another link was established between the intrinsic and extrinsic system when it was found that human factor VII could be directly activated by XIIa. However, factor VIIa still requires tissue thromboplastin to convert prothrombin to thrombin in maximal quantity. The binding of factor XII to an activating surface results in a change in the protein's conformation which exposes or makes more readily available the cleavage site for kallikrein and which enhances XII to XIIa conversion (Figure 4.3). Factor XI which circulates in plasma combined with high molecular weight kininogen is linked to the negatively charged surface by the high molecular weight kininogen, and is then attacked by factor XIIa to become XIa. Activated factor XII itself can activate prekallikrein which is attached to the negatively charged surface through the high molecular weight kininogen. Once prekallikrein is converted to kallikrein it passes from the surface into the fluid phase where it may convert the factor XIIa to a low molecular weight form which is then released into the supernate.

A key step in blood clotting is the activation of the zymogen prothrombin to form thrombin, an enzyme which has a multiplicity of effects and which attacks a number of the clotting factors. Its principal substrate is fibrinogen, a protein composed of a dimer of three polypeptide chains A, B and γ-chains which are linked by disulphide bonds. Thrombin attacks fibrinogen at specific sites on its A and B chains to release fibrinopeptides A and B. The fibrinogen molecules so altered polymerize with one another to form fibrin. Thrombin also activates another zymogen in blood called platelet factor XIII or the fibrin stabilizing factor. Factor XIII is a transglutaminase which forms peptide bonds between γ-carboxyl groups of glutamine and ϵ-amino groups of lysine, thus cross-linking the β- and γ- chains of fibrin. During coagulation in the test tube, prothrombin is almost completely converted to thrombin, but it is initially formed in amounts insufficient to result in the conversion of fibrinogen to fibrin. This small concentration of thrombin may be of physiological significance by activating other blood components such as factor V to Va and increasing the effect of factor Xa by activating antihaemophiliac globulin (factor VIII:C) to cause a five to ten fold increase in its clotting activity, and also by binding to the surface of platelets and triggering platelet aggregation (Table 4.5).

Table 4.5   Amounts of thrombin insufficient to produce fibrin in plasma may:

Cause platelet release reaction
Cause platelet aggregation
Activate V$\rightarrow$ Va
Activate VIII:C $\rightarrow$ VIII:C$_t$
Activates factor XIII
Activates protein C
Stimulates prostacyclin production of endothelial cells
Induces mitosis in fibroblasts

Thrombin also attacks prothrombin, and in an autocatalytic fashion increases its own production. This build-up in thrombin activity is well illustrated by its appearance either when whole blood is allowed to clot in a tube or where platelet-rich plasma is recalcified in a test called the 'thrombin generation test'. In this test the production of thrombin is measured by adding calcium to platelet-rich plasma in a glass tube and samples taken at 1 minute

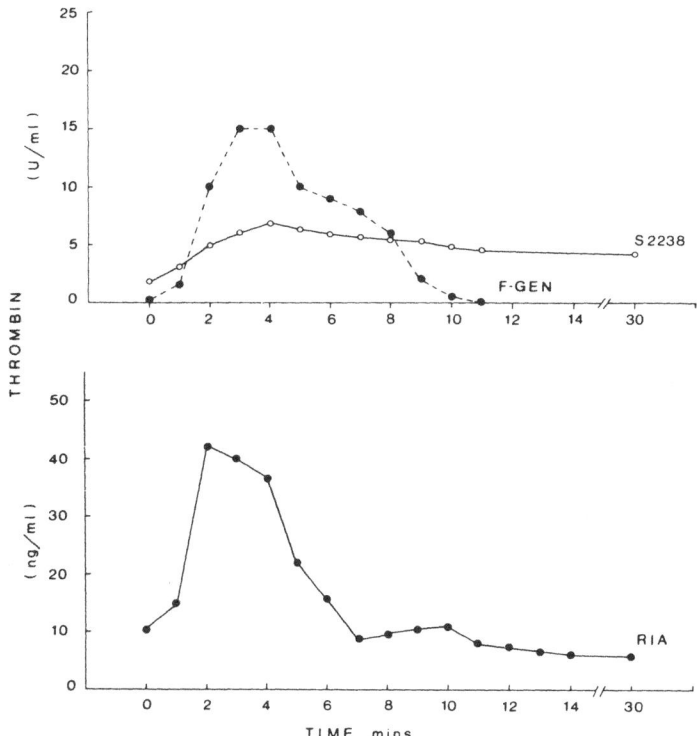

Figure 4.4 Generation of thrombin *in vitro* following the recalification of platelet-rich plasma (see text)

intervals, then added together with calcium to tubes containing fibrinogen and the clotting time measured. Using standard preparations of thrombin, the number of units needed to cause a particular clotting time can be calibrated and, therefore, the biological activity of the thrombin produced estimated in units (*see* Figure 4.4). Thrombin is a serine protease, but has esterolytic activities and other effects (*see* Table 4.5) including a mitotic stimulus on fibroblasts in culture and the stimulation of prostacyclin production by endothelial cells. This enzyme probably plays a wide role in the physiology of repair. Not only does it have the autocatalytic role mentioned above, but it also activates the recently recognized factor protein C, a serine protease which attacks and breaks down both factor V and factor VIII. Therefore, it may play a regulatory role as a safety mechanism in prohibiting an excessive formation of the active coagulant, and through its stimulation of PGI_2 production limit thrombus size. Three forms of thrombin have been identified which have been called α, β and γ. These have the respective molecular weights of 100 000, 80 000 and 70 000, the lower molecular weight species are derived from α-thrombin and are inactive biologically. The production of thrombin in blood is modulated by plasma proteins called antithrombin III (ATIII) or heparin cofactor II and α_2 macroglobulin, as well as by the binding of thrombin to fibrin, to platelets and to endothelial cells. Figure 4.4 shows the production of thrombin in recalcified platelet-rich plasma followed by its biological effects (clotting) on fibrinogen (F-GEN), its estimation employing radioimmunoassay techniques with a specific antithrombin antibody (RIA), and another technique which measures the enzyme's ability to split a specific low molecular weight chromagen (S2238). It will be seen that whilst its biological activity and radioimmunoassay peak at around 4–5 minutes, the chromogenic method shows a plateau effect which is due to the continued presence of thrombin which is not 'seen' by the antibody and is inert with fibrinogen, but which can still cleave the very low molecular weight chromagen substrate. The thrombin is bound to AT111 and α_2-macroglobulin, and its presence in such a combination is still detected by the small molecular weight chromagen. This modulation of thrombin production in the fluid phase is probably of importance in preventing the spread of thrombosis when the system is activated at an injury site *in vivo*, and also in neutralizing the slow release into the circulation of thrombin previously absorbed on fibrin and/or the endothelial cell surface. That these systems have a relevance to man is shown by the inherited anomaly of ATIII deficiency which is associated with a striking incidence of venous thrombosis. This safety mechanism is one of the many the body has to preserve the fluidity of blood and prevent widespread thrombosis. The other mechanisms which have so far been recognized include protein C, the fibrinolytic pathway which is present in blood and also in vessel walls, the clearance of activated clotting factors by the reticulo-endothelial system and the localization of clotting activation by its occurrence on the surface of the platelet itself (solid phase) rather than its free activation in the plasma (fluid phase).

Table 4.6 sets out the known clotting factors, and shows the current international nomenclature together with some of the common terms which have been used over the years, and which at times have led to considerable confusion. It will be noted that there is no factor VI and that most people prefer to use the term fibrinogen and not factor I; prothrombin, not factor II; tissue thromboplastin, not factor III; and calcium, not factor IV. Figures 4.1 and 4.2 show a schematic representation of a current model of the coagulation pathway. This represents a classically held concept of the coagulation process, outlining the extrinsic and intrinsic systems with a final common pathway which they both share by the formation of a complex 'prothrombinase'. This is thought to consist of a phospholipid micellar complex comprising phosphatidyl ethanolamine containing unsaturated fatty acids which binds factor V through calcium, a galactose residue on factor V is also important. This complex of Va, Xa, phospholipid and calcium rapidly converts prothrombin to thrombin. Factor Va does not have an enzymatic action but accelerates the prothrombin conversion by factor Xa, perhaps by some subtle configurational

50

Table 4.6 Coagulation nomenclature

International nomenclature	Terms commonly used in literature	Terms used in this book
I	Fibrinogen	Fibrinogen
II	Prothrombin	Prothrombin
	Prethrombin	
III	Tissue thromboplastin	Tissue thromboplastin
IV	Calcium	Calcium Ca^{2+}
V	Labile factor	V
	Ac globulin	
	Proaccelerin	
VII	Stable factor	VII
	Proconvertin	
VIII*	Anti-haemophiliac globulin (AHG)	VIII-C
	Anti-haemophiliac factor (AHF)	
	Anti-haemophiliac factor A	
	VIII-C	
IX	Christmas factor	IX
	Plasma thromboplastin	
	component (PTC), anti-haemophiliac factor B	
X	Stuart–Prower factor	X
XI	Plasma thromboplastin	XI
	antecedent (PTA)	
XII	Contact factor, Hageman factor	XII
XIII	Fibrin stabilizing factor (FSF)	XIII

The 'a' attached to the Roman numerals indicates that the factor has been activated
* VIII nomenclature is set out in the section on von Willebrand disease

change in prothrombin which greatly enhances factor Xa serine protease activity on prothrombin. Amino acid sequence studies of prothrombin have identified specific areas of the polypeptide which have an affinity for lipid and for factor V, respectively.

Whilst the evidence of the existence of these systems is extremely sound, difficulty may be experienced in trying to relate them to the actual process of haemostasis or thrombosis. This dilemma is best illustrated by considering the clinical effects of individual deficiencies of factors XII, XI, prekallikrein (Fletcher factor) and high molecular weight kininogen (see Figure 4.3). Even when these factors are virtually absent from a patient's blood, little or no haemostatic or other clinical problem is usually encountered. Indeed should these defects be detected in a patient who is having haemostatic difficulties, another cause should always be sought. Patients with factor XII deficiency such as the original proband, Mr Hageman, do not normally have any problems with haemostasis and can undergo major surgery quite safely. Factor XI deficiency rarely results in bleeding problems, and similarly patients with pre-kallikrein and high molecular weight kininogen deficiency, although having strikingly prolonged PTTKs, have no bleeding problems. It seems highly likely, therefore, that this portion of the intrinsic system with the exception of Factor XI is of little significance in haemostasis, although it is possible that it could be important in the production of thrombosis if it were activated in some fashion.

It has even been suggested that factor XII and factor XI deficiency may predispose to vascular disease and result in a higher incidence of coronary disorders, Mr Hageman himself died with a pulmonary embolus. One offered explanation is that the contact system also activates the fibrinolytic pathways, kininogen and complement systems, as well as the coagulation system. The low incidence of thrombosis and bleeding in such patients however, makes it much more likely that their presence or absence in plasma is of relatively little clinical significance.

If the intrinsic pathway is not a major one in haemostasis how then is this achieved, remembering that factors VIII and IX deficiency, factor VII deficiency together with X and V deficiencies, afibrinogenaemia and thrombocytopenia all can cause major haemostatic problems with spontaneous bruising and life threatening bleeding following the most minor trauma? One attractive explanation would be that platelets play an active role in coagulation rather than merely acting as a passive supplier of phospholipid as has sometimes been proposed. Although the clotting schemes outlined above (Figures 4.1 and 4.2) are of considerable value in the consideration and diagnosis of haemostatic and other factor defects, they are less relevant in the haemostatic process in man. They may be of more importance in immune and inflammatory response and perhaps are important back-up systems, both in the active clotting process and also in the modulation of coagulation in the body by activating fibrinolytic systems.

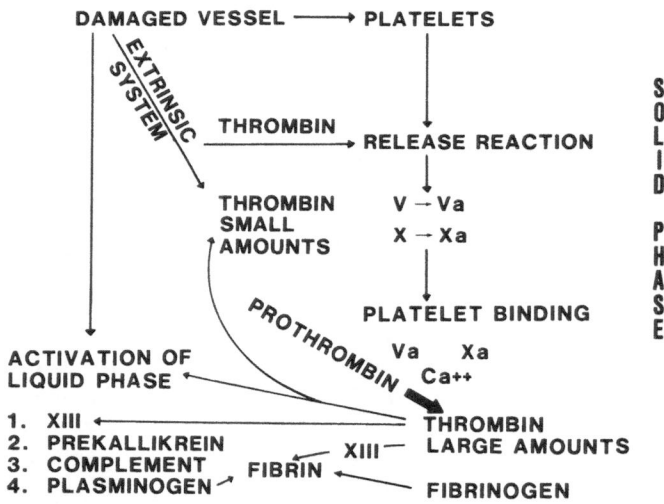

Figure 4.5 Events in haemostasis

It is the belief of many now that the important haemostatic mechanism is a solid phase one involving the platelet. Figure 4.5 summarizes the events leading to haemostasis. The platelet is seen as identifying the site of injury and being stimulated by a number of factors, e.g. the exposure to collagen tissue, or by the extrinsic system with the activation of tissue thromboplastin and factor VII producing small amounts of thrombin. Thrombin may enhance or induce platelet aggregation already occurring and also activate the platelet, producing a 'flip flop' of the membrane with exposure of coagulant active phospholipid sites which involve phosphatidyl ethanolamine now exposed on the external surface together with other receptors and contractile proteins such as actin and also fibronectin. Platelet factor V is released from the platelet to its surface, is activated to Va and establishes a specific receptor site for activated factor X (Xa). It is possible that the origin of Xa may be via the formation of small amounts of thrombin in the extrinsic pathway, and this mechanism may also cause the release and activation of platelet factor V. The reaction is localized to the platelet's surface, and thereby protected from the antithrombins present in the plasma enabling the explosive conversion of pro-thrombin to thrombin. This causes further platelet aggregation and fibrin formation, and establishes an effective haemostatic plug of fibrin stabilized by thrombin activated factor XIII and platelets. The roles of factors VIII and IX in this system are still uncertain, although IX may be activated directly by the alternate extrinsic pathway (see page 44); factor VIII has a specific binding site on the platelet which is related to glycoprotein Ib and/or other minor glyco-proteins missing in the Bernard–Soulier syndrome and which are important in the conversion of prothrombin to thrombin, in view of the abnormal serum prothrombin time in these patients. It may be that the high molecular weight components of factor VIII are important for the binding and localization of the prothrombinase on the surface of the platelet, while the VIII:C acts as a catalyst in the prothrombin–thrombin conversion, or acts by accelerating the effects of factor IXa on the activation of X. Apart from the demonstration by Majerus and his co-workers (1978) of these specific binding sites on the platelet surface, and that of Walsh (1974) and others showing that early contact phase can be greatly enhanced or bypassed by platelet activation, there is now evidence that the severity of the haemostatic defect in patients with factor V deficiency is not dependent on the level of factor V in the plasma (fluid phase), but relates more closely to the factor V levels in platelets (solid phase). Majerus and his colleagues have also shown that the conversion of prothrombin to thrombin is much more effective with these platelet receptor sites than can be achieved by any permutation or combination of added phospholipid to a platelet-free plasma system. Platelets, therefore, are not just passive in their role in clotting. Earlier studies which pointed to the importance of platelet factor V and VIII in generating adequate haemostatic plugs, were reported by Borchevink and Owren (1961) who infused normal platelets into patients with factor V deficiency and haemophilia (VIII:C deficiency), and converted the secondary bleeding time to normal for several days, but only for a few hours in those with factor X and IX deficiency.

Platelet factors in clotting

Table 4.7 sets out the nomenclature which has been used over the years with regard to platelets and blood coagulation. This table is included for the reader's convenience as except for platelet factor 3 and 4 most of this terminology is no longer used. Platelet factor 3 is often equated with platelet factor 3 release. This does not mean that a platelet procoagulant activity is released into the fluid phase with serotonin, its stored nucleotides and other components of release. The platelet's coagulant activity remains on its surface membrane, but this activity is enhanced if the platelet is subjected to stimuli which result in the release reaction and the associated changes in the surface membrane of the

Table 4.7 Platelet factors in coagulation

Platelet factor	
1	Factor V
2	Fibrinogen activator factor accelerating thrombin's conversion of fibrinogen to fibrin
3	Usually regarded as a phospholipid important in factor X activation
4	Anti-heparin factor
5	Fibrinogen
6	Plasmin inhibitor

Table 4.7 lists platelet factor terminology used over the years but only platelet factor 3 and 4 are now in common usage; others such as platelet factor 10 for serotonin (5-hydroxytryptamine) have dropped out of use completely

cell. One of the commonest systems for measuring this platelet coagulant activity is based on a recalcification of platelet-rich plasma in a two stage technique. Following the addition of calcium, an aliquot of the plasma, taken at appropriate time intervals, is added to the snake venom stypven with additional calcium and the clotting time observed. With incubation this time is shortened due to the platelet enhancing factor X activation. This test is also employed as an investigation of immune damage to the platelet, since the platelet's exposure to an antibody results in an alteration in its surface which enhances the clotting activity. Again this is frequently reported as the measurement of platelet factor 3 release by antibodies, although high speed centrifugation reveals that this activity is present in the platelet membrane components and not in the fluid phase. These tests are best regarded as screening tests for platelet procoagulant activity and/or activation of the platelet by mechanical or immune assault.

Platelet factor 4 (PF_4) is released from the platelet as a complex of two tetramers of PF_4 with two molecules of a proteoglycan carrier, giving an overall molecular weight of 350 000. PF_4 has an antiheparin activity, but its biological function is still unknown (see Chapter 3).

Coagulation factors and the platelet

Roskam and other earlier workers proposed that platelets were surrounded by a plasma atmosphere in which clotting factors were thought to be the most important. Suggestions were made that the affinity of the platelet for these factors might be of importance in its role in haemostasis, and a number of papers show that platelets exhibited clotting activities similar to prothrombin factors V, VII, VIII, IX, X, XI and XII. However, after washing platelets it becomes apparent that the only coagulation factors present in significant amounts are factors V, fibrinogen, VIII:Ag, factor XIII and calcium. In particular factors VIII:C, IX, X, XI and XII are readily removed with repeated washing. Other plasma proteins also remain after extensive washing of the platelets. These include albumin which constitutes 2% of the protein, and γ-globulin which is present in levels of 4.4 pg/mg of protein.

Factor XIII is located in the platelet cytosol, whereas fibrinogen and probably factor V are contained in the α-granules of the cell. Fibrinogen constitutes between 10 and 15% of the total protein of the cell, and is greatly diminished in patients with Glanzmann disease (*v. infra*) or congenital afibrinogenaemia. Fibrinogen receptors on the cell's surface are important in platelet aggregation (*v. infra*).

The factor VIII:Ag present in platelets, represents one fifth of the VIII:Ag content in blood; two thirds of platelet VIII:Ag is secreted by the platelets activated by collagen or thrombin, but the time of release is much more delayed than that of other substances released. The role of platelet factor V has already been discussed, but the function of the remaining clotting factors in the platelets is still uncertain.

Anti-thrombin III

This is an α_2-globulin, found in the platelet as well as in plasma; whose molecular weight is 63 000 and inhibits, in addition to thrombin, factors Xa, IXa, XIa and plasmin. One family has been described with a thrombotic tendency in which the only defect was a reduction in the platelet ATIII.

Platelet calcium

It is calculated that the platelet contains 10 μmol of calcium per 10^{11} cells, and that two thirds of this may be secreted during the release reaction; it is thought to be stored in the very dense granules. The remaining third is possibly located in the dense tubular system in the cell's cytosol and the membrane and by its modulation of free to bound forms, probably through the aegis of the enzyme regulating protein calmodulin, exerts a very important overall influence on the cell's metabolism. Since the amount of calcium secreted from a normal number of platelets has been calculated to give a level in blood of something in the order of 0.04 mmol/l compared with the plasma concentration of 2.5 mmol/l it seems unlikely that secreted platelet calcium would contribute greatly to any of the clotting processes. It is possible that its localization and even concentration in the cell's surface connecting system may reach much higher concentrations, and therefore be of importance in the atmosphere of the cell.

Summary of platelet function in blood coagulation

The three major functions of the platelet are: (1) to identify and localize the site of thrombus formation *in vivo*; (2) to provide specific receptor sites for activated clotting factors and the phospholipid milieu for optimal conversion of prothrombin to thrombin; and (3) to protect thrombin thus formed from plasma antithrombins. A major factor in the initiation and control of coagulation is the platelet, and the major events occur on the surface of this cell rather than on the damaged surface of the blood vessels or tissues (Walsh, 1974) and together with the work of Majerus and his colleagues (1978) quoted earlier, it would seem to make excellent sense that this cell orchestrates both the initiation and localization of thrombin production, and does not simply supply the lipid necessary for intrinsic factor clotting activity (platelet factor 3).

PLATELET AGGREGATION

Early histopathologists observed platelet clumps in thrombus formation. Platelet aggregation in whole blood and in citrated platelet-rich plasma was followed after the addition of calcium and/or thrombin by light microscopy. In 1960 Hellem reported a new factor which was derived from red cells involved in platelet aggregation. This was later identified as being adenosine diphosphate (ADP). It was the introduction of nephelometry by Born and Cross as a technique for investigating platelet aggregation which resulted in major advances in the study of platelet physiology, since it established for the first time a simple quantitative technique for examining the process of platelet aggregation. Apart from its importance in research it has become a keystone to the investigation and diagnosis of haemostatic and thrombotic problems. It has enabled the identification and study of both physiological and pharmacological agents which are both agonists and antagonists of platelet aggregation. Platelet-rich plasma usually anticoagulated with citrate is placed in a cuvette and stirred at a constant rate whilst being kept at a constant temperature, and to it is added an appropriate agonist or antagonist. Light is shone through the cuvette, and aggregation is measured by the increase in its transmission as the platelets change shape and aggregates form and enlarge, which result in the characteristic response. The change in amplitude of the trace immediately after adding an aggregating agent represents shape change in the platelet, and the increase in light transmission represents the degree of platelet aggregation. This technique can be employed not only to examine platelet function *per se*, but also to study the effects of antigen–antibody interactions on the cell, specific reaction of plasma components such as von Willebrand factor in the presence of the antibiotic ristocetin or the snake venom *Bothrops jararaca* and the interaction of platelets with lectins or with particulate matter such as latex, zymosan etc. Figure 4.6 illustrates the two phase platelet aggregation which occurs with adrenalin which unlike many agonists does not cause shape change. The primary wave of aggregation represents the initial interaction of the stimulus with the platelet surface prior to the induction of the release reaction which causes the second phase, or secondary wave of platelet aggregation. This form of aggregation is not seen when anticoagulants other than citrate are employed, e.g. heparin, when only one phase of aggregation is observed. It is in effect an artifact of the anticoagulant resulting in a relative lack of Ca^{2+} and perhaps Mg^{2+} ions, but it is a very useful phenomenon since it facilitates the recognition of release reaction abnormalities (*v. infra*). Some of the agonists employed in laboratories are listed in Table 4.8. Those designated in groups 1 and 2 and ristocetin in group 3 are standardly employed in routine laboratory screening tests of haemostatic function. Group 1 represents agents which are thought to be important physiological stimuli acting on a specific receptor site on the platelet surface and resulting in the initiation of aggregation as well as the release reaction by triggering the prostaglandin pathway. If the release reaction is blocked by drugs such as aspirin only the primary response will occur with adrenalin. There will be no aggregation induced by arachidonic acid but the response to the calcium ionophore will be normal. However, high concentrations of collagen and thrombin will still induce maximal aggregation, presumably by acting through alternative pathways.

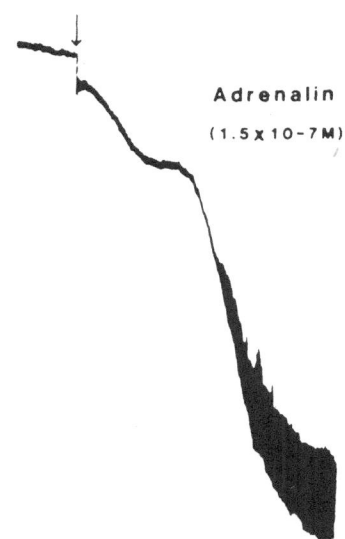

Adrenalin

$(1.5 \times 10^{-7}M)$

Figure 4.6 Two phase platelet aggregation following addition of adrenalin to citrated plateletrich plasma. Aspirin blocks the secondary wave of aggregation seen here

Table 4.8 Platelet aggregation agonists

Group 1	ADP
	Adrenalin (Epinephrine)
	Collagen
	Thrombin
Group 2	Arachidonic acid
	Calcium ionophore
Group 3	*Bothrops jararaca*
	Bovine fibrinogen
	Ristocetin
Group 4	1-0-alkyl-2 acetyl-glyceryl-3-phosphoryl choline
	(Platelet Aggregating Factor, PAF).
	Bacteria
	DNA
	Fibrin/fibrinogen monomers
Group 5	DNA
	Latex
	Lectins
	Polylysine (PLL)
	Zymosan

Other agonists such as stable analogues of thromboxane A_2 will undoubtedly soon be available, and increase the accuracy in defining individual platelet defects.

Group I agonists

Adenosine diphosphate (ADP)

The initial discovery that ADP induced platelet aggregation, and later that platelets contained a storage pool of ADP which was released, led to the belief that ADP was the final common pathway for platelet aggregation and the formation of a haemostatic plug.

It was found that platelet-rich plasma from patients with afibrinogenaemia did not respond normally to ADP, in contrast to thrombin aggregation of such platelets, perhaps explaining the prolonged skin bleeding time reported in some patients with afibrinogenaemia. Aggregation of washed platelets with ADP requires fibrinogen to be added to the suspending solution. The most immediate change on adding ADP to platelet-rich plasma is the conversion of the cell from a disc-like shape to a spiny sphere, in so doing fibrinogen binding sites on the cell are exposed, and fibrinogen so bound may bridge cell to cell and take part in the initial aggregate formation. Substances which inhibit the shape change, such as PGE_1 or treatment of the platelet to remove surface glycoprotein, abolish the uptake of fibrinogen onto the cell following exposure to ADP thus blocking ADP aggregation. ADP has been found to inhibit adenylate cyclase activity which in turn would lower the cAMP levels, predisposing to the release reaction and aggregation. Thromboxane A_2 appears to require ADP to cause aggregation (*see* Chapter 3). Platelets contain fibrinogen which may be released by ADP, and so it is possible that the cell's fibrinogen may itself be of importance in forming aggregates. ADP can act independently of the release reaction since at high concentrations it will still produce platelet aggregation when the prostaglandin pathway has been blocked by aspirin or where the release reaction has been inhibited by drugs, such as colchicine. Normally the concentration of ADP needed to cause aggregation is 10^{-6} mol/l, but previous exposure to suboptimal amounts of adrenalin will lower this to 10^{-7} mol/l, and similarly patients have been found with disorders such as diabetes and thrombotic states whose platelets are aggregable at these levels. The significance of this finding is still uncertain, although many think it is an indication of a hyperthrombotic state. ADP aggregation, in addition to fibrinogen, requires divalent cations, such as calcium and magnesium as well as the correct pH since both EDTA and lowering of the pH inhibits the ADP reaction.

Adrenalin

Platelets have approximately 100 α-adrenergic binding sites per cell, and it has been suggested that the lack of ability to saturate these sites may be due to their internalization during the study. The platelet α-adrenergic receptors have been classified as α_2 in type, since yohimbine is much more potent than prazosin in inhibiting binding with dihydrokryptine. This is an α-adrenergic antagonist which binds equally well to α_1- and α_2-receptors, and prazosin inhibits α_1-receptor binding while yohimbine inhibits α_2. It is interesting that guanosine nucleotides, e.g. GTP, convert high affinity α_2 sites to low affinity receptors, and may in this way modulate the platelets' response. The addition of adrenalin to platelets inhibits adenylate cyclase, and this may also explain how a small amount of adrenalin, which in itself is unable to cause aggregation, may potentiate the effects of other agents. The ability of small amounts of adrenalin to cause this effect may explain the reported enhancement of platelet aggregation in people under stress and in some cigarette smokers, although these particular studies apparently did not take into consideration the effect of minor changes in the haematocrit which may alter the plasma citrate concentration and thereby modify aggregation. Increased catecholamine levels in platelets have been documented in patients with phaeochromocytomas. Increased sensitivity of platelets to aggregation by adrenalin has been reported in patients with hyperlipoproteinaemia, e.g. diabetes, and this type of response can also be induced by deliberately raising the concentration of cholesterol in the platelets by incubating them in appropriately modified substrates with high cholesterol concentrations. The action of adrenalin on the platelet is unusual in that it does not induce a shape change and only $\frac{1}{3}$ the number of fibrinogen receptors are exposed on the surface when compared with ADP.

Collagen

Collagen is a fibrous protein which in mammals makes up approximately one third of the total body protein. Five major types of collagen have now been described, and collagen fibrils are arranged in different ways depending on the biological function of the connective tissue in which they are involved. In tendons they are arranged in parallel bundles, electron microscopy shows they have a characteristic periodicity of cross striations which have a spacing of 70 nm. The spacing is believed to be due to the heads of the tropocollagen molecules with repeating units constituting collagen fibrils. The tropocollagen molecule is made up of three single polypeptide chains arranged in a helical fashion and being 280×1.4 nm in length and width. The characteristic periodicity is due to the staggering of the heads of the tropocollagen molecules in the collagen fibrils where these are cross-linked covalently by dihydrolysine and leucine. The tropocollagen polypeptide chains are made up of repetitive groups of glycine, another amino acid, and either proline or hydroxyproline G–A–Pr or Hy, so that the polypeptide chains consist of 35% glycine, 11% alanine, 12% proline and 9% hydroxyproline. They are glycoproteins and usually have an oligosaccharide side chain attached to the hydroxyl group of hydroxylysine residues. These oligosaccharides are frequently glucose and galactose. In 1962 Hugues first demonstrated that platelets adhered to strands of connective tissue, which led to the recognition of collagen's importance in the initiating events of haemostasis. Collagen preparations induced platelet aggregation, and this was dependent on the type of collagen – Type 1 being greater than Type 2 – greater or equal to Type 3 – being greater than Type 4. Type 4 collagen, which is derived from basement membrane, was the weakest inducer of serotonin release of all four types. It was soon established that the tropocollagen was not capable of inducing platelet aggregation but had to be polymerized to form the quaternary structure to induce aggregation, and it was also found that agents which prevented the conversion of monomeric collagen to fibrillar collagen delayed or abolished collagen induced aggregation. Other workers found that collagen could activate factor XII and thus commence the clotting cascade. Nossel and his co-workers showed that the ε-amino groups of the N-terminal ends of the collagen molecule were important for its platelet aggregating function, whereas the carboxyl groups were important for its activation of factor XII. Further studies suggested that it was the helical portion of the collagen molecule (this comprises approximately 85% of the molecule) which is important in platelet aggregation and not the non-helical portion (telopeptides). The mechanism of collagen interaction with platelets is still debated, but specific receptor sites have been suggested, and one theory proposed that glucosyl transferase in the platelet membrane binds to the oligosaccharide portion of the collagen fibrils. Following the platelet's exposure to collagen its cGMP levels increase and the release reaction occurs. Whether platelet adherence and subsequently platelet aggregation occur through a similar receptor mechanism or differing receptor sites is still not known. It is known that platelet adhesion to collagen fibres requires calcium, and this can be prohibited by prostacyclin but not by aspirin. Platelets from patients with a storage pool defect or normal people following the ingestion of aspirin show an initial small aggregation on the addition of collagen but this is far less than normal. In normal people collagen aggregation is single phase, and one does not see the two-phase reactions that can be obtained with ADP or with adrenalin in citrated plasma.

Thrombin

Majerus has estimated that there are approximately 30–40 000 thrombin binding sites per platelet but only 500 are of a high affinity, and to induce the release reaction the thrombin needs to bind to 100–200 of these high affinity sites. Thrombin's serine protease activity is essential to the induction of the release reaction, since inactivation of thrombin by DFP does not alter its binding to the platelets, but no release follows. The actual protein or glycoprotein attacked by thrombin is still uncertain, although GPIb, GPIIIa and GPV have each been proposed. Monospecific antibodies have now been obtained to some of the platelet glycoproteins, and Polley and her colleagues (1981) using this technique have shown that normally the pattern of GPIb on the platelet surface occurs as small micro clusters. However, following exposure to thrombin, GPIIb and GPIIIa which normally occur in random fashion on the membrane aggregate and form clusters. These glycoproteins are the ones which are abnormal or missing in Glanzmann disease or thrombasthenia, where platelets do not aggregate with any of the physiological agonists including thrombin, but normal release occurs emphasizing the differences between release and aggregation. Circumstantial evidence has been produced by a number of laboratories which suggests that as well as stimulating the release reaction through activation of the prostaglandin pathway, thrombin has another mechanism of inducing aggregation.

It has been shown that after platelets have been exposed to thrombin they develop a lectin activity and can cause red cell agglutination, and that they have a much greater affinity for binding isolated platelet membranes than control platelets. Thrombin has been shown to activate the prostaglandin pathway by mobilizing arachidonic acid. Using radioimmunoassays small amounts of thrombin are present almost immediately in shed whole blood collected into glass tubes, and on recalcification of platelet-rich plasma in the earliest samples significant amounts of thrombin were present, in contrast to platelet-poor plasma where none could be detected on recalcification.

In view of the previous discussion of thrombin formation on the platelet membrane being physiologically important in coagulation, it may also be the initial step in *in vivo* platelet aggregation at the site of platelet plug formation, and may induce this reaction in a number of ways. Firstly thrombin may alter the properties of the membrane, making it stickier and hence adhering to other cells; secondly it may induce the release reaction with the generation of thromboxane A_2 and release of ADP. Thirdly by its action on fibrinogen, it may produce fibrinogen components which in themselves may cause platelet aggregation, and finally fibrin formation with its intimate relationship to platelets resulting in the phenomenon of clot retraction (*v. infra*). Unlike thromboxane A_2 thrombin does not require ADP to enable the induction of aggregation, and is a more potent agonist of aggregation of washed platelets suspended in buffer without added fibrinogen than it is in platelet-rich plasma, perhaps because plasma contains inhibiting factors such as ATIII and α_2 macroglobulin.

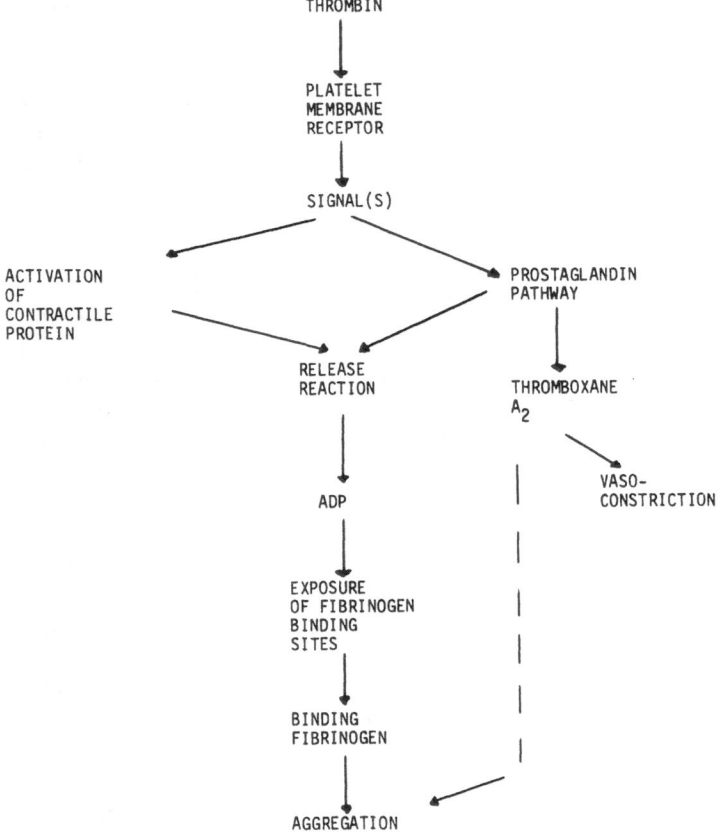

Figure 4.7 Steps in the interaction of thrombin with the platelet

Thrombin does not require the activation of the prostaglandin pathway to induce secretion, and appears to effect the release reaction via another mechanism so that there may be at least two independent pathways which induce the release reaction (Figure 4.7).

Huang and Detwiler have divided group 1 reagents into weak and strong agonists. They classify adrenalin and ADP as weak as they induce secretion by an aggregation mediated response, this secretion can be blocked by preventing aggregation by such circumstances as not stirring the platelet-rich plasma or by using inhibitors of the prostaglandin pathway. Strong agonists (collagen and thrombin) cause secretion without necessarily inducing aggregation. These agonists can induce aggregation even in the presence of blocked prostaglandin pathways.

A refractory aggregatory state may be induced by the addition of any of the group 1 agents to unstirred platelet-rich plasma, subsequent stirring will not induce aggregation, nor will this be overcome by the addition of increased amounts of the agent which has been used to induce this refractory state. This may be of physiological significance where stasis has been induced *in vivo*, and act as a safety mechanism in obstructed vessels by prohibiting further platelet aggregation. By analogy with other receptors, the first response of a receptor to its agonist could be the induction of clustering of the receptor sites, and lateral movement to activate a membrane effector protein or internalization as a part of the mechanism of producing aggregation. Thus the refractory state induced by not stirring platelets could relate to the internalization of receptor sites (down regulation) *without* clustering which may be essential for a positive stimulus.

Group 2 agonists

These agonists act by entering the platelet, and in the case of arachidonic acid, initiating the production of thromboxane A_2 by its conversion to PGG_2 (Figure 3.5). Calcium ionophore is believed to act by releasing calcium within the cytosol of the cell which, through the protein modulator, calmodulan, both initiates the prostaglandin pathway to produce thromboxane A_2 and also activates the contractile proteins in the cell directly to bring about release and to induce platelets aggregation (Figures 3.4 and 3.6). Calcium ionophores, therefore, are not blocked by aspirin.

Group 3 agonists

Group 3 lists reagents which react with a plasma factor, von Willebrand factor (vWf) and a specific platelet receptor site, but which do not require the platelets to be metabolically active since platelets fixed in formalin will agglutinate in response to the addition of any of the reagents in group 3 together with vWf. In the case of bovine fibrinogen and ristocetin, the platelet receptor involved is glycoprotein Ib, since platelets from patients with Bernard–Soulier syndrome (*v. infra*) or platelets treated with chymotrypsin do not react in the presence of vWf with either ristocetin or bovine fibrinogen. They do react, although in a significantly reduced fashion, to *Bothrops jararaca* (botrocetin) and vWf. A number of studies have shown a quantitative relationship between the number of platelets (receptor sites) present, the concentration of ristocetin (or botrocetin) and the concentration of von Willebrand factor, so this reaction is a quantitative one. Therefore, one can assay the amount of a plasma factor which reacts with fixed platelets in the presence of ristocetin or bothrops. Frequently this type of assay is called a von Willebrand factor assay, but by current knowledge it is more correct to term the result of such an assay as being VIII ristocetin co-factor (VIII:RCoF) when ristocetin is employed, and VIII bothrops co-factor (VIII:BCoF) when botrocetin is used in the assay. This will be discussed further in the section on von Willebrand disease. Bothrops and ristocetin will induce platelet aggregation in platelet-rich plasma, and in the case of ristocetin will induce a release reaction which can be blocked by the use of prostaglandin inhibitors, but platelet aggregation still results. Most routine laboratories use ristocetin in platelet-rich plasma as a screening test for Bernard–Soulier syndrome and von Willebrand disease. It is important to emphasize that mild forms of the latter disorder will react normally to ristocetin in platelet-rich plasma. There is one variant in which the addition of concentrations of ristocetin (which normally do not produce platelet aggregation in normal platelet-rich plasma) cause platelet aggregation (Chapter 6).

Group 4 agonists

These represent a miscellaneous list of agents which may have an important role in platelet aggregation *in vivo*, particularly in certain pathological states. Platelet aggregating factor (PAF) was first identified as playing a role in certain allergic responses such as acute anaphylactic reactions, where it was recovered from the blood of rabbits and identified in basophils, mast cells, polymorphonuclears and monocytes. This was released following exposure to ionophores, C5A or following phagocytosis. PAF has been characterized as having the chemical structure of 10-alkyl-2-acetyl-glyceryl-3-phosphoryl choline. It has been postulated that PAF released following various allergic situations, such as serum sickness and some autoimmune syndromes, may cause platelet agglutination to occur, and result in release of substances which may damage vessels or may result in obstruction of capillary networks, e.g. those in the lungs. This substance also causes aggregation and degranulation of polymorphonuclear leukocytes, and has been invoked as a reason that patients with serum sickness may develop coronary arteritis, which in animals has been shown to be blocked by rendering them neutropenic. In asthma, substances such as β-thromboglobulin and platelet factor 4 are increased during the acute attack, and it is postulated that this is a result of IgE mediated events causing the release of PAF from basophils or other tissues, and perhaps contributing to the circulatory problems in acute asthma by damaging capillary vessels. It has been suggested that this substance may be synthesized in platelets and account for a third platelet aggregating pathway independent of ADP and prostaglandin platelet aggregation, and explain mechanisms whereby thrombin and collagen can induce platelet aggregation when these other agonists are ineffective. PAF is synthesized in washed rabbit platelets following the addition of ionophore, thrombin or collagen whereas no synthesis occurs following the addition of ADP or arachidonic acid. It is a potent activator of platelet aggregation inducing both aggregation and release in platelet-rich plasma at concentrations of 1.9×10^{-8} mol/l, but studies by Marcus and his colleagues (1979) have not found the same synthesis of PAF by human pletelets following stimulation with thrombin or ionophore, casting doubt on the hypothesis that its synthesis by human platelets is an alternative pathway to platelet aggregation. Marcus' study showed that this agent is a potent agonist for platelet aggregation but was far less effective in inducing the release reaction, and was relatively weak in causing thromboxane production. Therefore, it seems possible in man that PAF, whilst it may be important in the pathogenesis and accentuation of some pathological conditions, is of little significance in the physiology of haemostasis.

Bacteria, particularly staphylococci, have been shown to induce platelet aggregation when added to platelet-rich plasma, and the extent of the aggregation is determined by the number of bacteria to that of platelets. This was at its maximum when the ratio was 1:1, but when the bacterial ratio was gradually reduced, a longer contact time was required before aggregation resulted. This aggregation was preceded by changes in the traces due to the platelets' shape change. Further reduction in the ratio, so that there was one bacterium to 70 platelets, resulted in a gradual narrowing of the trace secondary to shape change, but no aggregation took place. There were individual differences between bacteria. *E. coli* for example was a poor stimulus for platelet aggregation, whilst the β-haemolytic streptococcus was very similar but not quite as potent as staphylococcus. EDTA could completely block the response, and so presumably divalent cations are required; the platelet aggregation was also inhibited either by EDTA or by using an enzyme system which consumed released adenosine diphosphate. This phenomenon may account for the associated thrombocytopenia seen in septicaemia, although in most instances in the clinical situation of marked thrombocytopenia with septicaemia there is an associated severe degree of disseminated intravascular coagulation which might account for the thrombocytopenia. It has also been reported that fibrin/fibrinogen monomers may, in their own right, institute platelet aggregation, perhaps by interacting with the fibrinogen receptors on the platelet's surface.

Early studies reported that platelet aggregation and release of ADP and serotonin could be associated with the phagocytosis of antigen–antibody complexes. Later work has shown that antigen-antibody complexes can interact with the platelet surface through the platelet's Fc receptors, and in the case of rabbit platelets, will induce platelet aggregation and release reaction. In a number of studies with human platelets it has been shown that antigen–antibody complexes bind to the Fc receptor of the cell in situations where washed platelets are used, but that this is inhibited in platelet-rich plasma by the presence of plasma immunoglobulins. Immune complexes containing fibrinogen overcome this inhibition perhaps because they can react with both fibrinogen and Fc receptors.

Double stranded DNA (ds DNA) has been shown to be present in the plasma of patients with a number of conditions, in concentrations ranging from 5 to 100 μg/ml. It is therefore of interest that recent studies have shown that washed platelets suspended in saline will aggregate when ds DNA is added in this concentration range, and the aggregation is accompanied by serotonin release. This effect can be inhibited by treating the ds DNA with DNAase, but is not inhibited by equivalent concentrations of single stranded DNA or RNA. However, the addition of ds DNA to platelet-rich plasma does not induce aggregation, and indeed appears to inhibit aggregation induced by collagen and thrombin although not that induced by adrenalin or ADP. The inhibitory effect on thrombin and collagen does not seem to result from interference with the reaction of these substances with the platelet surface since the phenomenon of shape change occurs quite normally. DNA has been shown to bind to the surface of human platelets, and binding sites have also been demonstrated for single stranded DNA which can be enhanced by platelet activating agents such as ADP or immune complexes. Such interactions may be of fundamental importance in platelet physiology since there are many instances in man where there would be a combination of circumstances leading to increases in circulating DNA, immune complexes and disseminated intravascular clotting resulting in the release of fibrin/fibrinogen monomers. Fibrin/fibrinogen monomers may impair coagulation by inhibiting thrombin whilst others have been reported to induce platelet aggregation.

Group 5 agonists

The agents in Group 5 which have no known physiological or pathological counterparts, latex and zymosan, are discussed later.

Lectins are an interesting research tool, since they can interact with specific sugars on the cell's surface and in some cases cause agglutination of fixed platelets, therefore representing a purely surface phenomenon; whilst others do not produce agglutination or aggregation and yet induce the release reaction again demonstrating that these activities can be separated from each other. Two lectins which have been most extensively studied are wheat germ agglutinin which binds to *N*-acetyl glucosamine and which interacts with glycoprotein Ib, and concanavalin A which binds to mannose and glucose and interacts with glycoprotein IIb and IIIa.

Poly-l-lysine (PLL) induces both aggregation and release, but the aggregation proceeds where release is inhibited or where fixed platelets are employed and release cannot occur. This effect is, therefore, an agglutination phenomenon which has been shown to correlate with binding of PLL to the cell's surface. It is possibly due to a reduction in surface charge since the PLL aggregates are strongly cationic, and also possibly to interplatelet bridging by the PLL aggregates. PLL aggregate size is important and the ϵ-amino groups of the PLL are essential since succinylation abolishes the agglutinating effect.

More than one mechanism or pathway is involved in platelet aggregation. Collagen, thrombin and ionophores can induce platelet aggregation even when the prostaglandin pathway is completely blocked *in vitro*. In most instances shape change precedes aggregation, but this is not the case when adrenalin is used as the agonist. Aggregation and the release reaction can be clearly separated since one can obtain aggregation without release and *vice versa*. In most concepts of platelet aggregation the key events are regarded as first the perturbation of the cell's membrane resulting in message transmission, perhaps through enzyme activation or change in membrane permeability resulting in a calcium flux from outside to inside the cell, or secondly a stimulation of a calcium flux within the cell which triggers the activation of the platelet's contractile system, or perhaps acts through calmodulin thereby influencing or activating a variety of intracellular calcium dependent enzymes. These then result in further alterations on the surface of the cell exposing receptors for fibrinogen, for example, and perhaps translating actin to the platelet's surface where it may interact with ADP, and also altering the placement of phospholipids so that a surface more compatible for activation of coagulant proteins is developed. Changes in the glycolipid and perhaps glycoprotein and phospholipid exposure may support the released thrombospondin's lectin-like activity following thrombin.

Central to the cell's reaction is its overall metabolic state, and this appears to relate particularly to levels of cAMP and cGMP. Most reports indicate that elevated cAMP levels inhibit platelet aggregation, whilst cGMP levels have been noted to rise during the process of aggregation, and an opposing action of these two cyclic nucleotides has been put forward. This has recently been challenged by work which shows that the inhibitory effect of nitric oxide, nitroprusside and other vasodilator agents such as glycerol trinitrate is due to these compounds activating guanylate cyclase thereby resulting in an increase of 100–200 times cGMP above normal. Cyclic AMP levels are also increased, but only to twice the original level, and this contrasts to the effect of PGE_1, a potent inhibitor of platelet aggregation which when added in amounts to induce similar inhibition to that obtained with nitric oxide raises the cAMP level to 30 times its original value. Mellion and co-workers suggest that the increase in cGMP, seen normally in aggregation, may be a control safety mechanism to inhibit excessive formation of aggregates. A postulated role for the cyclic nucleotides ranges from the regulation of intracellular calcium in either free or stored forms to direct involvement in the activation or inhibition of actin and myosin interactions which are involved in both the release reactions and changes on the cells's surface (Figures 3.4 and 3.6). Mustard's group (1973) has shown that platelets may be treated with thrombin to deplete their releasable ADP and serotonin and then shown to undergo shape change and aggregation following exposure to ionophores. Shape change is not prevented by EDTA although aggregation is. This suggests that aggregation in this instance depends on external calcium ions. PGE_1 blocks the aggregation induced by ionophores in thrombin treated platelets, perhaps by increasing cAMP and thereby altering calcium availability within the platelet (Figure 3.6). Thrombin treated platelets may also be aggregated by adding ADP, provided fibrinogen is present. However, such cells show no response to thrombin itself. This group has shown that, thrombin treated cells which have been entirely exhausted of their dense bodies, and therefore ADP, serotonin and catecholamine stores, circulate for a normal lifespan and still retain a considerable metabolic capacity.

CLOT RETRACTION

This was one of the first properties of blood observed and was described by Hewson in his original studies on coagulation. The process is a relatively slow one, and when whole blood is collected into a glass tube, it is usually 30 minutes before some serum is observed around the periphery of the clot due to its retraction from the glass walls. The process continues until it reaches its maximum at 1.5–2 hours. The extent of the clot retraction depends on the platelet count, the fibrinogen concentration and the number of red cells present. Clot retraction is reduced in circumstances where the platelet count is less than 100×10^9/litre, where the fibrinogen concentration is high, and where the red cell numbers are increased as in polycythaemia. It is enhanced in thrombocytosis, hypofibrinogaemia and factor XIII deficiency. It is thought that the red cells become intermeshed in the interlacing fibrin strands, and polycythaemia prevents adequate retraction by its bulk physically impeding the fibrin retraction. Investigations of platelet-poor plasma have shown that washed platelets added to concentrations of over 50×10^9/litre can restore clot retraction which can be measured by the volume of fluid left after the clot is removed. The degree of retraction can be shown to be proportional to the numbers of platelets added to the platelet-poor plasma. Platelets which have been freeze–thawed or metabolically rendered inert, are incapable of restoring this property to platelet-poor plasma. If a solution of pure fibrinogen is made and clotted with thrombin, washed platelets on their own are not sufficient to restore clot retraction, but the addition of glucose will correct this defect. It is now realized that glucose is required by the platelets to generate ATP to enable activation of the contractile protein in the platelet.

Histological studies with the light and electron microscope have shown that if a clot is sectioned immediately after it is formed in platelet-rich plasma the platelets appear as single elements scattered like stars in the sky on a background of interwoven fibrin strands, and that as time proceeds the platelets swell and throw out more pseudopods, and by half an hour the swollen platelets are seen to be collected into groups of two or three as well as single cells, presumably reflecting retraction and apposition of the cells in a process similar to viscous metamorphosis. Early in the course of coagulation platelets are thought to throw out filopodia for considerable distances ($2-3\,\mu$m), and this phenomenon may continue for some time after the initiation of the clot. These filopodia attach at points in the fibrin network, and as the contractile protein of the cell becomes activated the filopodia contract pulling the strands together and producing the phenomenon of clot retraction. Inhibition of fibrin stabilizing factor (factor XIII) is known to enhance clot retraction.

The physiological significance of clot retraction is uncertain. It has been proposed that it may draw together the edges of traumatized or severed vessels, but this would seem unlikely when the measurement of the force developed in the clot is only 20 mm of water. It has been pointed out that this tensile strength may be greatly increased if one just examined the force generated by a platelet plug, rather than an *in vitro* clot. Measurements supporting this do not seem to be available. Another suggestion is that the retraction of the clot slowly releases thrombin which has been initially adsorbed to the fibrin and fibrinogen, and this enables its neutralization by passing plasma antithrombins. It may merely represent a process which was important in the haemostasis of lower forms of life, and thereby be a vestigial reminder of the evolution of this system.

PLATELET PHAGOCYTOSIS

The platelet's interaction with particulate matter was well recognized by early workers, and the injection of carbon particles into animals to produce thrombocytopenia experimentally was widely used. Since then it has been shown that platelets ingest a great variety of particles ranging from viruses, thorotrast, carbon, colloidal gold, technetium, fat and latex beads (from $0.1\,\mu$m to $0.3\,\mu$m in diameter). With some particles platelet aggregation results, and in certain circumstances the release reaction also occurs. Platelets also interact with particles such as zymosan and bacteria which are too large for the cell to take up.

The phenomenon differs from true phagocytosis since the particles enter the cell through the surface connecting system and not through the invagination of the surface membrane by a mechanism similar to pinocytosis in the case of small particles, or the indentation of the membrane with its subsequent

encirclement of the particle and production of a phagosome, as in true phagocytosis. In every instance that has been studied thus far, the particles enter the
cell through the surface connecting system, although a scalloping of the
external membrane by latex particles is frequently observed. Studies show that
after the engulfment of latex beads the addition of stains, which enter the
surface connecting system and stain its glycoprotein layer, demonstrates this
layer surrounding the engulfed particles. The use of a second particle such as
thorotrast also results in the appearance of these particles in the same areas of
the cell as the larger latex particles which therefore lie in an area of the cell
connected with the surface. Unlike phagocytosis the platelet releases its
contents to the exterior rather than into the compartment which is engulfing
the particles and the energy requirement and metabolic changes also differ.

The mechanism of uptake of particulate matter into the platelet differs
markedly between the two particles studied the most, namely thorotrast and
latex. Electronmicrograph studies show that thorotrast particles do not adhere
to the surface of the cell, but enter the surface connecting system, and
provided incubation continues for 30 minutes to 1 hour some of the particles
can be shown in α-granules, but the majority remain in the inner vesicles of the
cell which are part of the surface connecting system. The process of thorotrast
uptake is not inhibited by any of the standard biochemical metabolic inhibitors
blocking anaerobic or aerobic glycolysis or by sulphydryl inhibitors such as
N-ethyl maleimide. Indeed sodium flouride appears to greatly enhance the cell's
uptake of thorotrast. There is no difference in lactic acid or CO_2 production by
platelets incubated with thorotrast compared with normal control platelets.

In the case of latex particles, it has been shown that the particle must be
initially coated with a plasma protein, namely fibrinogen, then in the presence
of calcium the particle adheres to the surface of the cell causing a scalloped
appearance, and within 1–3 minutes other latex particles may be observed
within the surface connecting system of the cell; during this time platelet
adhesion to one another (aggregation) has commenced. This does not involve
the release reaction, and is not inhibited by aspirin, adenosine or enzyme
systems which remove ADP. It is, however, inhibited by EDTA, and a number
of metabolic inhibitors including sodium fluoride as well as classical inhibitors
of respiration such as KCN, and the combination of KCN and monoiodo-
acetate totally abolishes latex uptake whilst only reducing that of thorotrast.
Likewise, if the incubation is carried out at 4 °C there is some reduction in latex
particle uptake, but thorotrast uptake is normal or only slightly reduced. In the
initial stages of latex particle uptake, namely the first 5–10 minutes, there is
little or no change in lactic acid or CO_2 production by the cell. Subsequently at 30 minutes to 1 hour, there is a dramatic difference between
control platelets and platelets incubated with thorotrast compared with those
incubated with latex, in that there is a considerable increase in CO_2 and in
lactic acid production in the latter. It is thought that in these instances this is
due to the onset of the release reaction.

For latex particles to produce the release reaction they must have immunoglobulin in addition to fibrinogen on their surface, and it would seem that to induce this phenomenon, one requires both fibrinogen and Fc receptors on the cell to be stimulated. Both thorotrast and latex particle uptake are blocked completely by drugs such as cocaine and chlorpromazine which stabilize the membrane, and which under the electron microscope appear to cut off the surface connecting system or to close it down by the cells becoming spherical in shape.

The platelets' interactions with bacteria and zymosan are different again from that of latex and thorotrast particles, since they require not only the presence of immunoglobulin on the surface of the particle but also complement C3b. The latter requirement is surprising, since C3b receptors have been reported not to be present on human platelet membrane. Nonetheless, this is a prerequisite for these particles interacting with the platelet, resulting in platelet aggregation and the release reaction.

The physiological significance of this phenomenon is unknown, but it is consistently present in the thrombocytes of all submammalian species thus far studied, and one could speculate that it must represent some very fundamental aspect of the cell's function. Surface connecting systems are not evident in thrombocytes and so the mechanism of uptake may be different to the platelet. Behnke (1970) has proposed that there may be a constant movement of the platelet membrane which might transport attached particles such as latex. Perhaps there is also a similar but unrelated inflow of plasma to account for the uptake of thorotrast. Some authors have claimed that bactericidal substances are present in platelets, but recent studies examining bacteria causing platelet clumping and the subsequent measurement of bacterial viability showed that although the bacteria were enmeshed in the platelet aggregates they could grow normally in culture, and although collagen interaction with platelets produced substances which could clump bacteria no bactericidal effect could be shown.

References

ADELMAN, B., STEMERMAN, M. B., MENNELL, D. and HANDEN, R. I. (1981). The interaction of platelets with aortic sub-endothelium: Inhibition of adhesion and secretion of prostaglandin I_2. *Blood*, **58**, 198

BAUMGARTNER, H. R. (1972). Platelet interaction with vascular structures. *Thromb. Diath. Haemorrh. (Suppl)* **51**, 161

BORCHGREVINK, C. F. (1961). Platlet adhesion in vivo in patients with bleeding disorders. *Acta Med. Scand.,* **170**, 231

BORCHGREVINK, C. F. and OWREN, P. A. (1961). The haemostatic effect of normal platelets in haemophilia & factor V deficiency. The importance of clotting factors absorbed on platelets for normal haemostasis. *Acta Med. Scand.,* **170**, 375

BORN, G. V. R. and CROSS, M. J. (1963). *J. Physiol. (London)*, **168**, 178

BOWIE, E. J. W. and OWEN, C. A. (1971). Some factors influencing platelet retention in glass bead columns including the influence of plastics. *Am. J. Clin. Pathol.*, **56**, 479

CHIGNARD, M., LE COUEDIC, J. P., VARGAFTIG, B. F. and BENVENISTE, J. (1980).

Platelet-activating factor (PAF-Acether) secretion from platelets: Effect of aggregating agents. *Br. J. Haematol.*, **46**, 455

CLAWSON, C. C. and WHITE, J. G. (1971). Platelet interaction with bacteria. I. Reaction phases and effects of inhibitors. *Am. J. Pathol.*, **65**, 367

CLAWSON, C. C. and WHITE, J. G. (1971). Platelet interaction with bacteria. II. Fate of the bacteria. *Am. J. Path.*, **65**, 381

DAVIE, E. W. and RATNOFF, O. D. (1964). Waterfall sequence for intrinsic blood clotting. *Science*, **145**, 310

GRIFFIN, J. H. and COCHRANE, C. G. (1979). Recent Advances in the Understanding of Contact Activation Reactions. *Seminars in Thrombosis & Hemostasis*, Vol. V, p. 254

HELLEM, A. J. (1960). *Scand. J. Clin. Lab. Invest.*, **12**, (Suppl. 51)

HUANG, E. M. and DETWILER, T. C. (1981). Characteristics of the synergistic actions of platelet agonists. *Blood*, **57**, 685

HUGUES, J. (1962). Accolement des plaquette aux structures conjonctivis périvasculaires. *Thromb. Diath. Haemorrh.*, **8**, 241

MARCUS, A. J. (1979). The role of prostaglandins in platelet function. In Brown, E. B. (ed.). *Progress in Hematology*, Vol. XI, p. 147, (New York: Grune & Stratton)

MACFARLANE, R. G. An enzyme cascade in the blood clotting mechanism and its function as a biochemical amplifier. *Nature*, **202**, 498

MAJERUS, P. W. and MILETICH, J. P. (1978). Relationships between platelets and coagulation factors in hemostasis. *Ann. Rev. Med.*, **29**, 41

MARLER, R. A., KLEISS, A. J. and GRIFFIN, J. H. (1982). An alternative extrinsic pathway of human blood coagulation. *Blood*, **60**, 1353

MELLION, B. T., IGNARRO, L. J., OHLSTEIN, E. H., PONTECORVO, E. G., HYMAN, A. L. and KADOWITZ, P. J. (1981). Evidence for the inhibitory role of guanosine 3'5' monophosphate in ADP-induced human platelet aggregation in the presence of nitric oxide and related vasodilators. *Blood*, **57**, 946

MEYER, D. (1972). In vitro platelet adhesiveness. Methods of study and clinical significance. In Mannucci, P. M. and Gormi, S. (ed.). *Platelet Function and Thrombosis*. pp. 123–147. (New York: Plenum)

MOHAMMAD, S. F., CHUANG, H. Y. K., CROWTHER, P. E. and MASON, R. G. (1979). Interactions of poly (L-lysine) with human platelets. Correlation of binding with induction of platelet aggregation. *Thrombos. Res.*, **15**, 781

NEMERSON, Y. and PITLICK, F. A. (1972). Extrinsic clotting pathways. In Spaet, T. H. (ed.). *Progress in Hemostasis and Thrombosis*. Vol. I, p. 1, (New York: Grune & Stratton)

PACKHAM, M. A., GUCCIONE, M. A., GREENBERG, J. P., KINLOUGH-RATHBONE, R. L. and MUSTARD, J. F. (1977). Release of ^{14}C-serotonin during initial platelet changes induced by thrombin, collagen or A 23187. *Blood*, **50**, 915

PEEROCHKE, E. I. and ZUCKER, M. B. (1981). Fibrinogen receptor exposure and aggregation of human blood platelets produced by ADP and chilling. *Blood*, **57**, 663

POLLEY, M. J., LEUNG, L. L. K., CLARK, F. Y. and NACHMAN, R. L. Thrombin-induced platelet membrane glycoprotein IIb and IIIa complex formation: an electron microscope study. *J. Exp. Med.*, **154**, 1058

PROCKOP, D. J., KIVIRIKKO, K. I., TUDERMAN, L. and GUZMAN, N. A. (1979). The biosynthesis of collagen and its disorders. *New Engl. J. Med.*, **301**, 13

SHUMAN, M. A., BOTNEY, M. and FENTON, J. W. (1979). Thrombin-induced platelet secretion. *J. Clin. Invest.*, **63**, 1211

STEMERMAN, M. B. (1974). Vascular intimal components: precursors of thrombosis. In Spaet, T. H. (ed.). *Progress in Hemostasis and Thrombosis*. Vol. 2, p.1, (New York: Grune & Stratton)

TOCANTINS, L. M. (1938). The mammalian blood platelet in health and disease. *Medicine*, **17**, 155

WALSH, P. N. (1974). Platelet coagulant activities and hemostasis: A hypothesis. *Blood*, **43**, 597

WILNER, G. D., NOSSEL, H. L., LEROY, E. C. (1968). Activation of Hageman factor by collagen. *J. Clin. Invest.*, **47**, 2608

5
The physiology of haemostasis

Virchow triad is still a keystone in the current theories of haemostasis. The collaborative interaction of the vessel wall, the rheological properties of blood and the phenomenon of blood coagulation are universally accepted. The events triggering thrombosis, either venous or arterial, are less well documented although the common presence of phleboliths in the pelvic venous system together with the frequent demonstration of venous thrombi around the valves of veins in the lower limbs, show that *in vivo* such events are common and do not necessarily relate to standard processes of trauma.

Figure 5.1 illustrates the situation where a vessel wall has been ruptured.

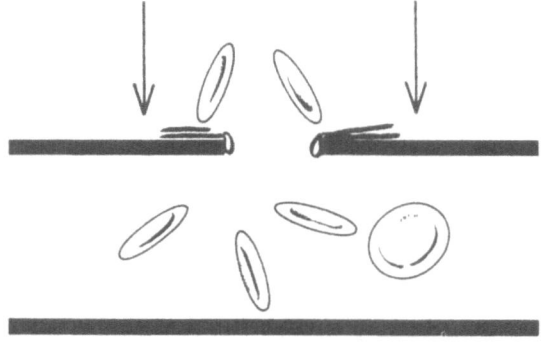

PLATELET ADHESION

1. BERNARD SOULIER RECEPTOR

2. VON WILLEBRAND'S FACTOR

3. COLLAGEN

Figure 5.1   4. MICROFIBRILS

73

This results in exudation of blood into the extravascular tissues, which in turn will result in the increased pressure on the vessel wall illustrated by the arrows. In the case of a vein or small vessel, such pressure can cause the vessel to collapse, with reduction in flow, therefore aiding in the staunching of the escape of blood. This mechanism clearly is more effective in situations where tissue is compartmentalized within some rigid structure. Apart from the physical escape of blood, the trauma causing the vessel rupture may sever or traumatize the nerve plexus which is adjacent to arterioles and sets up axonal reflexes which result in contraction with decrease in blood flow and loss. As blood flows past the damaged vessel wall, platelets adhere either to exposed collagen fibres or other microfibrils lying subjacent to the vessel. This adhesion requires the presence of a plasma factor called von Willebrand factor which resides particularly in the high molecular weight polymers of factor VIII which will be discussed in Chapter 6. Another requirement is a specific glycoprotein receptor on the cell's surface which is absent in Bernard–Soulier syndrome and which involves glycoprotein Ib. Both in von Willebrand disease, where the high molecular weight components of factor VIII are missing, and in Bernard–Soulier syndrome, there is a prolonged skin bleeding time because these initial events do not take place normally.

Figure 5.2 represents the next step where platelet aggregation has been initiated, for convenience this has been termed primary reversible aggregation.

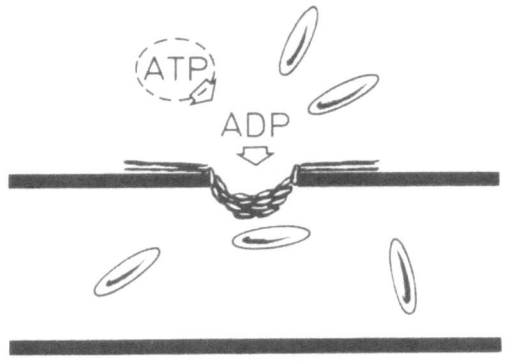

PRIMARY REVERSIBLE AGGREGATION

AGGREGATION INITIATED BY

a)   COLLAGEN

b)   ADP - FROM TISSUE OR RED CELL

c)   OTHER METABOLITES

     i)   ADRENALIN

    ii)   SEROTONIN

Figure 5.2

This is probably an artificial separation from the stage represented in Figure 5.3 since it is only clearly defined in artificial *in vitro* situations where citrate lowers the calcium concentration, or in some hereditary or acquired disease states. It envisages platelet aggregation before the onset of the release reaction, and this may be triggered either by the collagen fibres exposed on the traumatized vessel surface or by release of ADP either from the damaged tissue or from lysed red cells or perhaps even by small amounts of thrombin generated by the extrinsic clotting pathway. Other metabolites such as adrenalin or serotonin may potentiate the platelets' response to these factors, although whether the levels required to do this are achieved *in vivo* is uncertain. Fundamental to these events is the flow of blood, both through the vessel and initially through the wound. The term reversible is used for this initial stage since in the test tube, aggregation induced by ADP at low concentrations may revert without the release reaction occurring, and the platelets therefore remain morphologically entirely normal.

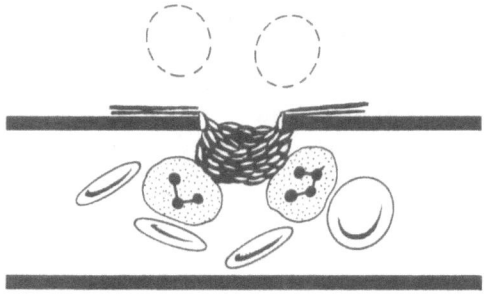

SECONDARY IRREVERSIBLE AGGREGATION

1. RELEASE REACTION ACTIVATED

2. PROSTAGLANDIN METABOLITE SECRETION
   a) HETE-CHEMOTACTIC
   b) THROMBOXANE A$_2$.   VASOCONSTRICTION

3. RELEASE OF PLATELET COMPONENTS
   a) ADP   g) FIBRINOGEN
   b) SEROTONIN   h) FIBRONECTIN
   c) β THROMBOGLOBULIN   i) WAG II
   d) PLATELET FACTOR 4   j) MITOGENIC FACTOR
   e) FACTOR V   k) ATP
   f) VIII-Ag

4. SOLID PHASE CLOTTING INITIATED AND AMPLIFIED

5. THROMBIN - INITIALLY SMALL AMOUNTS GIVING FURTHER AGGREGATION AND RELEASE.

6. FLOW - FURTHER AGGREGATION.

Figure 5.3

Figure 5.3 represents the onset of irreversible aggregation which results after the release reaction has occurred, and includes the secretion of a number of platelet components including the prostaglandin metabolites, in particular thromboxane A_2 which reinforces the aggregation process and is also a potent vasoconstrictor, therefore reducing the vessel diameter and flow. As is listed in Figure 5.3, a number of platelet components are released, the significance of many of which is still uncertain. The ADP release will reinforce the aggregation, perhaps in conjunction with thromboxane A_2 and serotonin may have some role in further vasoconstriction. The release of platelet factor V may be a very important step in providing the binding site for Xa and the activation and initiation of solid phase clotting discussed earlier. Small amounts of thrombin are initially formed which again reinforce aggregation. The release of the prostaglandin metabolites HETE and HHT results in the attraction of leukocytes to the platelet aggregate, which is a characteristic feature of histological sections of the platelet head of a thrombus. The platelet mitogenic factor is postulated to initiate smooth muscle proliferation which may be important in the initiation of atheroma.

Figure 5.4 represents the completed process where the thrombin produced by the solid phase clotting system has resulted in fibrin formation which, if sufficiently gross, may obstruct the vessel. The completed thrombus now consists of the clump of platelets at its head, with its surrounding neutrophils

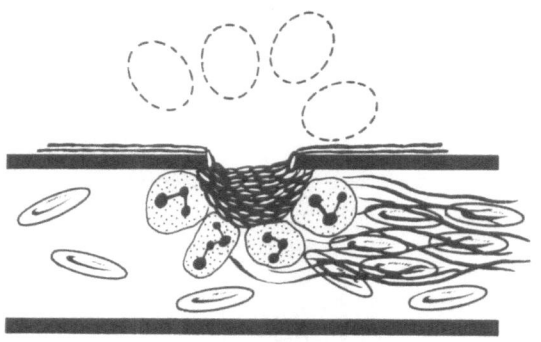

FIBRIN FORMATION

SAFETY MECHANISMS

STASIS

THROMBIN INACTIVATION

a)   FIBRIN

b)   ANTI-THROMBIN III

c) α_2 MACROGLOBULIN

PLASMINOGEN

Figure 5.4

PROTEIN C

and eosinophils, and its tail of fibrin in which the red cells and other platelets are enmeshed.

It is obviously of importance that thrombotic events should be localized to reduce the anoxic damage to the area supplied by the vessel, and also to prevent widespread thrombosis resulting in death. A number of safety mechanisms are thought to be important in this regard. First, stasis which will prevent fresh platelets arriving at the site of trauma and will also result in the local consumption of all the clotting factors so that further thrombin and fibrin cannot be produced and, as has already been emphasized, further flow is necessary to induce the phenomenon of platelet aggregation. ADP released by the platelet may be broken down by ADPase on the surface of the endothelial cell, as well as by plasma enzymes to substances such as adenosine and AMP which are in their own right inhibitory. During the process of platelet aggregation cAMP levels may become elevated, in part, following PGD_2 synthesis (Figure 3.6) and may act as a modulating system to limit the growth of the aggregate. 2,3-Diphosphoglycerate may be released from lysed red cells and this metabolite inhibits platelet aggregation. Thrombin inactivation may occur by binding to the platelet surface, to endothelial cells and to fibrin. The latter is reversible, and as time proceeds the thrombin is slowly released to be inactivated by plasma factors such as anti-thrombin III or α_2-macroglobulin. A recently discovered plasma component, called protein C, may be activated by thrombin together with activated factor V or an endothelial cell protein thrombomodulin; this protein attacks factor V and VIII:C destroying these important clotting components. Bound to the fibrin strands in the thrombus is the fibrinolytic precursor protein plasminogen, and during the clotting process this system is activated by the contact system and may cause the dissolution and/or reduction in size of the fibrin component of the thrombus. The damaged endothelial cell releases prostacyclin (PGI_2) and this inhibits platelet aggregation and clotting. Heparin-like components and plasminogen activator may be released also.

The leukocytes which are arranged around the head of the thrombus contain proteolytic enzymes which, if freed, will attack both the platelet aggregate and the fibrin strands. If a massive thrombosis has occurred these events will result in the presence in the systemic circulation of activated clotting factors, fibrin/fibrinogen monomers of varying size and specific platelet protein components such as β-thromboglobulin and platelet factor 4. Some of these may be inhibitory to coagulation, e.g. some fibrin monomers interfere with thrombin action on fibrinogen, whereas others may consist of activated clotting components such as factor Xa which would promote clotting elsewhere as would circulating platelet aggregates. It is believed, therefore, that one very important component in the prevention of the extension of thrombosis is a normally functioning reticulo-endothelial system which can remove activated components from the circulation.

Following the completion of the production of the thrombus, repair commences with the ingrowth of fibroblasts with subsequent recanalization of the thrombus, if it occluded the vessel lumen. The ingrowing fibroblast cells may repair a breach in the side of the vessel wall with eventual reconstitution of the surface by endothelial cells.

6
Von Willebrand disease

FACTOR VIII

Current evidence indicates that factor VIII is a glycoprotein complex of two distinct proteins or polypeptide components, which circulates as polymers ranging in size from 800 000 to 20×10^6 daltons. Lack of synthesis of whole or part of this complex results in a bleeding diathesis. One protein (VIII:C) is controlled by an X-linked gene, the other (VIII:vWf) is inherited autosomally. The two major biological functions of this molecular complex are participation in coagulation and involvement in adhesion of platelets to damaged surfaces. Unlike most other proteins involved in coagulation, factor VIII is not a serine protease and its structure and amino acid composition is unknown.

The concept that factor VIII is a complex of two distinct proteins or polypeptides has been derived from the following data.

Inheritance

The bleeding disorder, haemophilia A, is characterized by a lack of factor VIII procoagulant activity (VIII:C), but with normal levels of the factor VIII protein measured as factor VIII related antigen (VIII:Ag). This results from either synthesis of an inactive VIII:C molecule or its lack of synthesis. This condition is inherited as a sex linked recessive due to an abnormality located on the X chromosome. On the other hand, von Willebrand disease (vWd) results from a lack of production of the protein component (VIII:vWf). VIII:vWf is required for platelets to adhere to damaged surfaces and is present in normal amounts in haemophilia. In vWd there is usually an associated reduction in factor VIII:C. Synthesis of VIII:vWf is controlled by an autosomal gene or genes. It is thought that in the most severe forms of the disease in which both VIII:vWf and VIII:C are reduced to less than 5%, the abnormality is inherited

Table 6.1 Terms used to define aspects of factor VIII

Term	Meaning	Measurement
VIII:C	Procoagulant activity reduced in haemophilia and classical vWd	Coagulation assay using substrates lacking VIII:C
VIII:C$_t$	Transient increase in procoagulant activity on treatment with small amounts of thrombin	Add small amount of thrombin to VIII preparation and measure VIII:C
VIII:CAF	Activated VIII:C found in certain pathological circumstances such as some patients with glomerulonephritis	Shorten PTTK on addition to plasma
VIII:CAg	The antigen of the clotting component of VIII	Radio immunoassay using antisera which only recognize VIII:C
VIII:vWf	Blood component lacking in severe vWd. Absence results in poor platelet adhesion and a prolonged SBT. Present in normal levels in haemophilia	SBT, GBA, VIII:RCoF assayed by platelet agglutination in the presence of ristocetin
VIII:RCoF	Level of ristocetin, platelet agglutinating factor, ristocetin co-factor	Rate of agglutination of fixed platelet in the presence of ristocetin and known dilutions of plasma or VIII preparation
VIII:BCoF	Level of *Bothrops* platelet agglutinating factor	Rate of agglutination of fixed platelets in the presence of Botrocetin and known dilutions of plasma or VIII preparation
VIII:Ag	Antigen in blood identified by animal antibody raised against purified human factor VIII. Absent in severe vWd	Immunoelectrophoresis of plasma in agar containing the antibody *or* radioimmunoassay. Double imunoelectrophoresis (DIEP) is required to determine size of VIII multimers, since lower molecular weight components are more mobile
VIII:FMP	Piece of VIII:Ag which may follow proteolytic attack, most commonly observed in plasma of patients with disseminated intravascular coagulation. FMP means fast moving component.	

from both parents. In the majority of patients the disorder appears to be inherited as an autosomal dominant with varying degrees of penetrance, but in some instances a recessive pattern has been reported.

Synthesis

Patients with von Willebrand disease are capable of synthesizing VIII:C since the transfusion of haemophilic plasma or normal serum both deficient in

VIII:C cause a sustained rise in the VIII:C levels in the patient. There is good evidence that VIII:vWf is synthesized in the megakaryocytes and in endothelial cells lining blood vessels but the site of synthesis of VIII:C is still uncertain, although recent work indicates that it may be produced in the endothelial cells of the liver sinusoids.

Dissociation of activities

When purified human factor VIII is exposed to salt solutions of high ionic strength the VIII:vWf can be separated from VIII:C, the VIII:vWf is then retrieved in a high molecular weight fraction while VIII:C appears in a lower molecular weight fraction. Separated VIII:C is less stable than plasma VIII:C, but is still able to be activated by low concentrations of thrombin in the same way as VIII:C in plasma (*v. infra*).

Half-life of activities

Transfusion experiments in normal individuals and in patients with vWd show a striking disparity between the half-lives of VIII:vWf and VIII:C.

Against these points favouring two distinct proteins is a recent report that VIII:Ag synthesized by endothelial cells can develop the properties of VIII:C following exposure to phospholipase C. This suggests that factor VIII may be synthesized as a single molecule (VIII:vWf) which is enzymatically altered to express VIII:C activity.

Table 6.1 lists the various symbols used to express factor VIII and its components. This terminology has largely been derived by the evolution of different techniques for measuring Factor VIII (Table 6.2).

Table 6.2 Measurement of factor VIII

VIII: C
  1 Stage
  2 Stage
  CAg

VIII:Ag
  EIA – Laurell Rocket
  RIA – Liquid
       – Solid
  Cross
  Multimer analysis

VIII:vWf
  SBT
  GBA
  RCoF
  BCoF
  Endothelial cell adhesion
  VIII:C synthesis

VIII:C

Measurement of the clotting activity of the molecule is achieved by either a one stage or two stage technique. Most laboratories employ the one stage method which is based on the activated partial thromboplastin time with kaolin. VIII:C deficient plasma is used as a substrate and increasing concentrations of a standard VIII:C preparation are added to give a series of clotting times. These are used to prepare a standard curve. The patient's plasma is tested at various dilutions in a similar way to the standard, and the results expressed as units of VIII:C activity per millilitre of plasma. There have been claims that activation of labile clotting factors may be a source of error in the one stage technique. Activation of clotting factors is not a problem in the two stage method, however this is counterbalanced by the time consuming nature of the technique. Both methods give comparable results in VIII:C assays of normal and haemophiliac blood, however discrepancies have occurred in some clinical situations which are yet to be explained, and emphasize caution before equating these two techniques.

Investigation of VIII:C levels in patients with liver disease showed that the two stage technique gave higher values than the one stage assay. This higher level corresponded with the plasma VIII:Ag levels. A haemophiliac who contracted hepatitis had an increase in his VIII:C levels measured by the one stage technique but showed little change with the two stage assay. Artificially high levels of VIII:C are obtained with the one stage assay after tissue factor release following an inadequate venepuncture, or where there is disseminated intravascular coagulation, so that thrombin and activated factor X may be present in the circulation, whilst low levels are assayed when circulating anticoagulants are present. More recently a variant of vWd has been described, von Willebrand disease Denver, where there is a disparity between the one stage and two stage techniques for estimating VIII:C (v. infra).

VIII:CAg

VIII:CAg is a term used to denote the antigenic counterpart of VIII:C. Unlike VIII:C, VIII:CAg is stable and can be assayed in stored samples. Levels of VIII:CAg are measured by a radioimmunoassay. Antibodies specific for VIII:CAg are obtained from multi-transfused haemophiliacs, from patients in whom they have arisen spontaneously or are prepared by the monoclonal technique in mice. Generally, levels of VIII:CAg correlate well with the biological VIII:C activity in normal plasma, however there are some inconsistencies, notably in serum. In serum with no detectable VIII:C activity the level of VIII:CAg may be 50–80% of the plasma level, thus the antibody recognizes biologically inactive VIII:C antigen. Discrepancies between VIII:C and VIII:CAg levels are also noted in patients with haemophilia. In most patients with severe haemophilia, with an VIII:C activity of less than 1%,

VIII:CAg is absent, but in approximately 20% of cases measurable levels of VIII:CAg are obtained, even when the VIII:C coagulant activity is less than 1%. These two situations probably correspond to the CRM −ve and CRM +ve patients reported in the older literature by employing human anti-VIII:C antibodies in neutralization experiments.

When the levels of VIII:CAg are very low or absent there may be a lack of synthesis of the VIII:C antigen, alternatively an abnormal inactive protein may be formed which is not recognized by the antibody. Where the VIII:CAg level is higher than VIII:C activity, it is presumed that protein is synthesized which lacks biological activity (CRM +ve).

This technique for measuring VIII:CAg has proved to be useful for the prenatal diagnosis of haemophiliacs. The relative amounts of VIII:CAg and VIII:Ag are measured in a sample of fetal blood. Similar levels indicate the presence of a normal fetus, whilst lower levels of VIII:CAg than VIII:Ag indicate a fetus with haemophilia.

VIII:C_t

The addition of small amounts of thrombin (0.05 U/ml) to plasma or purified VIII:C produces a 10–40 fold increase in VIII:C activity. This reaction can be inhibited by DFP and is thought to result from the removal of a small peptide from the VIII:C molecule. The activation is shortlived, lasting only 10–60 minutes until the VIII:C activity is lost. Larger amounts of thrombin inactivate VIII:C in a matter of minutes. Many workers feel that thrombin activation plays a major role in the amplification of the coagulation system.

VIII:CAF

This denotes an activated form of factor VIII which is present in the plasma from some patients with renal disease, and when added to blood causes it to clot more rapidly. CAF stands for coagulation activating factor. These patients show a shortened partial thromboplastin time with kaolin and have a tendency to thrombosis. VIII:CAF, like VIII:C, is activated by small amounts of thrombin and on two-dimensional immunoelectrophoresis is identical to normal factor VIII. An additional protein band in the low molecular weight region is seen in plasma samples containing VIII:CAF when subjected to agarose-gel electrophoresis in the presence of sodium dodecyl sulphate (SDS).

VIII:Ag

Factor VIII antigen (VIII:Ag) is associated with the larger part of the factor VIII protein, and represents the antigenic counterpart of the functional VIII:vWf molecule. VIII:Ag is measured in most routine laboratories by an immunoelectrophoretic technique (Laurell) in which dilutions of plasma samples are electrophoresed into agarose containing rabbit anti-factor VIII antibody. Following electrophoresis the gels are stained for protein with Coomassie Blue, precipitant peaks are then visible, the height of which corresponds to the level of VIII:Ag. Normal levels are seen in classical haemophilia, but VIII:Ag is absent or greatly reduced in patients with severe vWd.

The nature of the VIII:Ag can be more closely examined by employing two dimensional immunoelectrophoresis (DIEP). The sensitivity of this technique is enhanced by the use of a radiolabelled anti-factor VIII antibody as developed by Zimmerman (*see* Figure 6.1). The characteristic broad, somewhat asymmetric arc of normal plasma VIII:Ag represents the differing electrophoretic migration of factor VIII polymers, the higher molecular weight polymers being closer to the starting well. The large number of different sized factor VIII polymers present in plasma is best demonstrated by SDS-agarose gel electrophoresis. The technique allows separation of the polymeric forms of factor VIII, which can be visualized by staining with Coomassie Blue or by overlaying the gel with ^{125}I rabbit anti-factor VIII followed by auto-radiography. This reveals the individual polymers which make up the broad arc seen by DIEP (Figures 6.1 and 6.2). Newer techniques demonstrate that the multimers are in the forms of triplets, but the significance of this is uncertain. The pattern of polymers is normal in haemophilia and they are usually normal, although greatly reduced in amount in the plasma from patients with vWd called classical or type I vWd.

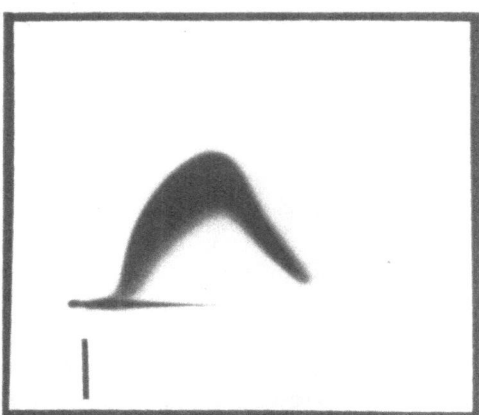

Figure 6.1 Two-dimensional immunoelectrophoresis (DIEP)

In other patients with vWd the VIII:Ag lacks some of the high molecular weight components, and therefore migrates faster on DIEP to give a more symmetrical peak which is further from the starting well than normal VIII:Ag. Using SDS-agarose gel electrophoresis the high molecular weight components are absent, but a normal complement of the low molecular weight components are present. Some of these patients may have a normal VIII:Ag by the standard Laurell technique. Such patients have been termed variant von Willebrand disease (Type II) (*v. infra*).

Normal

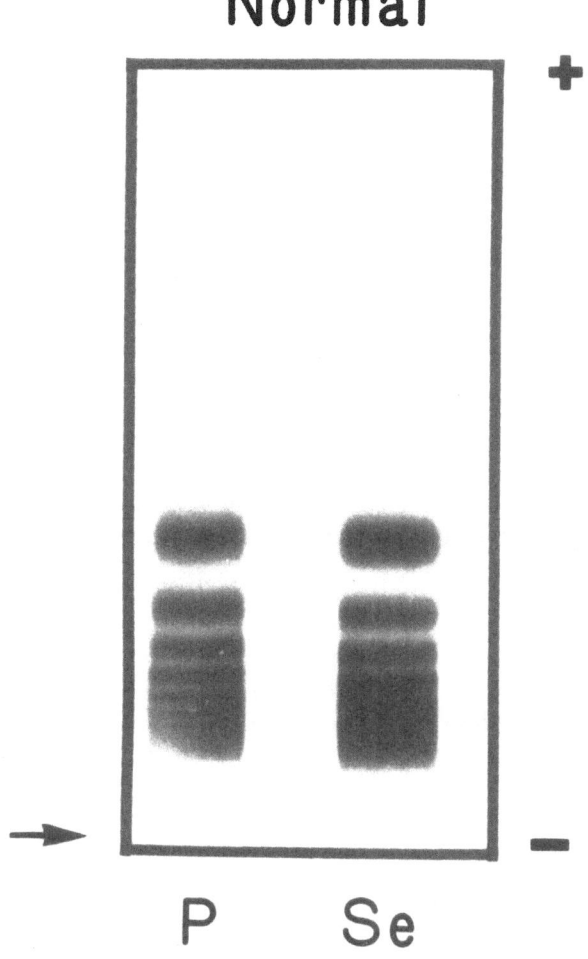

Figure 6.2   ^{125}I-anti-factor VIII binding to factor VIII multimers

VIII:FMP

VIII:FMP appears to be a proteolytic product of factor VIII, and is best detected by radio-DIEP where it appears as an additional precipitant arc migrating more rapidly than the main VIII:Ag arc. Its origin is still uncertain but it is present in higher amounts in serum than plasma. It is probably identical to VIII:FRAG described by Montgomery and his associates (1982), and is consistently observed in patients with disseminated intravascular coagulation and in some patients following a thrombotic episode.

VIII:RIA

This refers to the use of a radioimmunoassay using rabbit antibody to measure VIII:Ag, in contrast to the measurement of VIII:CAg with human antibody. Whilst in most circumstances this correlates closely with the VIII:Ag measurement by standard immunoelectrophoresis some differences have been noted between these two techniques in patients with variant von Willebrand disease. These differences possibly reflect the isolation technique used for preparing the antibody for the radioimmunoassay which may select out an antibody which is more reactive with some polymers than with others.

VIII:vWf

This is the component of the factor VIII molecule absent or abnormal in patients with vWd which is responsible for the prolonged skin bleeding time observed in these patients. The function and level of VIII:vWf are measured by the ability of platelets to adhere to glass beads in the presence of factor VIII, and by agglutination of platelets with the antibiotic ristocetin or with a snake venom *Bothrops jararaca* (botrocetin) in the presence of the plasma component (VIII:vWf). In normal plasma these three properties appear to be identical and to correspond with the VIII:vWf, but clearcut differences can be shown which suggest that the factor VIII components requisite for skin bleeding time, ristocetin induced agglutination and botrocetin induced agglutination may differ. The VIII:vWf level measured by ristocetin may become normal for a patient with vWd following transfusion of cryoprecipitate, while the skin bleeding time may remain prolonged. The platelet-rich plasma of a group of patients with variant vWd (Type IIB) (*v. infra*) reacts more strongly than normal to ristocetin, but they have a prolonged bleeding time. Another patient with variant vWd Type B has no detectable VIII:vWf activity by the ristocetin assay and a prolonged skin bleeding time, but has a normal assay using botrocetin.

Currently these various attributes are probably best recorded separately, so that ristocetin co-factor assay should be recorded as VIII:RCoF, and the botrocetin co-factor assay as VIII:BCoF.

vWag II

This is a recently identified plasma protein which is absent from the plasma of patients with severe von Willebrand disease. It is immunologically distinct from factor VIII and has a molecular weight of 140000 daltons. Approximately 70% of the circulating vWag II is present in platelets, and most of this is released during clotting so that the concentration of vWag II in serum is four times that of plasma. vWag II is released from platelets by collagen and thrombin, and this release is inhibited by aspirin. It is elevated in plasma from patients with conditions that cause *in vivo* platelet activation, such as disseminated intravascular coagulation, and thus it may be another useful marker protein for situations where platelets are activated intravascularly (*cf.* β-thromboglobulin and platelet factor 4). As yet no physiological function has been assigned to this protein which has only been identified by one group of workers.

COMPOSITION AND FUNCTIONS OF FACTOR VIII

Most laboratories which have examined the subunit structure of purified factor VIII, by reduction of the sulphydryl groups and electrophoresis on polyacrylamide gels in the presence of SDS, find a single protein band with a molecular weight of around 240–250 000 daltons. It has been suggested that this protein represents the basic subunit of VIII:vWf. The high molecular weight polymers of factor VIII appear to be involved in platelet adhesion, since they are absent from the plasma of patients with variant vWd with reduced platelet adhesion and normal VIII:Ag levels. Further, these polymers disappear following the addition of ristocetin to normal platelet-rich plasma, which in some respects mimics platelet adhesion. The role of VIII:C in clotting is believed to be to promote the activation of factor X by IXa in the presence of calcium and phospholipid. This effect is greatly enhanced by previous treatment of VIII:C with low concentrations of thrombin.

Several studies support the contention that the carbohydrate portion of the factor VIII molecule may be important in its function since many vWd variants have a reduced, or a less accessible carbohydrate moiety when examined by PAS staining techniques or concanavalin A binding. Removal of the sialic acid molecules from human factor VIII enables it to aggregate human platelets. This property is abolished by treatment of the asialo-factor VIII with galactose oxidase. It has been suggested by a number of workers that the penultimate galactose in the glycoprotein portion of factor VIII is vital for expressing VIII:vWf activity, although it is of no importance for VIII:C activity. Sulphydryl group reactivity is also thought to be important, since blocking it with appropriate chemicals results in the inhibition of VIII:C activity, but reducing agents such as 0.05 mol/l α,2-mercaptoethanol has little effect on VIII:C activity although it rapidly destroys VIII:RCoF.

When von Willebrand disease patients are transfused with plasma or cryoprecipitate, the infused high molecular weight multimers disappear first together with VIII:vWf activity leaving low molecular weight components and VIII:C circulating. Thus VIII:vWf/VIII:Ag may be important in stabilizing VIII:C activity, and perhaps act as a carrier molecule. The high molecular weight multimers are a stimulus to VIII:C synthesis, since the VIII:C levels in vWd patients are corrected following plasma infusions for longer periods, and to a greater degree than can be accounted for by the amount of VIII:C infused.

A number of *in vitro* studies have demonstrated that dynamic alterations can readily be affected in this glycoprotein complex. VIII:C can be removed from plasma factor VIII and readily rebound to the complex, although serum factor VIII does not have this ability. Cryoprecipitation of plasma results in separation of the polymeric forms of factor VIII. The low molecular weight forms remain in the supernate, while the larger polymers precipitate. The original composition of the multimers is re-established by re-combination of the precipitate and supernate. Reduction of purified factor VIII with dithio-threitol produces low molecular weight components which revert to their usual size and function by treatment with ε-aminocaproic acid. It seems likely, therefore, that a dynamic equilibrium takes place *in vivo* with an interchange of VIII:C molecules between molecules of VIII:Ag/VIII:vWf. The results of *in vitro* experiments also suggest an equilibrium between the various sized polymers of factor VIII found in the circulation.

VIII:Ag has been shown to be synthesized in both the endothelial cells and megakaryocytes by tissue culture and immunofluorescent anti-VIII antibody techniques. Howard *et al* (1974) demonstrated that VIII:Ag is present in platelets. Approximately 10–25% of the total circulating VIII:Ag is in platelets, and is probably located in the α granules. There seems to be little or no exchange between the platelet and the plasma. Following collagen or thrombin induced platelet aggregation, only 20% of the platelet VIII:Ag is released. When VIII:Ag levels are measured in serum, either following whole blood clotting or adding thrombin to platelet-poor plasma, the levels of VIII:Ag and VIII:vWf are usually somewhat reduced, suggesting either minimal consumption during the clotting process, or its absorption to the platelets or fibrin strands or to the surface of the containing vessel.

Numerous studies of lifespan of infused FVIII have shown that VIII:C has a $t_\frac{1}{2}$ of between 14–18 hours, and that in general terms the $t_\frac{1}{2}$ of VIII:C $>$ VIII:Ag $>$ VIII:RCoF $>$ VIII:vWf when the latter is determined by the skin bleeding time (SBT).

In normal plasma the ratio of VIII:C/VIII:Ag/VIII:RCoF is unity. Levels of all elements of factor VIII may be increased by exercise or the injection of adrenalin. The latter effect may be blocked by β-blockers, and is thought to result from release of stored factor VIII from the endothelial cells in the vessel wall or from the spleen. Other situations where an increase in the overall factor VIII levels is observed are pregnancy, thyrotoxicosis, liver disease, renal disease, malignancy and acute respiratory failure. Indeed, elderly sick people have higher levels of factor VIII than are seen in a control healthy population. The increase in the factor VIII levels in some of these disease states may be quite remarkable. We have seen factor VIII levels 8–10 times normal in the plasma from patients with renal disease.

Table 6.3

vWd	SBT	GBA	PRP$_R$	VIII:C	VIII:Ag	VIII:RCoF	VIII:BCoF	VIII:DIEP	Plasma VIII multimers	Platelet VIII multimers
I severe	↑	↓	0	<5%	<12%	<12%	<12%	Mainly normal distribution N↓	↓ all forms but normal distribution N↓	Reduced but normal
mod.	↑ or N	↓ or N	N↓	↓ or N	↓	↓	↓ or ↓			
IIA	↑	↓	↑s	N or mod reduced	N or mod reduced	<12% ↓	N or ↓	ABN	↓ HMW	↓ HMW
IIB	↑	↓		N or mod reduced	N	↓ ?	?	ABN	↓ HMW	N
IIC	↑	?	?	N	sl↓	?	?	ABN	↓ HMW	↓ HMW
B	↑↑	↓↑	0	N	N	<12% ↓	N	ABN	↓ HMW additional LMW	?
Denver	↑	↓	?	one stage N two stage ABN	↓	↓	?	?	?	?
*PvWd	↑	↓	↑s	N	N	↓	?	ABN	↓ HMW	N

Other associations

XIII deficiency – San Diego variant
Platelet release abnormality
Prolapsed mitral valve
Angiodysplasia

ABN	= abnormal
GBA	= glass bead adhesion
HMW	= high molecular weight multimer
LMW	= low molecular weight multimer
N	= normal
↓	= decreased
↑	= increased

↑s	=	platelet aggregation occurs in PRP at lower concentrations of ristocetin than is normally required.
PRP	=	platelet-rich plasma.
PRP$_2$	=	platelet rich plasma aggregated with ristocetin
mod	=	moderate
sl	=	slight

*The patients' platelets absorb HMW VIII:Ag and aggregate with normal purified VIII:Ag unlike vWd Type IIB

89

Factor VIII levels may be reduced in clinical situations such as disseminated intravascular clotting, although in some instances the levels are normal or even increased. Factor VIII is also reduced in myxoedema. The relationship between raised factor VIII levels and thrombosis is debatable since many people have high levels of factor VIII without necessarily having thrombosis. The VIII activator (VIII:CAF) which has been detected in some patients with glomerulonephritis warrants emphasis (v. supra).

VON WILLEBRAND DISEASE

Ever since its first description in families on the Åland islands by Eric von Willebrand (1931), this disorder has been subject to controversy.

Diagnosis of patients with severe vWd where the levels of factor VIII functions are very reduced or absent presents no problems, however patients with mild vWd and borderline factor VIII levels may be difficult to define. Clinically the bleeding problem is largely mucocutaneous, or follows trauma or operative procedures. Gastrointestinal blood loss can be particularly troublesome, and haemarthrosis and occasional deep haematomas are seen in the severe homozygous forms. Menorrhagia is frequently a problem in women and was the cause of death in some of von Willebrand's original families. Pregnancy results in an amelioration of the condition, and accounts for less frequent post-partum bleeding than might have been anticipated from the history of severe menorrhagia and nose bleeds observed in women with vWd. In most patients the oral contraceptives reduce menstrual loss to tolerable amounts. An improvement of the bleeding diathesis has been reported with ageing, but this is not always so.

Table 6.3 shows the classification of vWd. Diagnosis of classical Type I vWd rests on the demonstration of a prolonged skin bleeding time (SBT), reduced or absent glass bead adhesion (GBA), absent PRP, ristocetin-induced aggregation and absent VIII:RCof and VIII:BCof in platelet-poor plasma, severely reduced to undetectable levels of VIII:Ag by standard techniques, and less than 5% VIII:C. If VIII:Ag can be obtained from such patients it often appears normal on examination by DIEP but may show a lack of high molecular weight multimers. In the moderate forms of Type I the levels of factor VIII components may be variable and this may reflect the reproducibility of the various techniques employed. Exercise, adrenalin injection, administration of a vasopressin-like substance 1-deamino-8-D-arginine vasopressin (DDAVP) may result in the elevation of all factor VIII parameters in the mild but not the severe form. Therefore, it is important that measurements of the factor VIII levels be performed on a number of occasions, and that a careful family history is obtained and as many family members as possible investigated.

Von Willebrand disease Type IIA is probably the most frequent form of variant vWd. In this form of vWd the high molecular weight polymers of factor VIII are absent. This can be assessed by DIEP and SDS-agarose gel multimeric analysis. The patients' platelet factor VIII shows a similar lack of high molecular weight forms when multimeric analysis examination is performed. Laboratory findings show a prolonged bleeding time, low glass bead adhesion, reduced VIII:RCoF, moderately reduced to normal VIII:Ag and moderately reduced to normal VIII:C levels. Some of these patients react normally to botrocetin. The inheritance pattern of vWd in Type IIA is probably autosomal dominant.

Variant vWd Type IIB refers to a group of patients first reported from Italy. The PRP from these patients shows an enhanced sensitivity to ristocetin, so that platelet aggregation is induced by a lower concentration of ristocetin than required for normal PRP. The VIII:RCoF assay of the plasma is reduced, and thus the enhanced reaction to ristocetin in PRP results from an increased avidity for these patients' factor VIII multimers and platelets in the presence of ristocetin. DIEP and SDS-agarose gel analysis of plasma factor VIII is identical to that of Type IIA, but the platelet factor VIII in Type IIB has a normal concentration of high molecular weight multimers. It is thought that either the release of the high molecular weight forms of factor VIII tissues stores is defective or there is a greater tissue and/or platelet affinity for the heavy forms, resulting in the removal of high molecular weight forms from factor VIII from the plasma. DDVAP infusion into these patients, unlike Type IIA, results in an increase in the high molecular weight multimers in plasma, but these disappear more rapidly than in Type I either being more readily broken down or removed by the tissues.

The category variant Type IIC was defined in a patient who had a moderate bleeding tendency, a prolonged SBT and reduced plasma VIII:RCoF. Multimeric analysis of his VIII:Ag showed a striking reduction of high molecular weight forms with an increase in the lower molecular weight forms. The platelet factor VIII showed similar abnormalities. It differs from Type IIA in that the SDS-agarose gel factor VIII multimers were composed of doublets rather than showing the triplet formation normally seen with the technique employed. Type IIC is inherited as an autosomal recessive.

Von Willebrand type B is a patient first described in 1973. This patient has a prolonged SBT, glass bead adhesiveness is greatly reduced, ristocetin induced aggregation of the PRP is absent, VIII:Ag and VIII:C are normal. The DIEP shows normal high molecular weight components, but a hump on the descending limb. Multimer studies show an additional band in the low molecular weight region. Another interesting feature of this patient's plasma is a normal level of VIII:BCoF but absent VIII:RCoF suggesting a specific abnormality of factor VIII at the site of interaction with ristocetin.

Another variant is von Willebrand disease Denver. In this condition there is a great discrepancy in the level of VIII:C when measured by the one and two stage assays; the one stage giving a normal result and the two stage a reduced level for VIII:C. This discrepancy occurs because the VIII:C is more readily removed by Al(OH)$_3$ from plasma than normal. This could result from a reduced affinity between VIII:C and the carrier protein VIII:Ag or from some alteration in absorption properties of the VIII:C molecule.

Pseudo von Willebrand disease (PvWd) is a mild bleeding disorder characterized by intermittent thrombocytopenia and decreased plasma VIII:vWf, reduced high molecular weight VIII:Ag components and an increased sensitivity of the PRP to ristocetin as in Type IIB. Unlike the latter, the platelets appear to be defective in PvWd since they absorb high molecular weight VIII:Ag multimers more rapidly in the presence of ristocetin than normal platelets. The factor VIII molecule from patients with PvWd does not absorb to normal platelets at low concentrations of ristocetin, in contrast to the factor VIII from patients with vWd Type IIB. In addition, the PvWd platelets were aggregated by native human factor VIII in the absence of any other agent. A platelet membrane abnormality is probably the cause of the increased absorption of factor VIII, although initial analysis of the glycoproteins was normal, and in particular glycoprotein Ib was present in normal amounts (Weiss *et al*). The inheritance pattern of PvWd is probably autosomal dominant. There have been a number of reports of an association between thrombocytopenia and vWd. One report was of a family with large platelets and more consistent thrombocytopenia. The platelets of affected members displayed an increased affinity for VIII:vWf in the presence of ristocetin (Takahashi *et al.*, 1981).

The San Diego variant represents a joint defect of factor XII deficiency and von Willebrand disease, and may be suspected when the PTTK is more prolonged than would be expected for the degree of VIII:C deficiency. It is uncertain whether this variant represents a chance association or whether it is a separate hereditary syndrome.

The discovery that endothelial cells in culture synthesize VIII:Ag and VIII:vWf and reports of an associated VIII:vWf deficiency in patients with hereditary telangiectasia (Osler disease), angiodysplasia in the large bowel and Barlow syndrome has led to speculation that there may be some linkage between mesenchymal abnormalities and VIII:vWf disorders. In one study a 60% incidence of mitral valve prolapse was documented in patients with vWd compared to 15% in matched controls; telangiectasia was observed in 20%.

There have now been a number of reports of vWd associated with a platelet release abnormality. In the families we have studied the bleeding diathesis in these patients is mild. This association may be more common than previously realized since our families had been given a diagnosis of mild vWd. A further intriguing association is the observed correction of the bleeding problem by cryoprecipitate infusion in some patients with apparently pure release defects. This finding suggests that some subtle abnormality in the platelet factor VIII may be present and responsible for the bleeding diathesis.

There are numerous case reports of acquired vWd. These patients may have no apparent associated disease, but often they have some immunological disorder such as systemic lupus erythematosus, paraproteinaemia, lymphoma, chronic lymphatic leukaemia or angiodysplasia. Two children with Wilm tumour and acquired vWd have also been reported. Data from these reports are variable and in only some instances has an inhibitor of VIII:vWf, presumably an antibody, been demonstrated in the peripheral blood. When an antibody has been demonstrated the patient has usually had lupus erythematosus or paraproteinaemia. In other patients, absorption of VIII:vWf to lymphatic tissue has been demonstrated, and this is possibly also the result of an antibody. Absorption to the abnormal tumour tissue was not the case in a patient with Wilm tumour nor was a circulating inhibitor demonstrated. In this patient, when tissue containing endothelial cells was examined, using a fluorescent antibody technique, the VIII:vWf distribution was normal. Whether the endothelial cells are sometimes abnormal, resulting in faulty release of VIII:vWf, or cause excessive VIII:vWf catabolism is unclear, but the occasional reported association of structural abnormalities, angiodysplasia in the large bowel and vWd is intriguing.

The management of patients with von Willebrand disease currently rests on the use of oral contraceptives to control menorrhagia in females. Antifibrinolytic agents such as ε-aminocaproic acid and tranexamic acid are occasionally of value, particularly if the bleeding is gastrointestinal. Vasopressin-like agents such as DDAVP appear to be useful in mild to moderate forms of the disorder, and in Type IIB for a limited time until tissue stores of FVIII are depleted. Otherwise reliance has to be placed on the use of plasma, cryoprecipitate or purified preparations of FVIII. It is important to appreciate that some methods for the purification of FVIII result in the loss of high molecular weight components, and, therefore, are not effective in controlling haemorrhage in patients with vWd. It is necessary to check such preparations from time to time by DIEP or multimeric analysis. The wise policy is to use sufficient cryoprecipitate or FVIII concentrate to correct the SBT at the start of an operative procedure, then to cover the patient by 6 hourly infusions, maintaining an VIII:C level within the normal range, and if possible, keeping the VIII:RCof and SBT normal. Acquired vWd is resistant to correction by plasma or FVIII concentrate therapy even when combined with vigorous plasmapheresis, although this should be tried as an emergency measure. Treatment of the underlying condition should be commenced, and as this responds there is an accompanying resolution of the acquired vWd.

Table 6.4 Haemophilia

(1) Autosomal haemophilia
(2) Combined V and VIII deficiency
(3) Combined VII and VIII deficiency
(4) Heckathorn disease
(5) Classical haemophilia
   Mild
   Moderate
   Severe

Table 6.4 shows a classification of haemophilia. Autosomal haemo-philia could be regarded as being truly a variant form of vWd because it is inherited as a dominant trait, however there are no reports of any abnormality of FVIII other than VIII:C levels reduced to between 2 and 5%. The bleeding diathesis is usually mild and VIII:Ag and VIII:vWf levels are normal, but crosses and multimeric studies have not been reported.

Combined factor V and VIII deficiency is probably an autosomal recessive condition, and although it was suggested to be due to the excessive destruction of factor V and VIII by protein C because of a lack of a specific protein C inhibitor normally present in blood, recent evidence is against this explanation.

The single patient reported with factor VII and VIII deficiency inherited it as an autosomal dominant disease.

Only one family has been reported with Heckathorn disease. This disorder may be particularly important since the bleeding problem seen in these patients may provide direct evidence of the interaction between platelets and FVIII in the clotting system. The inheritance pattern in this family was consistent with a sex-linked recessive. Investigated symptomatic family members showed a remarkable variation in the levels of VIII:C, but the pro-thrombin consumption time was consistently abnormal. It is well recognized that in true haemophilia, the prothrombin consumption time is not nearly as sensitive an index of VIII:C activity as specific VIII:C assay, and this could imply that in patients with Heckathorn disease there is some abnormality in the interaction between FVIII and the platelet.

True haemophilia has been well reviewed (Koutts *et al.*, 1979); Hoyer, 1976, 1981). It is classified as mild, moderate or severe based on both the clinical features of the disorder and the levels of VIII:C and VIII:CAg. Since the degree of severity runs true in individual families, it has been proposed that the genetic loci for VIII:C on the X chromosome must have multiple alleles.

Acquired disorders of FVIII most commonly relate to overall increases in its plasma level, with the exception of disseminated intravascular coagulation where the VIII:C level may be strikingly reduced. FVIII has been regarded as an acute reactant protein which is elevated in all acute inflammatory situations, and is also increased following exercise and the injection of adrenalin, an increase which can be blocked by β-blockers such as propanolol. Apart from these rather artificial situations, overall increases in VIII:Ag and VIII:vWf in particular are seen in any disorder in which the endothelial layer of the vessels is diseased or damaged. This may in part explain the very high levels seen in patients with renal disease and in acute respiratory distress states, as well as patients with peripheral vascular disease and atheroma. Very high levels have also been seen in patients with severe liver disease. In all of these instances there have been abnormalities in the multimeric distribution of factor VIII which have most frequently shown a reduction in the high molecular weight component, and may also account for a number of reports of low VIII:vWf in patients with uraemia and the subsequent correction of the bleeding diathesis and SBT by infusions of cryoprecipitate.

Low levels of VIII:C due to the development of a circulating antibody may arise spontaneously in mothers post-partum and in elderly people of either sex. This usually presents as a severe bleeding diathesis, and fortunately frequently remits after some months with or without immunosuppressive treatment. Very rarely the patient may have lupus erythematosus. The antibody resembles that which develops in some haemophiliacs during replacement therapy.

References

HOYER, L. W. (1981). The Factor VIII complex: structure and function. *Blood*, **58,** 1

HOYER, L. W. (1976). Von Willebrand's disease. In SPAET, E. H. (ed.). *Progress in Hemostasis and Thrombosis*. Vol. 3, p. 231. (New York: Grune & Stratton)

HOWARD, M. A., MONTGOMERY, D. C., HARDISTY, R. M. (1974). Factor VIII-related antigen in platelets. *Thromb. Res.*, **4,** 617

ITALIAN WORKING GROUP. (1977). Spectrum of von Willebrand's disease: A study of 100 cases. *Br. J. Haematol.*, **35,** 101

KOUTTS, J., HOWARD, M. A. and FIRKIN, B. G. (1979). Factor VIII physiology and pathology in man. In *Progress in Hematology*, Vol. XI, p. 115. (New York: Grune & Stratton)

MONTGOMERY, R. R., HATHAWAY, W. E., JOHNSON, J., JACOBSON, L. and MUNTEAN, W. (1982). A variant of von Willebrand's disease with abnormal expression of Factor VIII procoagulant activity. *Blood*, **60,** 201

PICKERING, N. J., BRODY, J. I. and BARROT, T. (1981). Von Willebrand syndromes and mitral valve prolapse. Linked mesenchymal dysplasias. *N. Engl. J. Med.*, **305,** 131

RUGGERI, Z. M., MANNUCCI, P. M., LOMBARDI, R., FEDERKI, A. B. and ZIMMERMAN, T. S. (1982). Multimeric composition of factor VIII/von Willebrand factor following administration of DDAVP. Implications for pathophysiology and therapy of von Willebrand's disease subtypes. *Blood,* **59,** 1271

RUGGERI, Z. M., NILSSON, I. M., LOMBARDI, R., HOLMBERG, L. and ZIMMERMAN, T. S. (1982). Aberrant multimeric structure of von Willebrand factor in a new variant of von Willebrand's disease (Type IIC). *J. Clin. Invest.*, **70,** 1124

TAKAHASHI, H., NAGAYAMA, R., HATTORI, A., IHZUMJ, T., TSOKADA, T. and SHIBATA, A. (1981). Von Willebrand disease associated with familial thrombocytopenia and increased ristocetin-induced platelet aggregation. *Am. J. Hematol.*, **10,** 89

VON WILLEBRAND, E. A. (1931). Über hereditäre pseudohämophilie. *Acta Med. Scand.*, **76,** 522

WEISS, H. J. (1975). Abnormalities of factor VIII and platelet aggregation – use of ristocetin in diagnosing the von Willebrand syndrome. *Blood*, **45,** 403

7
Qualitative platelet disorders

HEREDITARY QUALITATIVE PLATELET DISORDERS

Qualitative platelet disorders may cause bleeding due to platelet dysfunction when the platelet count is normal. In some instances both qualitative and quantitative defects may coincide. Table 7.1 lists the hereditary forms of qualitative platelet defects, and indicates those which may have an associated thrombocytopenia. There are instances where platelet function abnormalities have been established *ex vivo*, but no accompanying bleeding disorder is present. The majority of these disorders are extremely rare, the exception

Table 7.1 Hereditary qualitative platelet disorders

(1) Bernard–Soulier syndrome*	(4) Alport syndrome*
(2) Glanzmann disease	(5) May–Hegglin anomaly*
(3) Platelet release disorders	(6) Gray platelet syndrome
(a) Membrane defect	(7) Ehlers–Danlos syndrome
(b) Defect of metabolic pathway of release reaction	(8) Osteogenesis imperfecta
(c) Storage pool defect	(9) Marfan syndrome
– δ	(10) Pseudo-xanthoma elasticum
– $\alpha\delta$	(11) Glycogen storage disease Type I
– Hermansky–Pudlak syndrome	(12) Miscellaneous
– Wiskott–Aldrich syndrome*	
– Chediak–Higashi anomaly*	
– Foetal and neonatal platelets	
(d) Associated with von Willebrand disease	

*May also have thrombocytopenia.

being release-reaction anomalies which are the cause for many previously undiagnosed mild bleeding diatheses.

The Bernard–Soulier syndrome (BSS) or hereditary giant platelet syndrome was first described by Bernard and Soulier in 1948. The defect is inherited as an autosomal recessive, and first cousin marriages and consanguinity are, therefore, often a feature. The bleeding diathesis is moderate to severe with spontaneous bruising, nose bleeds and sometimes fatal haemorrhage after minor operative procedures. Epistaxis is common and menorrhagia is usually seen in the female and often difficult to control. Physical examination is unrewarding apart from the presence of ecchymoses. Examination of a peripheral blood film may show a platelet count which is markedly to moderately reduced or normal. The most significant feature on the film is the presence of platelets which may be as big or bigger than lymphocytes. The skin bleeding time is markedly prolonged regardless of the platelet count. Standard coagulation screens are normal, but tests which examine the platelets' interaction with the clotting factors such as the prothrombin consumption test or the thrombin generation time are abnormal, in contrast to platelet factor 3 activation which is usually normal. Glass bead adhesion is reduced, but platelet aggregation studies with collagen, ADP, thrombin, calcium ionophore, arachidonic acid and adrenalin are normal. Platelet agglutination is absent with ristocetin or bovine factor VIII and is reduced with botrocetin. The ristocetin and botrocetin responses are not corrected by the addition of normal plasma or factor VIII. Studies in systems examining platelet adherence to subendothelial layers show a similar lack of adhesion to that seen in platelets from patients with von Willebrand disease (vWd). Detailed analysis of the membrane protein of BSS platelets shows a reduction in glycoprotein Ib and often other less evident glycoprotein components, whereas vWd platelets are normal. Electron microscopic pictures show extreme variation of size, confirming light microscopic findings, and demonstrate the presence of all the characteristic platelet organelles. The reduced or absent surface glycoprotein(s) is requisite for the platelet's reaction with von Willebrand factor to enable its adherence to damaged surfaces *in vivo*. It may also be important for binding of V, VIII and XI to the cells' surface since Bernard–Soulier platelets are more readily depleted of these factors on washing compared with normal platelets. When thrombin generation is studied in recalcified platelet-rich plasma the amount of thrombin generated over the ensuing 10–15 minutes, measured by its reaction with plasma or fibrinogen, is markedly reduced. This is consistent with the findings in the prothrombin consumption test. If the thrombin generated is measured by the chromogenic substrate technique, a slightly delayed but overall normal thrombin generation is noted suggesting that a normal amount of thrombin is produced. However, this surface glycoprotein may be important in stabilizing the solid phase clotting reaction localizing it to the cell's surface and preventing inhibition by inhibitors in the liquid phase. The chromagen measures the presence of thrombin whether it be bound or not to ATIII or α_2-macroglobulin, and so although a similar amount of thrombin is generated to normal in Bernard–Soulier platelet-rich plasma the thrombin may be more readily available for inactivation (*see* chapter 3). It seems possible that the platelet glycoprotein, together with the high molecular weight polymers of factor VIII, may protect thrombin generation on the platelet surface. The glycoprotein lacking in Bernard–Soulier syndrome is a requisite for the reaction of most quinine/quinidine antibodies with platelets. The thrombocytopenia which is frequently seen in the Bernard–Soulier syndrome is not significantly improved by splenectomy.

Glanzmann disease, or hereditary thrombasthenia, was first described by Glanzmann in 1918. This is another autosomal recessive defect and has similar clinical features to that described for the Bernard–Soulier syndrome, the moderate to severe bleeding diathesis causes the males to avoid contact sports and the females to have troublesome menorrhagia. Epistaxes are a common problem with both sexes. Any surgical procedure is dangerous and requires cover with platelet transfusions.

Investigation of the patient shows a strikingly prolonged bleeding time and absent or very minimal clot retraction. The remainder of the clotting screen is normal except platelet factor 3 activation is reduced, and factor IX levels when measured in serum are often lower than normal. Both these findings are probably related to the inability of the cell in this disorder to activate factor XII normally on glass contact. The remainder of the clotting tests are normal, but virtually all of the platelet function studies are strikingly abnormal. Glass bead adhesion is greatly reduced, the platelets do not aggregate with collagen, ADP, arachidonic acid, calcium ionophore, thrombin or adrenalin. Platelets will react with ristocetin, although in some the response is less than normal which probably reflects the contribution of the release reaction to this test when it is performed in platelet-rich plasma. The ristocetin reaction is abnormal in that the platelets disaggregate much more rapidly despite a normal initial response. The platelets react normally to botrocetin, but also disaggregate more rapidly than normal. There is a low platelet fibrinogen level and a striking reduction in the platelets' surface glycoproteins IIb and IIIa, as well as the platelet antigen PI[A1] which is on IIIa. It has been claimed that the glycoprotein IIIa and α-actinin are identical, and that this protein may act as an anchor for actin inside the membrane. Glycoproteins IIb and IIIa are thought to be major components of the fibrinogen receptor site for the cell, and may explain the low fibrinogen content normally found in Glanzmann platelets, and perhaps their inability to interact with fibrin and cause clot retraction. Studies with lectin Con A have shown a lack of binding sites for this lectin in platelets from patients with Glanzmann disease compared with normal platelets. Although platelets from patients with Glanzmann disease will agglutinate well with lectins such as phytohaemagglutinin or ricinis communis I, they show no response to Con A. There is also an abnormal interaction and uptake of latex particles by some patients with this disorder although other particles such as thorotrast readily enter. It has been postulated that there may be subsets of Glanzmann disease but these are yet to be defined, although in one series glutathione peroxidase deficiency was documented with reduced glutathione levels.

PLATELET RELEASE DISORDERS

These probably constitute one of the most common and heterogeneous forms of hereditary platelet anomaly. First recognized in 1967, they are still poorly defined. Most patients have a mild bleeding diathesis with troublesome bleeding after trauma or operations such as tooth extraction or tonsillectomy, and menorrhagia is frequently a problem in women, although it is often well controlled by the use of the oral contraceptive pill. Theoretically these disorders should fall into three major categories. The first relates to a membrane defect where there may be an abnormality of a specific receptor for signals which induce the release reaction, or an abnormality resulting in faulty signal transmission or a lack of another specific surface receptor to the products of the release reaction. The second category is an abnormality in the metabolic pathways which are required for release, sometimes termed the aspirin-like deficiency since the basic laboratory platelet function tests are similar to that seen in people who have ingested aspirin. The third is an abnormality of the storage granule, the very dense granule, of the cell and this is usually termed a storage pool disorder.

In the routine laboratory examination these patients most commonly show increased or normal bleeding time, a normal platelet count and clot retraction, decreased availability of platelet factor 3, absence of the second wave of aggregation seen when adrenalin or ADP is added at the appropriate concentrations to platelet-rich plasma prepared by blood anticoagulated with citrate. Aggregation to other agonists especially collagen may be greatly reduced. Subsequent studies with serotonin show a normal uptake, but a reduced or absent serotonin release following the addition of appropriate agonists, e.g. collagen or thrombin. Serotonin studies distinguish the first two categories from that of storage pool disease because serotonin uptake in the latter, although initially normal, rapidly reaches saturation and does not attain normal levels because the organelles concerned are abnormal or missing.

Specific membrane defects have not yet been identified, but one patient with a defective or missing surface receptor for thromboxane A_2 has been reported.

The second category, namely that of the metabolic pathways involved in the release reaction, appears to be the most common form of disorder, and families have been described with cyclo-oxygenase deficiency and thromboxane synthetase deficiency (*see* Chapter 3, Figure 3.5). There are also reports of defective calcium mobilization resulting in a reduced production of thromboxane A_2. A mild form of this disorder has been called 'Intermediate syndrome of platelet dysfunction', and consists of intermittent bleeding episodes in patients who have ingested medicine which is known to interfere with platelet function, but who are now off the drug. These patients had a normal to very slightly prolonged skin bleeding time, a normal platelet count and glass bead adhesion and normal platelet serotonin content, but they had variable abnormalities in their prothrombin consumption time and platelet factor 3 abnormalities, and all showed abnormal platelet aggregation using adrenalin, collagen and ADP. In view of the various dietary constituents which have now been shown to cause minor platelet abnormalities (see Table 7.3) and of the increasing use of non-steroidal anti-inflammatory agents which usually have similar effects to that of aspirin, this particular problem may be recognized more frequently. An advocated method for ready identification of such a problem is the use of the aspirin tolerance test, in which 975 mg aspirin is administered to patients following a skin bleeding time test and then 2 hours later the skin bleeding time is repeated. Although this disorder can be identified by platelet aggregation studies, it has been advocated that the aspirin tolerance test represents the cheapest and simplest way to identify this problem.

Storage Pool Defect (SPD)

This abnormality can appear in isolation or associated with a number of other unusual syndromes. In some instances the mode of inheritance appears to be autosomal dominant. The routine findings are similar to the other release abnormalities and two types of disorder have been identified by Weiss (1967, 1981). One group he calls δSPD in which the sole abnormality appears to lie in the very dense granules (δ-granules) which are either absent or incapable of function, so that electron microscopy reveals platelets which do not contain dense granules and the platelets have a very low content of serotonin and ADP with a resultantly high ATP-ADP ratio. Serotonin uptake studies show a rapid initial uptake, but the platelets become saturated far below the normal level and the serotonin so taken up is more rapidly metabolized than in the normal cell, perhaps due to its exposure to mono-amine oxidase enzymes in the mito-chondria or other parts of the cell instead of being protected in the very dense granule. The release mechanism in some of these patients may also be abnormal, since although the level of platelet factor 4 is normal, a reduced quantity is released when the cells are reacted with collagen or adrenalin. Others believe that in these instances there may be some abnormality with phospholipase A_2 activation releasing arachidonic acid from phospholipid in the cell's membrane, since malondialdehyde (MDA) production of the platelets is normal with arachidonic acid, but not to adrenalin or collagen, presumably due to a difficulty in releasing endogenous arachidonic acid by these agents in this disorder (see Chapter 3, Figure 3.5). Aggregation response to arachidonic acid is reduced, but this appears to relate to the intrinsic ADP content of the platelet since the degree of aggregation with arachidonic acid (AA) correlates with this.

The other group termed $\alpha\delta$SPD by Weiss is one in which there is a deficiency of the very dense granules and also a lack or decrease in the numbers of the α granules. In these patients there is not only an abnormality to aggregation when using collagen, ADP or adrenalin, but the platelets do not respond with arachidonic acid. The ADP level in patients with $\alpha\delta$SPD is not as low as that in δSPD and here the defect appears to lie in the arachidonic acid pathway since MDA production is also reduced when AA is added to platelets. platelets.

Hermansky–Pudlak syndrome (HPS)

This is an autosomal recessive condition in which the patient is an albino, commonly termed tyrosinase positive oculocutaneous albinism. There is often a reduction in visual acuity and sometimes nystagmus, and some patients have a bleeding tendency. Platelet function studies are consistent with a storage pool deficiency, and δ-granules are not seen when the platelets are examined by the electron microscope. Analysis of the platelets shows a striking reduction of ADP, Ca^{2+}, pyrophosphate and serotonin, all constituents of the δ-granule.

Wiskott–Aldrich syndrome

The Wiskott–Aldrich syndrome has also been reported to have a storage pool defect, but may have other metabolic abnormalities since mild thrombocytopenia is often present. This syndrome is a sex-linked recessive disorder which has associated features of eczema and low levels of IgA and IgM, with decreased numbers of lymphocytes in the spleen and lymph nodes but not in the bone marrow. The principal clinical problems are those of recurrent infections as well as a mild bleeding diathesis. The thrombocytopenia is corrected by splenectomy, but this increases the risk of infection, and when undertaken must be accompanied by prophylactic antibiotic therapy and vaccination against pneumococcal infections.

Chediak–Higashi anomaly

The Chediak–Higashi anomaly is inherited as an autosomal recessive and was first recognized by giant granules in the cytoplasm of neutrophils and eosinophils. Its clinical features are that of recurrent pyogenic infections and an associated oculocutaneous albinism frequently with photophobia and nystagmus. The basic cellular defect appears to be some impairment of microtubule function or formation, and the condition often terminates in an accelerated lymphoma-like phase with pancytopenia, hepatosplenomegaly and lymphadenopathy. Patients with the storage pool defects have a history of easy bruising prior to any thrombocytopenia. Despite normal platelet counts they have prolonged bleeding times and platelet aggregation studies typical of storage pool disease with increased ATP–ADP ratios and impairment of serotonin uptake by the platelets.

Foetal and neonatal platelets

A physiological version of storage pool disease may be seen in platelets obtained from fetus' blood following abortion and from the new-born.

Associated with von Willebrand disease

Another hereditary platelet release anomaly occurs in some families with vWd (*see* Chapter 6). This association is of interest because cryoprecipitate infusion has been found to ameliorate the bleeding diathesis in some patients with storage pool disease.

Alport syndrome

Alport syndrome is the association of interstitial nephritis and nerve deafness which is inherited in a dominant autosomal fashion, generally affecting males more severely than females. Other associations such as cataracts have been reported. Many patients have a lifelong history of a mild bleeding diathesis, such as recurrent epistaxis and post-operative haemorrhages. Peripheral blood examination reveals a mild thrombocytopenia associated with giant platelets which appear normal on electron microscopic study. The thrombocytopenia is due to reduced platelet production with normal platelet survival. The average diameter of the platelet was 4.4 μm compared with a control of 2.4 μm in one study, but no investigations on membrane glycoprotein are yet reported. The platelet abnormality resembles a release abnormality but is unlikely to be a storage pool defect since the ultrastructural studies show normal δ-granules. The findings show a prolonged skin bleeding time, reduced glass bead adhesion and reduced aggregation in response to collagen, adrenalin and an impaired release of nucleotide following reaction with collagen. Platelet factor 3 availability is also reduced. In one family platelet function studies were normal, and we have investigated two families with Alport syndrome in whom the platelet count and platelet function was normal.

May–Hegglin anomaly

May–Hegglin anomaly is characterized by an autosomal dominant inheritance pattern with giant platelets which usually vary greatly in size, and Döhle inclusion bodies seen in granulocytes. These inclusions are diffuse blue areas in the cytoplasm and consist of RNA. There are usually no associated clinical manifestations, although a bleeding disorder has been reported which is disproportionate to the thrombocytopenia frequently seen. The skin bleeding time and capillary fragility test may be normal, platelet adhesion and aggregation responses to collagen, adrenalin, ADP and release reaction are also usually normal. The serum prothrombin time (prothrombin consumption time) and the contributions platelets make to thromboplastin formation in the classical thromboplastin generation test may be reduced. Platelets can be up to 8 μm in diameter. Approximately 25% of these patients are reported to have a bleeding tendency. Since the skin bleeding time is normal, it is probable that this relates more to the abnormal platelet coagulant function seen in these platelets. Clot retraction is normal or proportional to the platelet count, and the capillary fragility test is normal unless the platelet count is reduced. The abnormal prothrombin consumption time is similar to that seen in Bernard–Soulier syndrome, but so far there are no reports of studies on the platelet membrane, and electron microscopy has shown no gross abnormalities other than the size of the platelets. There have been conflicting reports on the platlet lifespan but in some it has been reduced and this would concur with the increased numbers of megakaryocytes usually reported on bone marrow examination.

The Gray platelet syndrome

The first patient who presented with this disorder was diagnosed as having thrombocytopenia which initially responded to steroid therapy and subsequent splenectomy. When his peripheral blood was examined, platelets were found to be large in size and deficient in granules. The bleeding diathesis with this syndrome is very mild. The platelets are devoid of α-granules and contain normal numbers of mitochondria, very dense bodies and peroxisomes. It is thought that this disorder arises through some abnormality in the Golgi apparatus in the megakaryocyte. This syndrome could imply that α-granules have little importance in the overall physiology of haemostasis since the patient reached adulthood in excellent health and participated in contact sports without problems.

Ehlers–Danlos syndrome

This condition presents clinically with hyperelasticity of the skin, joint hyperextensibility and sometimes easy bruising. So far, eight types have been recognized and the biochemical defect which has been identified in most cases is that of abnormal collagen synthesis. Mitral valve prolapse is a common association and there are often other congenital cardiac defects. Most forms are autosomal dominant, but some are recessive including one which has recently been described with abnormal platelet function. The propositus presented with the characteristic features of double jointedness, she also had a mitral valve prolapse and had bruised easily all her life. She had noted petechiae after coughing, and also after drying herself following a shower. Teeth had been extracted without problems and her menstrual periods were not remarkable. The inheritance pattern in her family suggested an autosomal recessive type of inheritance. Her platelet count was normal as was her skin bleeding time and standard coagulation screen. Her platelets and those of her affected relatives failed to aggregate or aggregated very poorly with collagen and did not show a second wave response to ADP. Aggregation to serotonin, thrombin and adrenalin was less than normal, but not markedly so. The abnormality in the collagen and ADP aggregation could be corrected by the addition of cryoprecipitate or pure human plasma fibronectin. No correction was observed by the addition of fibrinogen free of fibronectin. The correction with the addition of fibronectin or cryoprecipitate was not complete. Storage pool abnormality was excluded by showing that the patient's platelet serotonin and ATP and ADP levels were normal and her platelets were also morphologically normal. Immunological measurement of fibronectin in the patients' plasma and immunohistological studies of fibronectin in her platelets' α-granules were normal. It was postulated that fibronectin is present but is biologically ineffective. The Ehlers–Danlos group of disorders should be very interesting to study further, both in regards to collagen and fibronectin interaction. Isolated patients have been reported with a mild bleeding diathesis in which the tissue collagen has been reported to be abnormal (without Ehlers–Danlos syndrome), and it is postulated that their bleeding diathesis is due to an inability of their platelets (normal) to interact with the abnormal collagen in their tissues. A family with prothrombin Cardeza has been reported in whom some of the members have the Ehlers–Danlos syndrome, but this may be a chance relationship.

Osteogenesis imperfecta

This is an autosomal dominant disorder whose primary clinical manifestation is that of recurrent fractures of the bone and blue sclera. A few patients have a mild bleeding diathesis due to a release anomaly, although this has yet to be defined. The bleeding time is rarely prolonged, but capillary fragility is often increased and platelet adhesiveness may also be reduced. One of the more consistent findings is a reduction in platelet factor 3 availability, and an abnormality with the second phase of aggregation of platelet-rich plasma in citrate collected blood with ADP and adrenalin. Collagen aggregation may be impaired but thrombin aggregation is normal.

Marfan syndrome

An associated bleeding tendency with a prolonged skin bleeding time and ill-defined platelet abnormalities has been reported in some patients with Marfan syndrome. This is a disorder of connective tissue, and is characterized by the patient being tall with a long narrow face, a high arched palate, and an arm span greater than height. There is often joint hyperextensibility and there is an associated incidence of subluxation of the lens, aortic regurgitation and dissection of the aorta.

Pseudo-xanthoma elasticum

This is an autosomal recessive disorder which may involve the skin, eyes and vessels. The skin lesions usually develop after the second decade and progress with age. They have a characteristic appearance of 'chicken skin' and are usually best evidenced in the neck, axilla and groin. There is an association with angioid streaks in the retina, and gastrointestinal bleeding has been said to occur in 10% of patients. Arterial calcification is found at an early age and there appears to be a risk of both haemostatic defects and thrombosis. The bleeding time may be prolonged, but the most common defect has been an abnormality in the platelets' response to collagen. An association of factor XI deficiency and a prolonged skin bleeding time with abnormality in the release reaction has also been described, but whether this represents a real syndrome or a chance association will have to await further reports.

Glycogen storage disease Type I

This disorder has been reported to be associated with an haemorrhagic diathesis. Affected individuals have been reported with easy bruising, a history of epistaxis and bleeding following teeth extractions and following surgery. Skin bleeding time is prolonged, platelet adhesion decreased and prothrombin consumption and platelet factor 3 availability is abnormal. The platelets respond poorly to collagen, ADP and adrenalin. These abnormalities are believed to be due to the general metabolic state of the patient rather than the specific biochemical defect in this disorder, namely glucose-6-phosphatase deficiency. When the patient's metabolic problems were corrected by hyperalimentation, the platelet function returned to normal.

Miscellaneous

Platelet function studies resembling release defects have also been described in patients with factor VIII abnormalities, such as von Willebrand disease and haemophilia, a family with bisalbuminaemia and a patient with cavernous haemangioma, without overt disseminated intravascular coagulation.

Platelet functional abnormalities have been described in adenosine deaminase deficiency, Bartter syndrome, Duchenne muscular dystrophy, glucose-6-phosphate dehydrogenase deficiency and idiopathic scoliosis, but there has been no associated bleeding diathesis (Table 7.2). In the first two instances, the abnormality in platelet aggregation is secondary to an elevation of cAMP levels in the platelets.

Table 7.2 Hereditary qualitative platelet disorders without a bleeding tendency

Adenosine deaminase deficiency
Bartter syndrome
Duchenne muscular dystrophy
Glucose-6-phosphate dehydrogenase deficiency
Idiopathic scoliosis

Bartter syndrome

In the case of Bartter syndrome, this is part of a general metabolic problem created by the hyper-renninaemia, hyper-aldosteronism and hypokalaemia secondary to juxtaglomerular cell hyperplasia. It is associated with the increased synthesis of various prostaglandins. When the patients were treated with ibuprofen or indomethacin (inhibitors of prostaglandin synthesis), there was a reduction in the urinary excretion of prostaglandin E_1 and a return of platelet aggregation towards normal. The defect lies in the patients' plasma since platelet-free plasma from patients with Bartter syndrome rapidly induces the aggregation defect in normal platelets, and platelets from subjects with Bartter syndrome improve when suspended in normal plasma. The skin bleeding time was normal and the aggregation responses were most markedly abnormal to adrenalin and ADP and less to collagen and thrombin. The defect appeared to involve both primary and secondary phases of aggregation and serotonin release was absent in all the patients studied, even when there was some degree of second phase aggregation. Patients with hypokalaemia, similar in extent to that seen in the above patients, were also studied and their platelet function and aggregation was quite normal.

Adenosine deaminase deficiency

Also called combined immune deficiency because there are defects in both B and T cell parameters in this disorder with a history of recurrent infections. There is no associated bleeding diathesis and the skin bleeding time is normal. Studies with platelet aggregation, however, show a diminished response to ADP, adrenalin, collagen and thrombin. This correlates with the increased cAMP levels in the patient's cells. It was shown that adenosine, when added to the patient's platelet-rich plasma, was less rapidly broken down than normally, and that the patient's platelet-rich plasma responded normally to adrenalin and collagen, but not to ADP. The addition of adenosine deaminase to the patient's platelet-rich plasma restored the aggregation to normal.

Duchenne muscular dystrophy (DMD)

Platelets from DMD patients have impaired serotonin transport, and increased calcium and phosphate levels in the very dense granules, but no haemostatic abnormality has been reported.

Glucose-6-phosphate dehydrogenase deficiency (G6PD)

No bleeding diathesis has been reported with this deficiency, but Caucasian patients with G6PD deficiency have approximately 25% the normal level of this enzyme in their platelets and consistently show a reduction in platelet factor 3 activity and abnormal prothrombin consumption time. The skin bleeding time and platelet count are normal and platelet aggregation with ADP, collagen and adrenalin are also normal.

Idiopathic scoliosis

Platelets from these patients have increased membrane structures and are larger than normal as well as having increased calcium and phosphorus concentrations, both overall and in the individual dense bodies and α-granules. The platelets show defective aggregation responses to adrenalin and ADP, but not to collagen or ristocetin. There are no clinical haemostatic problems.

ACQUIRED QUALITATIVE PLATELET DEFECTS

One of the earliest examples recognized and best documented is that occurring with uraemia, but as Table 7.3 indicates, there are many causes to be considered. These defects are important to recognize and to investigate:

(1) To ensure that the patient's diet or intake of drugs does not impair platelet function. This could lead to incorrectly attributing the resultant platelet impairment, being investigated by platelet function tests as the cause of a bleeding diathesis.

(2) To warn patients with any form of bleeding diathesis to avoid certain drugs and dietary fads which may increase their tendency to bleed or to

Table 7.3 Acquired qualitative platelet defects

(1)	Nutritional	(4)	Acquired storage pool disease
	19- or 21-chain fatty acids	(5)	Disseminated intravascular coagulation (D.I.C.)
	Mo–Er or black fungus		
	onions and garlic		
	folic acid and B_{12} deficiency	(6)	Infectious causes
	vitamin C	(7)	Autoimmune causes
	vitamin E		
(2)	Uraemia	(8)	Paraproteinaemia
(3)	Dyshaematopoiesis	(9)	Liver disease
		(10)	Hypothyroidism
		(11)	Eosinophilic purpura
		(12)	Drugs

improve a bleeding diathesis by removal of possible aggravating causes.

(3) To improve understanding of the basic mechanisms of platelet dysfunction as well as to provide an approach to patient management when the pathogenesis of the clinical problem involves platelet activation.

Nutritional causes

Epidemiological studies amongst the Eskimos in Greenland revealed a lower incidence of atheroma, and this was related to their diet which was almost exclusively fish. It was postulated that this could be due to the lipid components of this diet, which were distinctive from that of the western world since it consisted of a preponderance of 21-carbon unsaturated fatty acids. The ingestion, by volunteers, of high concentrations of salmon oil, with the exclusion of animal fats in the diet, resulted in an alteration in the fatty acid content of plasma lipid and also the lipid contained in platelet membranes. Some of the parameters of platelet function are altered by such a diet, the platelets aggregate less to standard agonists and occasional subjects develop a mild thrombocytopenia. It is thought that such diets or the intake of eicopentoic acid result in the replacement of arachidonic acid, which is a 20-chain fatty acid, by 19- or 21-chain fatty acids. These result in the production of inactive prostaglandins such as TXA_3, and it is postulated that such diets may reduce platelet aggregation and platelet aggregate formation with a concomitant reduction in atheroma.

Another dietary component which has recently been shown to induce mild platelet defects is a herb, frequently used in Schezwanese cooking, called Mo-Er which on ingestion produces a mild prolongation of the skin bleeding time, together with abnormalities in the platelets' release reaction.

Onions and garlic have an extractable component which inhibits platelet aggregation, and it has been reported that eating onions will inhibit hyperaggregable platelets secondary to a high fat meal.

Vitamin B_{12} and folic acid deficiency both lead to qualitative disorders and sometimes to overt thrombocytopenia. There is a generalized reduction in response to aggregating agents, and these defects may contribute to retinal haemorrhages which seem more prevalent in anaemia caused by these nutritional defects than with other anaemias of similar degree in which the platelet count is not reduced.

Although vitamin C deficiency is characterized by a bleeding tendency, the role of the platelet in this is still doubtful although there have been some reports of a qualitative defect. Most people believe that the disorder relates to a vascular anomaly illustrated by a strongly positive Hess test when the skin bleeding time is normal.

Vitamin E administration has been shown to produce a platelet abnormality which is thought to be due to the lipid peroxidation with resultant abnormalities in the prostaglandin pathways. On dosage of 1800 International Units daily, a 40–50% reduction in collagen-induced release–reaction has been demonstrated. In view of the current advocacy of this vitamin by the popular press, a careful enquiry of the patient's intake should always be made.

Uraemia

Although specific haemostatic defects are occasionally seen in renal disease such as factor X deficiency in amyloidosis or factor IX deficiency with the nephrotic syndrome, the most common bleeding diathesis seen in uraemia relates to an acquired platelet defect which can be corrected by dialysis. Two types of acquired defects are identified. One has an abnormality in platelet aggregation and abnormal responses to collagen, adrenalin, and ADP with an associated prolonged skin bleeding time, diminished platelet adhesiveness and abnormal platelet factor 3 activation. This may be caused by an increased concentration of guanidinosuccinic acid, which when added to platelet-rich plasma *ex vivo* gives similar changes. An abnormality in the release mechanism has been postulated, and as in some other release abnormalities, cryoprecipitate infusions may correct uraemic bleeding. Other workers have shown this defect in some patients, but a reduction of the platelet coagulant activity in others. This has been attributed to the presence in blood of phenol and several hydroxy-phenylacetic acids. When these are incubated with plate-let-rich plasma, the platelets' coagulant activity in the thromboplastin generation test is reduced. In the same concentration as that seen in uraemic plasma, phenol and hydroxy-phenylacetic acid will also reduce adrenalin and ADP aggregation. The defects seen in uraemic platelets may be due to the accumulation of guanidinosuccinic acid and hydroxy-phenylacetic acid or both, and the combination of the two would explain both the platelet coagulant abnormality and the platelet aggregation dysfunction in uraemia. The correction of the bleeding defect in uraemia by the administration of DDVP (*see* Chapter 6) and cryoprecipitate supports the suggestion that factor VIII abnormalities may be a cause of the problem in some patients, and that some defect in uraemia may result in either a decreased or defective formation of the high molecular weight polymers of factor VIII with a consequent abnormality in vWf activity. There are several reports in the literature of reduced VIII:RCoF activity compared with VIII:Ag and VIII:C levels but how consistently this is related to uraemic bleeding remains debatable.

Other investigators have reported diminished prostaglandin synthesis in platelets in uraemia and an increase in prostacyclin produced by vessel endothelial cells, and incubation of uraemic plasma with normal platelets and vessels has produced similar results.

Dyshaematopoiesis

Numerous platelet abnormalities occur in acute non-lymphocytic leukaemia, including defects in the cell's glycoprotein membrane constituents and release abnormalities. As might be expected by the various chromosomal abnormalities detected in acute leukaemias, these defects appear to be diverse and vary from patient to patient. Any one or all of the mechanisms of the platelet plug formation may be found to be abnormal. Morphologically there may be increased numbers of giant platelets and abnormal cytoplasmic granules with decreased numbers of dense granules and a reduced storage pool content as measured biochemically with or without defective prostaglandin pathways. There is also the high incidence of disseminated intravascular coagulation in patients with acute promyelocytic leukaemia, acute non-lymphocytic leukaemia M3 in the FAB classification.

The defect in chronic myeloid leukaemia more closely resembles that of myelofibrosis, polycythaemia and essential thrombocythaemia, and is usually an abnormality in the release reaction as expressed by poor aggregation with adrenalin and collagen. These abnormalities have been attributed to the circulation of 'exhausted' platelets to account for reduction in storage granules (*v. infra*), or to biochemical abnormalities in the membrane of granules secondary to the cell's chromosomal abnormalities. One report stresses a high incidence of lipo-oxygenase deficiency in chronic myeloid leukaemic platelets which results in a reduction in HETE production (*see* Chapter 3, Figure 3.5), and this pathway may be important in irreversible platelet aggregation. Another report in essential thrombocythaemia has stressed a specific reduction in α-adrenergic receptors which might explain the poor response to adrenalin in other myeloproliferative conditions. More global abnormalities may be seen in individual patients with these disorders. Platelet abnormalities have also been documented in patients with refractory anaemia, either refractory anaemia with excess blasts or sideroblastic refractory anaemia; it has been speculated that these abnormalities reflect a more widespread involvement of the haematopoietic tissues in such patients, and perhaps therefore a greater propensity for them to develop leukaemia. This is unproven.

Acquired storage pool disease

Both experimental and clinical studies show that platelets may be activated and undergo a release reaction so that they now have a storage pool 'lesion' and circulate for a relatively normal lifespan *in vivo*. Such platelets, therefore, have an acquired storage pool 'lesion'. It is believed that the most common pathology causing this is disseminated intravascular coagulation, and so one would expect to see such a problem associated with other laboratory findings of this condition. However, acquired storage pool disease has been reported without overt evidence of disseminated intravascular coagulation. The most common clinical associations appear to be that of disseminated lupus erythematosus and cavernous haemangiomas. It would not be surprising to find reports of this situation in disseminated carcinoma and/or sepsis. The laboratory findings of the platelets in this syndrome are identical to those seen with inherited storage pool disease. Such an abnormality must be distinguished from the inhibitory effects of fibrin and fibrinogen breakdown products seen in classical disseminated intravascular coagulation.

Another situation where granule depletion may occur is that following open heart surgery, where bleeding defects are multi-factorial and may include:

(1) Decreased level of clotting factors,
(2) Over heparinization or inadequate neutralization with protamine,
(3) Increased fibrinolytic activity,
(4) Thrombocytopenia, and
(5) Acquired platelet defects.

The latter now seem to be the major problem encountered, and at the end of bypass surgery most studies show that the platelets are partially depleted of α-granules although their dense granules have not been changed. It is interesting that this is associated with a prolonged skin bleeding time, and when a bleeding diathesis occurs this is promptly corrected by the administration of platelet transfusions.

Disseminated intravascular coagulation (DIC) (*see* Chapter 9)

Apart from the intrinsic platelet defect mentioned above, the degradation products of fibrin and fibrinogen (FDP) may themselves inhibit platelet plug formation and also interfere with the clotting pathways. FDPs *in vitro* may impair ADP aggregation and the release reaction. Similar situations can be seen after fibrinolytic therapy and in liver disease, and are thought to be a manifestation of the fibrin fragments interfering with thrombin's actions, both in the clotting pathway and on platelets. DIC is most commonly seen secondary to shock, sepsis, disseminated carcinomatosis, systemic lupus and obstetrical situations (*see* Chapter 9).

Infectious causes

Viral, rickettsial, protozoal and bacterial infections have all been associated with haemorrhagic diatheses. In many instances this appears to be secondary to disseminated intravascular coagulation or to platelet activation. One of these two explanations may result in the reported platelet abnormalities. Qualitative platelet defects are common in patients with infective mononucleosis whose platelet count is normal and in other childhood exanthemata. However a haemorrhagic diathesis is very unusual unless there is an associated thrombocytopenia. Nonetheless, these qualitative platelet defects may explain some of the clinical manifestations such as palatal petechiae which may be seen early in patients with infective mononucleosis.

Dengue haemorrhagic fever is viral induced and is geographically confined to the far East, particularly Thailand and other Asian countries, usually appearing as epidemics in children and young adults but also occurring sporadically. The thrombocytopenia is often accompanied by hypofibrinogenaemia and disseminated intravascular coagulation has been implicated, but the FDPs are usually only minimally elevated and the demonstration of a shortened platelet survival and the presence of Dengue antigen, human immunoglobulin and complement together or singly, in platelets of 48% of those affected suggests an immunological explanation, e.g. immune complexes.

Autoimmune causes

A common conundrum in clinical medicine is why some patients have bleeding problems with a platelet count of $40–50 \times 10^9/l$ and others do not. Indeed platelet counts between $5–10 \times 10^9/l$ can be tolerated without spontaneous bleeding episodes, unless the platelets are in some way qualitatively defective. A subset of patients with idiopathic or auto-immune thrombocytopenic purpura have now been identified, in whom the skin bleeding time is sometimes greater than one would expect for the platelet count, whose platelet adhesiveness is often reduced and whose response to aggregating agents, adrenalin, collagen, ADP, thrombin and ristocetin, is impaired to some or all of these agonists. A similar situation has been identified in patients with systemic lupus erythematosus. In one study the defect appears to be identified as due to an acquired abnormality in release reaction, a form of acquired storage pool disease. Whether this is the case in all instances awaits further study, but homologous antibodies against platelets can inhibit platelet function, and this is reinforced by the development of specific antibodies in patients with inherited platelet membrane defects such as Bernard–Soulier syndrome and Glanzmann disease. Such antibodies produce similar defects when reacted against normal platelets to those with the inherited anomaly. Two explanations appear possible in the clinical situation. Firstly that the patients' platelets have been activated to induce an acquired storage pool defect, or secondly that the antibodies themselves, perhaps by combining with the platelet membrane, inhibit the platelet response to the various aggregating agents. Either explanation is possible, and the fact that ristocetin aggregation is reduced could be explained by the finding that pretreatment of platelets *in vitro* with ADP renders normal platelets insensitive to ristocetin. Another possibility is that the antibody is directed against glycoprotein Ib, thereby interfering with the VIII:vWf interaction with Ib and ristocetin.

Paraproteinaemia

Numerous haemostatic defects can occur in patients with monoclonal gammo-pathies, and the mechanism of bleeding in these situations is often multi-factorial, c.f. renal failure. However, in some instances the paraprotein may interfere with the platelet's surface reactions, perhaps by creating an abnormal atmosphere or coating its surface, and impair the platelet adhesion to damaged vessels (collagen) or the platelet–platelet interaction required in normal plug formation. Faulty fibrin polymerization and abnormal clot retraction have been reported even when platelet numbers and function were normal.

It has been proposed that the prolonged skin bleeding times seen in patients treated with dextran, given as a prophylaxis (60-100 g i.v.) against deep venous thrombosis formation during surgery, may be due to the dextran coating the platelet membrane or altering the plasma proteins required for aggregation. Reduced platelet glass bead adhesion and decreased platelet factor 3 release are also observed. Heparin has similarly been reported by some to cause prolonged skin bleeding times and to impair serotonin release from the platelet. This has not been the experience of all investigators.

Liver disease

The bleeding diathesis in hepatic disorders is multi-factorial, and includes platelet functional abnormalities. These are most probably extrinsic to the platelet relating to an imbalance of fibrinogen and fibrin degradation products, some components of which inhibit platelet aggregation. However, a platelet glycoprotein I defect has been reported in patients with cirrhosis. Alcohol itself may induce a qualitative abnormality (*v. infra*). It is remarkable how few problems are seen in the chronic cirrhotic situation following invasive techniques, such as liver biopsy. The qualitative platelet defect is rarely significant compared to the thrombocytopenia, the low levels of clotting factors synthesized by the liver together with faulty fibrinogen synthesis resulting in a prolonged thrombin time, imbalance of the plasminogen-plasmin system together with abnormalities of the reticuloendothelial system which result in poor clearance of activated clotting components.

Hypothyroidism

Reduced platelet adhesiveness and low factor VIII levels are seen in patients with myxoedema. These appear to have little clinical significance although easy bruising and menorrhagia have been reported.

Eosinophilic purpura

One of the commonest paediatric causes of spontaneous ecchymoses in Eastern countries, such as Thailand and Singapore, is due to a qualitative platelet defect which occurs in children who have an eosinophilia, usually secondary to parasitic infestation. This syndrome has also been reported in adults. It usually presents with ecchymoses or bleeding following trauma or surgery. The platelet count is normal but the peripheral blood film shows an eosinophilia with an absolute count often in excess of $3 \times 10^9/l$. The skin bleeding time is usually prolonged and platelet aggregation to collagen, adrenalin and ristocetin is often reduced, platelet factor 3 availability is abnormal in approximately 50%. The bruising and platelet function tests resolve when treatment of the cause reduces the eosinophil count to normal.

Drugs

Table 7.4 and 7.5 list the drugs which have been reported to cause platelet functional abnormalities. Of these drugs only aspirin, alcohol, the penicillins (especially carbenicillin), dextran and heparin have been reported to cause bleeding problems clinically, but with the latter two drugs this was probably not related to their platelet effect. It is theoretically possible that any or all of

Table 7.4 Drugs employed in trials to reduce thrombosis

Aspirin

Dipyridamole

Sulphinpyrazone

Hydroxychloroquine

Clofibrate

Table 7.5 Drugs which affect platelet function and which may increase bleeding diathesis although they often have no effect

(1) Alcohol

(2) Antibacterial agents
The penicillins
Carbenicillin
Nitrofurantoin

(3) Anti-inflammatory agents
Aspirin
Indomethacin
Ibuprofen
Flurbiprofen
Butazolidine etc.

(4) Adrenergic receptor blockers
(a) *α-adrenergic*
phentolamine
dihydro-ergotamine
(b) *β-adrenergic*
propanolol

(5) Membrane stabilizing drugs
(a) *Anaesthetics*
cocaine
lidocaine
(b) *Antidepressives*
tricyclic agents
imipramine
amitriptyline

(6) Corticosteroids

(7) Diuretics
Frusemide

(8) Serotonin antagonists

(9) Glyceryl guaiacolate

these drugs could have an additive effect on some underlying bleeding diathesis. Obviously, it is important to know of these effects when attempting to assess platelet function studies in a patient who is being studied with a bleeding problem, and to ensure that drugs are not being administered which might affect the investigations.

Table 7.4 lists a number of drugs which have been employed in trials in endeavours to reduce thrombotic complications of one form or another. The first and most extensively studied is aspirin. It has the theoretical advantage that it irreversibly inhibits platelet cyclo-oxygenase thereby preventing formation of thromboxane A_2, but it is less effective in its inhibitor effects on the endothelial cell since this cell is capable of resynthesizing cyclo-oxygenase. It could be predicted that a dosage of aspirin could be achieved which completely blocks the platelet prostaglandin pathway, but which is ineffective or has no effect on the production of prostacyclin by the vessel wall. Initial studies with this compound used dosages of 1.2 g/day which may be too high, thereby inhibiting prostacyclin production in the endothelial cell, although many of these studies showed beneficial effects. Currently, a dose of 300–600 mg a day of aspirin in combination with dipyridamole is one of the most favoured programmes of inhibiting platelet aggregation *in vivo*. Such a regime appears to be effective in increasing cAMP levels in the platelet and in preventing some thrombotic events. Aspirin on its own has been reported to be effective in relieving platelet aggregates causing amaurosis fugax, leg cramps in patients with thrombocythaemia and reducing the incidence of transient ischaemic attacks in males but not females. In combination with dipyridamole, aspirin has been claimed to reduce thrombotic events following surgery, to prevent embolism when given to patients with prosthetic valve replacements and to return platelet survival time to normal in situations such as myocardial ischaemia and infarction. The effectiveness of other non-steroidal anti-inflammatories has not been thoroughly assessed, although anecdotally both indomethacin and butazolidine have been effective in the treatment of superficial thrombophlebitis. All the non-steroidal anti-inflammatories inhibit cyclo-oxygenase activity, but unlike aspirin the effect is reversible and is transient in nature. These, therefore, seem less likely to be useful pharmacological agents.

Dipyridamole's mechanism of action is still uncertain, although it is a phosphodiesterase inhibitor and it does potentiate the endogenous production of prostacyclin by endothelial cells. As a single agent it seems to be of little value in the management of thrombotic problems, but may enhance the action of aspirin and together they have maintained graft patency in patients following coronary artery surgery.

Sulphinpyrazone is another agent which has frequently been employed in an effort to reduce thrombosis. Its mode of action is still uncertain, although *in vitro* it does act as a competitive inhibitor of platelet cyclo-oxygenase, the levels required are never reached *in vivo*. Clinical trials have suggested that it is of benefit in reducing occlusions in extracorporeal shunts and also in reducing mortality in myocardial infarction, although this trial has been subject to controversy.

Hydroxychloroquine has been used as an anti-inflammatory agent and has been shown to affect platelet aggregation to ADP and collagen, but not to alter the bleeding time in man. It has been claimed to reduce deep venous thromboses following operative procedures, but has not been successful in other situations.

Clofibrate, an agent which reduces cholesterol levels, has also been shown to reduce platelet glass bead adhesion, and to weakly inhibit ADP-induced aggregation. It has been claimed to prolong platelet survival in situations where it has been reduced, such as disseminated atheromatous disease. Another hypolipidaemic, beclobrinic acid, which has a much greater hypo-cholesterolaemic and hypotriglyceraemic effect, is also more potent in *in vitro* testing in platelet-rich plasma, where it appears to act by inhibiting prosta-glandin biosynthesis and interfering with the release of arachidonic acid from platelets. From studies to hand it seems unlikely that these agents will prove to be of practical value in the prophylaxis of thrombosis.

There are many anti-platelet agents which are currently on trial and are not generally available for therapeutic use. Many of these agents may be more potent in their anti-platelet activities but it is too early to judge how effective they will be as therapeutic measures. Table 7.5 lists drugs which are not generally used specifically for anti-platelet purposes. Dextran and heparin are referred to later in Chapters 8 & 9.

Alcohol has been shown to cause a prolonged skin bleeding time, impaired platelet factor 3 release and reduced secondary aggregation, and in some individuals a decreased platelet survival. These effects required sustained exposure and may be further complicated by the production of a thrombo-cytopenia. In some instances at least, nutritional problems may be associated and increase the qualitative defect of the platelet. One suggested mechanism of the defect is a reduction in prostaglandin synthesis, since malondialdehyde production is reduced *in vitro* when platelets are subjected to alcohol in concentrations which can be readily achieved by its ingestion.

Antibacterial agents. All the penicillins at sufficient concentrations affect platelet function, carbenicillin being the most potent. It exerts this effect by interacting with the platelet membrane causing a prolonged skin bleeding time and a reduction of the platelet's response to all the aggregating agents, in parti-cular collagen, adrenalin, ADP and even ristocetin. It has been postulated that the penicillins may bind to specific glycoproteins in the platelet membrane in the same way as they bind to the bacterial membrane. Penicillins can also be shown *in vitro* to reduce the platelet's ability to interact with coagulation proteins, and to reduce the amount of thrombin produced when platelet-rich plasma is recalcified.

Nitrofurantoin causes some prolongation of skin bleeding time in therapeutic dosages, and inhibits collagen-induced release as well as primary platelet aggregation with ADP. Unlike carbenicillin there are no reports of any bleeding problems.

The anti-inflammatory agents have attracted especial attention because they block prostaglandin synthetic pathways. The majority block cyclo-oxygenase, but some may also block lipoxygenase. Unlike aspirin they bind reversibly, but care should be taken in their use in patients with a bleeding diathesis.

Adrenergic receptor blocking agent. The adrenergic receptors on the platelet surface are α in character. The α-adrenergic inhibitors phentolamine and dihydro-ergotamine both inhibit platelet aggregation *in vitro* to adrenalin, as well as causing a reduction in response to adrenalin when they are administered to patients *in vivo*. Propranolol does not inhibit platelet aggregation *in vitro* unless dosages are used which are far greater than that achieved *in vivo*, but one study has shown that it does inhibit aggregation in normal patients by mechanisms other than the β-blocking effects. This may be due to its local anaesthetic-like activity causing inhibition of secondary aggregation and release reaction.

Membrane stabilizing drugs. These inhibit secondary aggregation *in vitro*, and may work by preventing the release of arachidonic acid from membrane phospholipids. These drugs include the phenathiazines, the H_1-antihistamines, the local anaesthetics, e.g. lidocaine and cocaine, and the tricyclic antidepressives, e.g. imipramine and amitriptyline. These agents have little effect *in vivo*. They may affect primary ADP aggregation at concentrations higher than is required to suppress the release reaction.

Corticosteroids have been reported to inhibit platelet adhesion as well as platelet aggregation and release to endotoxin. These effects seem to have little practical importance since steroids have been used for decades in the prevention of bleeding in patients with severe thrombocytopenia without any clinical reports of them potentiating bleeding, although there has been considerable controversy as to whether they may induce or aggravate peptic ulceration and perhaps instigate bleeding from a peptic ulcer. More prolonged administration leads to the production of steroid purpura which is similar in appearance to senile purpura, and appears to be secondary to the catabolic effects of steroids on the support and connective tissues rather than an effect on the platelets or clotting mechanism.

Frusemide. This diuretic has been reported to competitively inhibit ADP's action on platelets, and perhaps to inhibit the prostaglandin pathway.

Although gastrointestinal blood loss has been reported with ethycrinic acid, there are no reports in the literature incriminating frusemide.

Serotonin antagonists such as reserpine, methysergide and cyproheptadine can all be shown to reduce the serotonin content in the platelet, but have not been shown to cause any clinical bleeding problems: although cyproheptadine has been reported to be useful in the prevention of kidney graft rejection, and these effects have been attributed to its antiplatelet action.

Glycerol guaiacolate is present in a number of antitussive mixtures, and has been reported to give mild platelet functional defects. Therefore, it should be avoided in patients with lowered platelet counts or qualitative platelet abnormalities.

MANAGEMENT OF QUALITATIVE PLATELET DEFECTS

Patients should be advised to avoid the dietary fads and drugs which have been discussed already, and which are known to produce platelet abnormalities. They should also be advised to have prophylaxis before surgery, including dental extractions. Where the clinical manifestations are moderate to severe, e.g. Glanzmann disease or the Bernard–Souler syndrome, surgical procedures should be covered with a combination of platelet concentrates and cryoprecipitate. We would recommend 6 units of platelet concentrate immediately prior to surgery together with 6 units of cryoprecipitate. In the case of patients with Bernard–Soulier or Glanzmann disease we would repeat the platelet infusions at 12 hourly intervals for the next 48 hours and then daily for another 2 days. Further treatment depends on the clinical situation and the type of surgery undertaken. The possibility that platelet antibodies may arise during therapy must be remembered, as this is particularly common in patients who have membrane glycoprotein abnormalities. This problem may be checked prior to surgery by examining the patient's plasma for antibodies and a panel of platelet donors screened to select ones which react less to the patient's plasma.

Patients with milder bleeding diatheses, notably the release–reaction abnormalities, can usually be treated with cryoprecipitate alone. In these patients we usually use 6 units of cryoprecipitate immediately pre-operatively, then give 6 units 12 hourly for 48 hours and then daily for another 48 hours. The patient is then re-assessed but usually further treatment is not necessary.

A recent study has shown that prednisolone, in doses of 20–50 mg daily given for 3 days pre-operatively and for 3 days post-operatively, is also an effective prophylaxis against bleeding in surgery undertaken in these circumstances.

Acute bleeding problems which may be encountered are epistaxes, gastro-intestinal bleeding and menorrhagia. The acute bleeding episode, from whatever site, should be treated with platelets and/or cryoprecipitate initially. Epistaxes are usually best managed by local treatment. In gastro-intestinal bleeding the local lesion should always be searched for and treated in the appropriate fashion. If no bleeding site can be found and the bleeding is believed to be upper gastro-intestinal in origin, cimetidine 200 mg t.i.d. and at night can be used, either alone or in combination with tranexamic acid 500 mg t.i.d. If the site is believed to be lower than the stomach or duodenum, tranexamic acid 500 mg t.i.d. may be used alone.

Menorrhagia should be managed in concert with a gynaecologist, but standard oral contraceptive therapy is often successful and tranexamic acid may also be helpful.

A careful assessment of iron status by measuring serum iron and ferritin levels is essential, and if reduced a course of iron therapy given.

References

BERNARD, J. and SOULIER, J.P. (1948). Sur une nouvelle variété de dystrophie thrombocytaire hémorragipare congénitale. *Sem. Hôp. Paris,* **24,** 217

CAEN, J.P., CASTALDI, P.A., LECLERC, J.C., INCEMAN, S., LARRIEU, M.J., PROBST, M. and BERNARD, J. (1966). Congenital Bleeding Disorders with Long Bleeding Time and Normal Platelet Count. I. Glanzmann's Thrombasthenia (Report of Fifteen Patients) *Am. J. Med.,* **41,** 4

CZAPEK, E.C., DEYKIN, D., SALZMAN, E., LIAN, E.C., HELLERSTEIN, L.J. and ROSOFF, C.B. (1978). Intermediate syndrome of platelet dysfunction. *Blood,* **52,** 103

GLANZMANN, E. (1918). Hereditäre hämorrhagische thrombasthenie. Ein beitrag zur pathologie der blut plättchen. *J. Kinderkr.* **88,** 1

HARDISTY, R.M. and HUTTON, R.A. (1967). Bleeding tendency associated with 'new' abnormality of platelet behaviour. *Lancet,* i, 983

LAGES, B., MALMSTEN, C., WEISS, H.J. and SAMUELSSON (1981). Impaired platelet response to thromboxane A_2 and defective calcium mobilization in a patient with a bleeding disorder. *Blood,* **57,** 545

PACKHAM, M.A. and MUSTARD, J.F. (1977). Clinical pharmacology of platelets. *Blood,* **50,** 555

PATRIGNANI, P., FILABOZZI, P. and PATRONO, C. (1982). Selective cumulative inhibition of platelet thromboxane production by low-dose aspirin in healthy adults. *J. Clin. Invest.,* **69,** 1366

SCHWARTZ, J.P., COOPERBERG, A.A. and ROSENBERG, A. (1974). Platelet-function studies in patient with glucose-6-phosphate dehydrogenase deficiency. *Br. J. Haematol.,* **27,** 273

WEISS, H.J. (1967). Platelet aggregation, adhesion and ADP release in thrombopathies (platelet factor 3 deficiency): a comparison between Glanzmann's thrombasthenia and von Willebrand's disease. *Am. J. Med.,* **47,** 579

WEISS, H.J. and LAGES, B. (1981). Platelet malondialdehyde production and aggregation responses induced by arachidonate, prostaglandin-G_2, collagen, and epinephrine in 12 patients with storage pool deficiency. *Blood,* **58,** 27

YAROM, R., MUHLRAD, A., HODGES, S. and ROBIN, G.C. (1980). Platelet pathology in patients with idiopathic scoliosis. *Lab. Invest.,* **43,** 208

8
Quantitative platelet disorders

THROMBOCYTOPENIA

Most laboratories define thrombocytopenia as being a platelet count of less than $150 \times 10^9/l$. In view of the inaccuracies of the platelet count whether done by eye or a machine, it is mandatory to repeat this investigation a few times when the count is only slightly reduced, e.g. $130 \times 10^9/l$, to ensure that the patient does have mild thrombocytopenia. Increasing numbers of patients are being discovered as a result of chance observation during routine blood counts for problems not directly related to thrombocytopenia. Apart from chance observation, the modes of presentation are easy bruising, epistaxis, excessive menstrual losses, haematuria, blood loss in the gastrointestinal tract, and anaemia consequent upon unnoticed blood loss.

There are four basic causes of thrombocytopenia:

(1)   Excessive pooling of platelets,
(2)   Decreased production of platelets,
(3)   Increased destruction of platelets, and
(4)   A combination of one or all of the above.

Thrombocytopenia secondary to excessive pooling of platelets has only been described in patients with splenomegaly, and it may be discounted if one cannot palpate the patient's spleen. This type of thrombocytopenia does not cause haemostatic problems, and should there be excessive bruising or evidence of platelet dysfunction, such as a prolonged skin bleeding time, other reasons should be sought. The most common causes of platelet pooling are splenomegaly secondary to liver disease and portal hypertension due to excessive alcohol intake. That splenic pooling is the cause of thrombocytopenia, may be confirmed by undertaking a platelet survival study which should demonstrate a normal lifespan of autologous platelets, but a reduction in platelet recovery from the normal of 80% to 20–40%. In some circumstances, e.g. chronic active hepatitis, the thrombocytopenia may be due to a reduction in platelet survival, possibly related to an associated autoimmune response, or the effects of circulating immune complexes as well as excessive pooling of platelets in the spleen.

Studies from several laboratories have demonstrated that platelets pooled in the spleen may become available in the peripheral circulation following the injection of adrenalin. This explains the lack of bleeding problems associated with this particular mechanism, since the pooled platelets are available on demand. It also accounts for the lack of complications when liver biopsies and/or other invasive or operative procedures are undertaken on these patients, unless they have other associated coagulation or platelet problems. Most centres undertaking liver biopsies are happy to proceed when the platelet count is above $50 \times 10^9/l$ and the prothrombin time and skin bleeding time are normal, provided there is no history of any bruising or bleeding.

Problems of diminished production are usually identified by bone marrow aspiration and trephine revealing a reduction in megakaryocyte number or morphological abnormalities associated with haematopoietic dysfunction, or replacement of the marrow by abnormal cells or tissue. Platelet lifespan studies will be normal. In contra-distinction, marrow examinations in patients with thrombocytopenia due to increased destruction reveal increased numbers of megakaryocytes and the platelet lifespan is reduced.

Compensated thrombocytopenia is a term which has been used to describe patients with reduced platelet survival whose platelet count is normal due to increased platelet production, and has been documented in a number of clinical situations including lupus erythematosus and some 'non haematological' conditions described in Chapter 9.

Spurious thrombocytopenia

Spurious thrombocytopenia may result from a faulty blood sampling technique initiating clotting, and by contaminants in the collecting tubes causing platelet adherence or clumping. Cold agglutinins of platelets with a thermal range of up to 34 °C have been reported to cause pseudothrombocytopenia and these were not dependent on the type of anticoagulant. Other platelet agglutinins, some with and some without thermal dependence, require the presence of EDTA and cause falsely low platelet counts when blood is collected into that anticoagulant. Heparin is not used since it commonly agglutinates normal platelets. Another curious phenomenon which may cause spurious thrombocytopenia is platelet 'satellism' in which platelets adhere to leukocytes giving a halo appearance. Again this is usually dependent on the presence of EDTA. These conditions should be suspected when the platelet count does not match the clinical picture or the peripheral blood film, and may

Table 8.1 Familial thrombocytopenia

Autosomal recessive
    Thrombocytopenia with absent radius (TAR)
    Large platelet thrombocytopenia
    Hereditary thrombocytopenia
    Upshaw–Shulman syndrome
    Afibrinogenaemia

Autosomal dominant
    Alport syndrome
    Bernard–Soulier syndrome
    Bis-albuminaemia
    Hereditary autoimmune thrombocytopenia
    Hypogranular thrombocytopenia
    May–Hegglin anomaly
    With platelet function abnormalities
    Without platelet function abnormalities
    Pseudo von Willebrand syndrome

Sex-linked recessive
    Wiskott–Aldrich syndrome
    Incomplete Wiskott–Aldrich
    Associated with renal abnormality

be checked by performing a platelet count using blood from a lanced finger tip.

Table 8.1 lists the forms of hereditary thrombocytopenia. These types of thrombocytopenia are more common than previously appreciated, and their importance lies in distinguishing such patients from those with acquired forms of thrombocytopenia since the hereditary thrombocytopenias frequently do not respond to glucocorticoid therapy or splenectomy. The classification listed in Table 8.1 is an endeavour to place these disorders according to their modes of inheritance. In some instances, such as the Upshaw–Shulman syndrome, the condition is so rare that it is difficult to know the true form of inheritance, and perhaps it would be better described as a congenital form of thrombocytopenia rather than familial. Similarly, the thrombocytopenia associated with bis-albuminaemia has only been reported in one family and may represent a chance association of these anomalies.

Autosomal recessive

Thrombocytopenia with absent radius (TAR)

This is characterized by a bilateral absence of the radius together with reduced numbers of megakaryocytes. In most of the patients clinical features such as purpura, melaena, haemoptysis, haematemesis or epistaxis occur before the age of 4 months and frequently within the first week of life. Over half the patients have associated leukaemoid reactions with high white cell counts, splenomegaly and hepatomegaly, and this often coincides with worsening thrombocytopenia and sometimes death. When cases were examined, the organ enlargement was found to be due to extramedullary haematopoiesis, and true leukaemia has not been documented. Anaemia when present was due to blood loss. Cardiac abnormalities were present in a third of the patients and a number of other anomalies were noted, but were much less frequent. Chromosome studies with one exception were normal. Splenectomy rarely helped, but 4 of 18 patients treated with steroids showed definite improvement. In some instances infections appeared to precipitate both the thrombocytopenia and the leukaemoid reactions, and the most critical period was from birth to one year of age when most deaths occurred. Bone marrow examination in the main showed normal erythroid and myeloid precursors with absent, reduced or morphologically abnormal megakaryocytes. This disorder is probably inherited as an autosomal recessive.

There have been a number of other patients reported in the literature with congenital thrombocytopenia secondary to a reduction or absence of megakaryocytes in the newborn, and in many of these instances some congenital anomalies such as Fallot tetralogy and cleft palate have been reported and so may relate to this syndrome.

Large platelet thrombocytopenia

Murphy has reported a family with giant platelets and thrombocytopenia in whom the autologous platelet survival was normal, and thus is secondary to a reduction in platelet production. The inheritance in this family was autosomal recessive in type. Other families with an autosomal recessive hereditary thrombocytopenia have been described in whom the platelet size was apparently normal. There is no information concerning platelet lifespan studies in the latter.

Upshaw-Shulman syndrome

This interesting but extremely rare congenital disorder consists of thrombocytopenia with intermittent microangiopathic haemolytic anaemia which may be overlooked. The condition responds to infusions of plasma, and in the first patient reported was thought to be due to a lack of thrombopoietin because the episodes of thrombocytopenia occurred at regular intervals, and responded to plasma infusions. This condition may begin in infancy or develop in early adult life, and consists of recurrent episodes of intravascular haemolysis with thrombocytopenia and may be accompanied by fever, abdominal pain and neurological manifestations including transient central neuropathy as well as peripheral nerve involvement. The episodes may be precipitated by infection trauma or in later life pregnancy. Examination of their plasma has shown an unusual proportion of large factor VIII multimers which are similar to the large VIII multimers secreted by cultured human venous endothelial cells. During relapse it has been found that these large multimers are diminished, and it has been postulated that this is due to their consumption triggered by some other factor which induces the platelets to bind the large factor VIII multimers and agglutinate in a similar way to the ristocetin response (chapter 6). This co-factor may be some positively charged component which is released following tissue necrosis since each of the clinical relapses in four patients occurred in association with injury, infection, surgery and pregnancy. Normal plasma may contain the necessary factor to reduce the abnormally large VIII von Willebrand multimers and explain its curative action. Investigations in one patient have shown a low level of cold insoluble globulin (fibronectin), although measurements of fibronectin in two other patients were normal.

Congenital afibrinogenaemia

This autosomal recessive condition has frequently been reported to be associated with a prolonged bleeding time, perhaps related to the platelet's lack of response to ADP or a requirement for fibrinogen in platelet adhesion since the abnormalities in aggregation are seen in citrated, but not heparinized plasma. Some of these patients, however, do have an associated mild thrombocytopenia, the pathogenesis of which is uncertain.

Autosomal dominant

Alport syndrome (v. supra)

Bernard–Soulier syndrome (v. supra)

Bis-albuminaemia

One family has been described in which there appears to be a linkage between bis-albuminaemia and a hereditary thrombocytopenia with some associated platelet functional defects. The pathogenesis of the thrombocytopenia in this instance has not been absolutely proven as only isologous platelet survivals were undertaken which were normal. The bone marrow did show normal to increased megakaryocytes which would suggest that the functionally abnormal platelets might have a reduced lifespan. These platelets showed functional abnormalities which would be compatible with a release reaction problem.

Hereditary auto-immune thrombocytopenia

Although there have been a number of reports of this entity, they are all subject to criticism since platelet lifespan studies were not undertaken, and the tests to establish the auto-immune aetiology were ones which may be seen in situations other than auto-immune thrombocytopenia. As many other auto-immune disorders have now been convincingly reported in families, it seems likely that some or all of these reports are correct, but further studies will have to be done to establish this entity.

Hypogranular thrombocytopenia

These patients exhibit a moderate to severe bleeding diathesis, and the megakaryocytes were found to be normal in numbers but abnormal morphologically. Platelet function studies showed defective aggregation and nucleotide release. Electron microscopic studies showed a reduction in the number of dense granules in the circulating platelets and platelet survival time in one family was normal, suggesting that thrombocytopenia was due to reduced platelet production. Platelets adhered normally to collagen but did not aggregate, and the functional defect in the cells resulted in a prolonged skin bleeding time > 30 minutes in one family where the platelet counts ranged from $60-129 \times 10^9/l$. There was a very marked abnormality with the prothrombin consumption and platelet factor 3 release tests. Unfortunately, studies of serotonin uptake and release have not as yet been reported. This entity may be a variant of the Gray platelet syndrome (*v. supra*).

The May–Hegglin anomaly (v. supra)

With platelet function abnormalities

Where autosomal dominant thrombocytopenia has been reported together with functional abnormalities, the latter has usually been consistent with a platelet release abnormality. Unfortunately, most of this evidence relies on the fact that the platelets aggregate abnormally with collagen and/or do not have second phase with ADP and adrenalin, since in few instances have serotonin release studies been undertaken. In most, the platelet lifespan with isologous cells has been normal, but it is reduced to the order of 1–2 days when autologous cells are employed. Although there are both decreased platelet numbers and function, the bleeding diathesis is quite mild and usually consists of epistaxis in childhood, some menorrhagia in the females which is usually readily controlled by hormonal means, and excessive bleeding after operative procedures or trauma. In one family the author has studied, in three generations the propositus died at the age of 82 years with a rectal carcinoma.

Without platelet function abnormalities

Clinically these patients have a mild to moderate bleeding diathesis as in the group described above, and the degree of bleeding diathesis correlates well with the platelet count. Again the majority of patients studied show a reduced autologous but normal isologous platelet lifespan and splenectomy in both these groups has rarely been of benefit. Bone marrow examination shows a normal marrow, unless there is an associated reduction in iron stores through blood loss such as menorrhagia and a normal to increased number of megakaryocytes without gross morphological abnormalities.

Thrombocytopenia with von Willebrand disease (pseudo von Willebrand disease (see chapter 6)

A condition called pseudo von Willebrand disease has only very recently been described, and it is uncertain whether a number of case reports in the past of von Willebrand disease associated with intermittent thrombocytopenia represent a similar entity. The patient presents with a moderate to severe bleeding tendency, and plasma factor VIII investigations are identical to the von Willebrand disease Type IIB (see Chapter 6). The thrombocytopenia is intermittent in nature. It is important to recognize this group of patients since care must be taken when correcting the factor VIII defect with cryoprecipitate not to depress the platelet count further.

Sex-linked recessive states

Wiskott–Aldrich syndrome

The Wiskott–Aldrich syndrome, originally described in children with otitis, eczema, recurrent pyogenic infections and bloody diarrhoea, has now been recognized to have the classical triad of recurrent infectious episodes, eczema and thrombocytopenia. Investigations show that the IgM level is usually reduced and the IgG and IgA levels are normal or increased. *Pari passu* with the reduction in IgM levels is also the reduction in isohaemagglutinin titres. Treatment of such children with transfer factor has been reported to improve their immune state, and to correct their thrombocytopenia to some degree.

The platelets in Wiskott–Aldrich syndrome have been shown to be smaller than normal and to have reduced levels of glycogen and hexosekinase. When examined with the electron microscope, the plasma membrane has an unusual wavy appearance with small indentations, and α-granules and mitochondria are reduced in numbers. Often the mitochondria are larger and more elongated than usual. Very dense bodies are rarely seen but there is often an increase in the number of dense tubules. The platelets adhere poorly to collagen and do not aggregate or show a markedly reduced aggregation, with collagen, adrenalin, and ADP. They aggregate and release nucleotides normally with thrombin, and have a normal release reaction with collagen. Autologous platelet survivals are short, less than 24 hours in some, and in one study the platelet survival of Wiskott–Aldrich platelets was short when transfused into a normal volunteer. There is, therefore, an intrinsic metabolic defect in these platelets. Splenectomy improves the thrombocytopenia, but is initially avoided because of the increased risks of death due to overwhelming septic-aemia. A recent study in which the splenectomy has been combined with prophylactic antibiotics suggests that splenectomy may sometimes be indicated where bleeding is marked and the thrombocytopenia has not responded to transfer factor. An increased incidence of lymphoma has been reported, and one patient died with myeloid leukaemia but the majority of deaths have resulted from either septicaemia or bleeding.

Incomplete Wiskott–Aldrich syndrome

This refers to families whose major problem is that of a moderate bleeding diathesis secondary to thrombocytopenia, in which the platelets are small in size and which have similar functional findings to those reported in the Wiskott–Aldrich syndrome. There is sometimes an associated eczema but not the other immunoglobulin problems or recurrent infective episodes seen in the classical syndrome. These patients have a decreased autologous platelet survival, and thrombocytopenia is corrected by splenectomy.

Associated with renal abnormality

Two families have been reported with a sex-linked recessive pattern who have elevated IgA levels and glomerulonephritis. None of the patients had any history of recurrent infection and immunological response tested by lympho-cyte *in vitro* reactivity to phytohaemagglutinin, tetanus toxoid and allogenic cells were normal. Delayed sensitivity skin tests were found to be normal as were isohaemagglutinin titres. Bone marrow examination showed decreased numbers of megakaryocytes, and the administration of fresh frozen plasma did not result in any alteration in the number (compare Upshaw–Shulman syndrome). Percutaneous renal biopsies were performed in some of these patients following infusion of platelet-rich plasma, without any bleeding problems. This family also showed little bleeding following dental extractions, and some had undergone major surgical procedures without any problems and without any particular cover for haemostasis. The thrombocytopenia varied from $30–100 \times 10^9/l$ and the platelets looked morphologically normal on the peripheral film. In one instance bone marrow was reported as showing an absence of megakaryocytes and an homologous platelet survival was normal. Treatment of one patient with prednisone and azathioprine was unsuccessful.

ACQUIRED THROMBOCYTOPENIA

The distinction between acquired and hereditary thrombocytopenia can be particularly difficult in the neonatal period. Table 8.2 lists the causes of neonatal thrombocytopenia. Of particular interest and importance to the physician looking after adults, are the drugs which can cause thrombo-

Table 8.2 Acquired thrombocytopenia – neonatal

Diminished production
  Amegakaryocytic
  TAR syndrome
  Drugs
    – tolbutamide

  Drugs ingested by mother
    Chlorthiazide
    Chloramphenicol

  Congenital leukaemia

  Reticuloendotheliosis

  Associated with generalized marrow hypoplasia

  Idiopathic

Increased destruction
  Congenital infection
    Rubella
    Cytomegalovirus
    Toxoplasmosis
    Disseminated herpes
    Syphilis

  Drugs ingested by mother
  (see Tables 8.3 and 8.5)

  Disseminated intravascular coagulation

  Isoimmune
    Mother has unusual platelet group (e.g. Pl^{A-}ve)
    Mother has ITP

cytopenia in the baby without necessarily affecting the mother. Isoimmune thrombocytopenia can occur when the mother has an unusual platelet blood group such as Pl^A negative and develops antibodies to her baby's Pl^A positive platelets similar to the Rh problem. Fortunately this is a very rare form of thrombocytopenia but it is important to recognize it, since the use of the mother's platelets will rapidly correct the baby's thrombocytopenia. If the mother is known to be Pl^A – ve it is easy to monitor, since platelet antibodies can be readily detected in the mother's plasma when incubated with normal Pl^A + ve platelets. A more common problem is a mother who has had idiopathic or auto-immune thrombocytopenia in the past and this will be discussed later.

Table 8.3 lists the causes of acquired thrombocytopenia due to reduced production, and Table 8.4 lists those due to increased platelet destruction. In many instances there may be a combination of the two factors.

Clinically acquired thrombocytopenia is usually divided into acute and chronic forms. Acute is when a patient presents with a sudden onset of widespread purpura and bruising, sometimes associated with bleeding, epistaxis, haematuria or menorrhagia, and on examination blood blisters may be noted

Table 8.3   Acquired thrombocytopenia – reduced production

Selective suppression of megakaryocytes
Drugs
  Chlorthiazide
  Oestrogen
  Alcohol
  Glucocorticoids

  Cyclical thrombocytopenia

  Lupus erythematosus

  Idiopathic

Marrow hypoplasia
Primary

Secondary
  Drugs
        – Chemotherapy
        – Chloramphenicol
        – Phenylbutazone
        – Gold salts
        – Methyl phenylethylhydantoin
        – Trimethadione
        – Quinacrine
        – Organic arsenicals

  Radiation

  Chemical exposure and poison
        – Benzene
        – Alcohol
        – Heavy metals

  Virus
        – Viral hepatitis
        – Dengue haemorrhagic fever

  Paroxysmal nocturnal haemoglobinuria

Bone marrow replacement
Leukaemia
  Acute
  Chronic

  Refractory sideroblastic anaemia with excess blasts

  Myelofibrosis

  Myeloma

  'Hairy' cell leukaemia or leukaemic reticuloendotheliosis

  Macroglobulinaemia

  Lymphoma
    Hodgkin
    Non-Hodgkin

  Disseminated malignancy

Megaloblastic anaemia

Iron deficiency

Table 8.4 Acquired thrombocytopenia – increased destruction

Infections

Drugs and chemicals

Thrombosis
  DIC
  Vascular malformation
  Massive thrombosis

Antibodies
 (a) Autoantibody
      Idiopathic
      Secondary – CLL
               – Lymphoma and cancer
               – SLE
               – Drugs
      Evan syndrome
 (b) Pregnancy
      Transfusion

Miscellaneous
      Thrombotic thrombocytopenic purpura (TTP)
      Haemolytic uraemic syndrome (HUS)

Acquired biochemical defects

in the mouth and haemorrhages in the retina. The presence of the latter signals an emergency, since such lesions may cause permanent visual defects and may be a harbinger of an intracranial bleeding episode. Immediate careful assessment is essential and this should include a skin bleeding time, examination of the peripheral blood and a bone marrow aspirate and trephine. From these investigations and consideration of the clinical history and physical examination, a provisional diagnosis can usually be made, although further appropriate tests may have to be undertaken to clinch the diagnosis. Acute thrombocytopenia is most commonly seen secondary to drug ingestion or a viral illness, especially in children; however all forms of thrombocytopenia may present in this fashion.

Most regard chronic thrombocytopenia as being a state which has lasted 3–6 months or longer. In most instances, the clinical manifestations and the thrombocytopenia is not as severe as that seen in acute thrombocytopenia. The reason for distinguishing between acute and chronic thrombocytopenia is the difference in clinical course. Acute thrombocytopenia, particularly that occurring in children, very frequently remits although the patients may have to be treated if the bleeding and bruising problems are severe. Chronic thrombocytopenia rarely remits without treatment, although it may pursue an intermittent course with clinical exacerbations and remissions. The bone marrow will distinguish thrombocytopenia secondary to reduced production or increased destruction in most instances, but a platelet survival may be occasionally required to firmly establish whether there is increased platelet destruction.

Table 8.3 lists a number of drugs which have been implicated in causing thrombocytopenia due to suppression of platelet production, and a history of drug ingestion should be sought. The peripheral blood examination will usually disclose only thrombocytopenia; however in the case of a chronic alcoholic, there may be accompanying red cell changes, in particular macrocytosis and target cells, often causing a strikingly elevated mean corpuscular volume. Glucocorticoid administration may be accompanied by an eosinopenia and lymphopenia.

Since these drugs are thought to act by suppression of platelet production, their withdrawal from the patient may not result in an immediate recovery of the platelet count, unlike drugs which cause increased platelet destruction. Chlorthiazide has been reported to give an immune antibody response similar to quinine, but this is less common than its marrow suppressant effect. Mild thrombocytopenia has been reported in a number of series with chlorthiazide, and it is probably a drug which should be avoided during pregnancy since it could cause thrombocytopenia in the baby.

There have been a number of reports of thrombocytopenia following the administration of oestrogens such as diethyl-stilboestrol, and recovery may not occur for 1–2 months following the withdrawal of the drug. Oestrogens have been shown to be quite a potent marrow suppressant in some animals, and have been postulated to play a role in the increased incidence of thrombocytopenia in women and the recrudescence of idiopathic thrombocytopenia in pregnancy.

Alcohol may have both a suppressant effect and a destructive effect on platelets, and in the chronic alcoholic there may be added nutritional problems with folic acid or less commonly B_{12} deficiency. Alcohol is a general marrow suppressant, and it is common to have alcoholic patients admitted with mild to moderate thrombocytopenia who, following the withdrawal of alcohol, develop a modest thrombocytosis. Even alcoholics with portal hypertension and resultant thrombocytopenia due to pooling, may demonstrate this effect. They often enter hospital with a platelet count of $30–60 \times 10^9/l$ and after a few days this rises to, what is a normal level for them of $90–120 \times 10^9/l$.

In the author's experience, glucocorticoids are responsible for thrombocytopenia in one restricted clinical setting, *viz.* a patient who is receiving large doses of glucocorticoids for idiopathic thrombocytopenic purpura. The bruising and bleeding problems have usually resolved, but the platelet count has made little or no progress. The dosage level is usually in the order of 40–80 mg prednisolone daily. Reduction of the prednisolone dose results in a gradual rise in platelet count and may enable the total withdrawal of glucocorticoid therapy. This phenomenon was first noted by Cohen and Gardner in 1961, and is a rare complication of glucocorticoid therapy in thrombocytopenia. Steroid purpura on the other hand is a common problem especially in old people. This purpura is identical in its site and nature to senile purpura and will exaggerate the latter if it is already present. It is largely a cosmetic problem, but it must not be mistaken for a recrudescence of the thrombocytopenia since an increase in glucocorticoid dose will worsen the purpura.

Cyclical thrombocytopenia is a rare condition which more commonly occurs in women than men. There is normally a variation in platelet count during a woman's menstrual cycle in which there is an average of a 20% drop in the count in the 2 weeks prior to menstruation. Cyclical thrombocytopenia in females is usually not related to menstrual cycle and may occur in women after the menopause. The most frequently noted cycles are 28–30 days with the platelet count falling to $10–20 \times 10^9/1$. In some instances isologous platelet survivals have been found to be normal, and the infusion of the patient's plasma into normal recipients has also not resulted in any change in platelet count. Bone marrow studies, done at appropriate time intervals, have also been reported to show a reduction in megakaryocyte numbers to account for the thrombocytopenia. In some cases there is a rebound thrombocytosis to platelet levels of $500–600 \times 10^9/1$. In one instance, the patient later developed aplastic anaemia. Steroid treatment and splenectomy have been of little value when tried. The pathogenesis of the problem is uncertain, although in one patient thrombopoietin levels were consistently reduced. Should there be any severe or life threatening bleeding, platelet transfusion should be given, and later glucocorticoids and/or antifibrinolytic agents such as tranexamic acid should be considered a few days prior to the predicted fall in count.

Lupus erythematosus rarely causes thrombocytopenia through a selective suppression of megakaryocytes, although the association is now well recorded. This condition will be considered with its more common pathogenesis of thrombocytopenia, namely auto-antibodies to platelets later.

Table 8.3 also lists the causes of more generalized bone marrow hypoplasia, in which the major problem may be thrombocytopenia rather than leukopenia or anaemia. Idiopathic marrow hypoplasia is an uncommon condition and rarely presents with thrombocytopenia alone. Secondary forms, particularly with the increasing use of chemotherapeutic agents in oncology practice, are far more common and other drugs which have been reported to cause this problem are listed in the table.

Virus infections are common causes of mild to moderate but less commonly very severe thrombocytopenia. In most cases this is due to a reduction in lifespan, but depression of megakaryocyte production of platelets has been documented both in viral hepatitis and dengue fever. The latter is a particularly common form of thrombocytopenia in South East Asia and constitutes the commonest form of recurrent infectious thrombocytopenia in the world, termed dengue haemorrhagic fever. It has a high incidence in young children, but epidemics are seen in older age groups including young adults. The patient usually presents with fever, headache, gastrointestinal symptoms of nausea, vomiting and abdominal pain, myalgia and abnormal taste sensations. Examination at the commencement of illness shows lymphadenopathy, conjunctival injection and sometimes some petechial eruptions a macular rash and a positive Hess test. The liver may be enlarged. In the haemorrhagic form there is often an abrupt worsening of the patient's clinical status several days after the onset of the disorder with increased abdominal pain and irritability, with generalized haemorrhagic phenomena and sometimes hypoalbuminaemia and shock. Peripheral blood examination may show a striking leukopenia and the presence of transformed lymphocytes or plasma cells, as well as a thrombocytopenia. The skin bleeding time will be prolonged and there may be evidence of disseminated intravascular coagulation. Currently it is believed that patients who develop dengue haemorrhagic fever and dengue shock syndrome, are individuals who have had a previous dengue infection or have acquired maternal dengue antibody. The disorder runs a course which lasts 10–15 days. Most haematological studies and bone marrow examinations show that there is an overall depression of marrow function early in the course of the infection, and this is often associated with quite a striking reduction of megakaryocytes so that initial investigations concluded that its pathogenesis was largely that of reduced platelet production. More recent studies, using platelet survival and measurement of platelet complement and IgG employing immune fluorescent techniques, have suggested that in many instances at least, there is an important contribution by peripheral destruction. There is often associated evidence for disseminated intravascular coagulation when the shock syndrome occurs. The overall cause of thrombocytopenia in these patients may therefore be due to a number of mechanisms which may vary from epidemic to epidemic. It is still difficult to ascertain the precise incidence of this condition, but in Eastern countries, many practitioners believe that it is endemic and that they regularly see a number of such patients in young adults every year.

Paroxysmal nocturnal haemoglobinuria may rarely present as a bleeding problem. This diagnosis is usually considered in any thrombocytopenic patient who has features of haemolytic anaemia, and can be excluded confidently by undertaking a sucrose haemolysis and Ham test, and examining the urine for haemosiderin which is often positive even when the haemolytic features of this disorder are not prominent. More difficult are the rare patients who present with menorrhagia and thrombocytopenia whose bone marrow appears hyperactive and deficient in iron. These findings may be attributed to the blood loss, and the correct diagnosis can only be reached when features of intravascular haemolysis occur. The basic defect in this problem appears to be that of the plasma membrane since, just like the red cells, the platelet is exquisitely sensitive to the effects of complement activation. However, most investigations of platelet survival in these patients using either isologous or autologous platelets have been normal, so that even in circumstances where the marrow is normo- to hypercellular and with normal numbers of megakaryocytes, there is an apparent defect in platelet production. Even when there is significant thrombocytopenia, the patients may not suffer from bruising problems, and indeed may present with a thrombotic episode such as a deep venous thrombosis or some other thrombotic event such as hepatic vein thrombosis (the Budd–Chiari syndrome). The reason for the 'hypercoagulability' in this condition has been much discussed and investigated over the years, and for some time was believed to relate to abnormal membrane phospholipids in the red cells. More recent evidence suggests that it is due to an increased sensitivity of platelets to normal physiological aggregating processes. The precise mechanism remains uncertain.

Situations of thrombocytopenia secondary to bone marrow replacement are also listed in Table 8.3. Often there will be a clue as to this problem from the peripheral blood examination where a leukoerythroblastic anaemia may be reported. This type of blood picture can be seen in any of the diagnoses listed in Table 8.3 under 'bone marrow replacement', but the presence of premature red cell and white cell precursors is more commonly seen in situations of myelofibrosis and secondary malignancy. Myelofibrosis is more likely when tear drop red cell morphology is a striking feature and when splenomegaly is present.

Acute leukaemia frequently presents as a bleeding problem, examination of the peripheral film usually shows the presence of lymphoblasts, myeloblasts or monoblasts, where the leukaemia is acute lymphoblastic, myeloblastic or monoblastic respectively. The diagnosis is confirmed by bone marrow examination with the appropriate cytochemical stains and chromosome studies. Bleeding problems frequently complicate the course of both chronic myeloid and chronic lymphatic leukaemia due to thrombocytopenia secondary to therapy or progression of the disease. Splenomegaly is usually a striking feature, and the peripheral blood and bone marrow examination make the diagnosis. Successful therapy of the leukaemia often improves the platelet counts. If not, splenectomy should be considered, and steroid therapy given if investigations suggest an auto-immune element, which is common in chronic lymphatic leukaemia (v. infra).

Somewhat more difficult may be the diagnosis of refractory anaemia with excess blasts or preleukaemia. In this situation the peripheral blood may only show anaemia and thrombocytopenia, whilst the bone marrow usually reveals a hypocellular marrow with the presence of blasts usually less than 10% of the total marrow population. There may also be accompanying dyshaematopoietic features due to abnormal maturation of the red and white cell series. Chromosome studies may also be helpful, and there is commonly an increase in bone marrow iron and sometimes sideroblasts are prominent. A particularly common chromosome abnormality is a 21, 8 translocation. One variety is associated with abnormal megakaryocyte morphology with reduced lobe formation, and usually an accompanying thrombocytosis rather than thrombocytopenia. This is called the 5q anomaly. These conditions are frequently referred to as pre-leukaemic although it is impossible on presentation to predict the 10% of patients who will develop leukaemia.

Multiple myeloma may be suspected when the thrombocytopenia is associated with marked rouleaux formation in the blood, especially if circulating plasma cells are also noted. The diagnosis is clinched by serum and urine protein studies looking for monoclonal paraproteinaemia and Bence Jones proteinuria. Bone marrow biopsy may display sheets of abnormal plasma cells. Occasionally, the diagnosis will not be revealed until the bone marrow biopsy is performed in patients who have non-secretory forms of the disorder. The patient is often anaemic and may present with any of the other features of this disorder such as low back pain and bony tenderness secondary to associated osteoporosis, compression fractures of the vertebrae and bone infiltration by plasma cells.

Myelofibrosis often presents with a mild to moderate thrombocytosis, rather than thrombocytopenia which usually develops later in the course of the illness. When thrombocytopenia is a presenting feature there is usually, but not always, a mild to marked anaemia. The peripheral blood reveals a leuko-erythroblastic picture and tear drop morphology of the red cells is often prominent. The patient almost invariably has a considerably enlarged spleen and often accompanying hepatomegaly. Bone marrow biopsy results in a dry tap, and the formal diagnosis is made on the trephine which reveals a variable degree of cellularity with a striking increase in collagen and fibrous tissue.

It is important to consider leukaemic reticulo-endotheliosis or hairy cell leukaemia since it may mimic myelofibrosis in many respects, but is usually excluded by examining a wet peripheral film and undertaking acid phosphatase stains both on the peripheral film and the bone marrow. Often the patient has an enormous spleen and there may be a 'dry tap' as in myelofibrosis. It is an important diagnosis to make since some patients respond well to splenectomy and/or androgen therapy.

Macroglobulinaemia frequently presents with mucosal bleeding and often has an accompanying thrombocytopenia. Quite frequently this is associated with the hyperviscosity syndrome so that the patient also complains of failing vision and on fundoscopic examination, the classical cattle truck appearance or 'string of sausages' sign in the retinal veins is seen together with widespread fundal haemorrhages. The skin bleeding time is characteristically prolonged and equally characteristically is often rapidly corrected following plasmapheresis since it is secondary, not only to the thrombocytopenia, but also to an acquired platelet defect due to the macroglobulin. Very frequently the patient has associated hepatosplenomegaly and often lymphadenopathy. The peripheral blood may be similar to myeloma with rouleaux formation and sometimes shows the presence of transforming lymphocytes. Serum electrophoretic analysis reveals the presence of a paraprotein, which is IgM, and which ultracentrifuge studies show is a macromolecule of 19S molecular weight. Bone marrow biopsy commonly reveals a dense lymphocyte infiltrate with a cell intermediate between a lymphocyte and a plasma cell.

Lymphoma rarely presents purely as a bleeding problem, but thrombocytopenia is a frequent accompaniment and may be on the basis of marrow replacement or increased peripheral destruction. The patient usually presents with enlarged lymph nodes and often accompanying hepatosplenomegaly and the other clinical features which go with the various forms of Hodgkin and non-Hodgkin lymphoma.

Disseminated malignancy also rarely presents purely as a bruising problem, but when associated with thrombocytopenia secondary to marrow replacement, often has a leukoerythroblastic blood film, and a bone marrow biopsy may reveal the presence of cancer cells. A more common form of thrombocytopenia is seen with chronic disseminated intravascular coagulation which will be discussed later. An unusual association is that of an auto-immune thrombocytopenia with a malignancy. Whether this is a chance association or is related to some immune defect predisposing to or resultant upon the malignancy is unknown.

It is unusual for megaloblastic anaemias to present primarily with bruising and bleeding problems, but in some exceptional instances, marked thrombocytopenia and bruising may be the dominant feature, although usually it is accompanied by a moderate to severe anaemia. If the megaloblastosis is secondary to folic acid deficiency, the possibility of alcohol playing an aetiological part in both the folate deficiency and the thrombocytopenia should be kept in mind. The diagnosis is readily made by observing a high mean corpuscular volume, an accompanying hypersegmentation of the neutrophils in the peripheral blood and a bone marrow showing megaloblastic maturation features. Serum B_{12} and serum and red cell folate levels will serve to pinpoint which of these two major causes is involved and also indicate the direction for further investigations. It should be remembered that there are an increasing number of drugs related to the aetiology of megaloblastic maturation as well as a number of very uncommon hereditary anomalies.

Finally iron deficiency anaemia is usually quoted in the textbooks as a cause of thrombocytopenia, and there are papers in the paediatric literature which have established this as a definite cause. The author has not seen such an instance in an adult. It is far more common to see an associated thrombocytosis in the setting of iron deficiency.

ACQUIRED THROMBOCYTOPENIA DUE TO INCREASED DESTRUCTION

Table 8.4 classifies conditions which cause thrombocytopenia by shortening the platelet lifespan.

Early descriptions of pestilence associated with purpura appear in the Decameron, and in the 20th century there have been numerous reports of thrombocytopenia with viral illness, following vaccination with cowpox, with septicaemia and other disorders such as malaria. Platelets react and in many instances take up foreign particles which, even if they are inert in nature such as carbon, produce thrombocytopenia. One explanation of these forms of thrombocytopenia is that the platelet is altered by uptake or interaction with particles which result in its earlier removal from the circulation by the reticulo-endothelial system. These interactions are discussed in Chapter 4. The nature of the increased platelet destruction has been further complicated by the appreciation that in many instances disseminated intravascular coagulation is also triggered by the infective agents, and thus results in thrombocytopenia from so-called consumptive coagulopathy. As has been discussed, there is good evidence to suggest that there is an element of marrow suppression and resultant depressed platelet production, but platelet survival studies make it clear that in many instances the major cause of the thrombocytopenia is a reduction in platelet lifespan. This may result from actual particle uptake by the platelet, as has been documented in viral infections and even in malaria, or may be due to platelet interaction with the infective particles, resulting in their stimulation with consequent surface and metabolic changes in the cell, or result from disseminated intravascular clotting in their involvement in fibrin interactions throughout the body. In a recent study of patients with thrombo-cytopenia, secondary to septicaemia, it was found that a very high percentage of patients with Gram-negative septicaemia and a small majority of those with Gram-positive septicaemia had thrombocytopenia, with one exception these showed a diminished platelet survival. It was also found that patients whose platelet counts were below $50 \times 10^9/1$ usually had associated intravascular coagulation as indicated by standard tests for fibrin degradation products or circulating fibrin monomers. A number of reports have now shown that patients with thrombocytopenia and septicaemia have elevated platelet associated IgG levels in their platelets, and it has consequently been postulated that the shortened platelet survival results from some interaction of the platelets with immune complexes which would bind to the platelet Fc receptors, thereby altering the surface membrane as well as being taken up into the cell. It seems highly likely that infections often result in an increased platelet turnover, but that overt thrombocytopenia with its clinical mani-festations is relatively uncommon. Surveys of children with acute exanthe-mata and of patients with infective mononucleosis have frequently shown a lower platelet count at the time of the illness compared with subsequent platelet counts undertaken on the same group of patients some months after recovery. There is a frequent association of platelet functional defects during the acute phase of infectious mononucleosis supporting the concept that the viraemia or its consequent antigen–antibody complexes, altered the patient's platelets. Thrombocytopenia and disseminated intravascular coagulation have been reported in malaria, and thrombocytopenia of mild degree is a common complication of the active disease. Experimental animal studies and studies in man have now shown the presence of merozoite and trophozoite stages of the parasite in mammalian platelets. So far these have not been seen in the megakaryocytes. Only a small proportion of platelets which are circulating have been found to contain the parasites, which may reflect an early culling of platelets which are so invaded from the blood, or such platelets with inclusions may have the parasites removed by the reticulo-endothelial system in the spleen in the same way as this organ monitors red cell nuclear inclusions and removes Howell–Jolly bodies from red cells. Since many patients with malaria have enlarged spleens, there may also be an element of pooling in that organ to explain the thrombocytopenia as the spleen can enlarge rapidly during acute episodes.

Drug and chemical induction

Table 8.5 lists drugs which have most commonly caused thrombocytopenia due to increased platelet destruction. Many other drugs have been implicated in the literature, and all drugs should be regarded as possible aetiological causes. The commonest mechanism of this has been antibody production, although the documentation of this rarely entails more than one or two case reports. Indeed the only instances in the author's practice where a drug antibody causing thrombocytopenia has been well documented, have been in patients with quinine or quinidine purpura or where the thrombocytopenia was secondary to heparin. In other instances, acute thrombocytopenia has been corrected by the withdrawal of one of the drugs listed in Table 8.5, but no absolute proof obtained of the presence of an antibody related to the drug in *in vitro* tests. This identification may improve with the introduction of immunofluorescent techniques for detecting surface immunoglobulins and also by radioimmunoassay and ELISA techniques, by which total platelet

Table 8.5 Drugs causing thrombocytopenia by increased destruction

Antibody production
  Quinine
  Quinidine
  Heparin
  Sedormid – allylisopropyl acetyl carbamide*

Direct effect on platelet
  Heparin
  Ristocetin*

Miscellaneous ? Antibody production
  Gold salts
  Aldomet
  Penicillin and cephalosporin
  Trimethoprim
  Chlorthiazide
  Digitoxin
  Aspirin*
  Isoptin
  Rifampicin

*The author has not seen patients with thrombocytopenia due to these drugs, but they are included in the table because they all have been reported with considerable frequency. The first two have not been used in clinical practice for some years

gammaglobulin may be compared with that of platelet immunoglobulin (IgG, IgA, IgM) on the surface with or without the suspected drug. It seems clear that in some cases, such as heparin, only some of the instances of thrombocytopenia are related to a drug dependent antibody, and that in other instances some direct chemical action may be involved such as is the case for ristocetin.

In general terms, with an analogy to red cell Coombs +ve haemolytic anaemia one would expect there to be four mechanisms by which a drug could produce a platelet antibody:

(1) Penicillin has been shown to bind to the surface of the red cell and act as a hapten with resultant antibody production which then binds to the drug on the cell surface.

(2) A plasma component binds with the drug, e.g. stibophen, to form the drug hapten, make an antibody which then combines to form an immune complex which in turn binds to the surface of the red cell – the so called 'innocent bystander' reaction, and fixes complement with consequent damage and cell removal.

(3) The drug causes the lymphatic system to produce an antibody, as with aldomet, and the antibody is directed against components of the red cell membrane. There is some evidence suggesting that the mechanism whereby the drug causes this effect is by inhibiting suppressor T cells which release a clone of normally suppressed lymphocytes and allows them to produce the red cell antigen antibody.

(4) The antibody may be induced by a metabolite of the drug and not the drug itself as is the case with para amino salicylic acid antibodies in Coombs positive haemolytic anaemias.

In the case of drug induced thrombocytopenia, there is remarkably little evidence available as to which mechanism is operative, with the exception of quinine and quinidine. Clinically, drug dependent purpura should be suspected in any patient who has an acute form of thrombocytopenia, and since most drugs can be readily substituted with others of different chemical structure but similar effect, most clinicians adopt the policy of immediately ceasing any drug which may be an offender and substituting it with another clinically unrelated compound. Frequently the thrombocytopenia is quite severe and is often associated with widespread purpura and in particular buccal and mucosal haemorrhages and blood blisters. Fundoscopic examination usually is normal, unless there are associated illnesses such as diabetes and/or hypertension. The presence of fundal haemorrhages represents an emergency for which immediate platelet transfusion should be given, as well as instituting prednisolone treatment (v. infra). Microscopic haematuria is not uncommon. The remainder of the examination is usually unrewarding, and any other evidence of involvement of the haematopoietic system such as lymphadenopathy or splenomegaly should point to other causes. Once the drug has been withdrawn, the thrombocytopenia usually responds rapidly and indeed the skin bleeding time may revert to normal in the first 24–48 hours. There are, however, some instances where there is a much longer delay in improvement, and in these instances the mechanism is probably not that of a drug dependent antibody reaction (since most drugs are rapidly cleared from the body) but rather a mechanism similar to that with aldomet red cell antibody production. A notable exception is gold, but whether this produces a drug dependent antibody reaction is still uncertain, since frequently the patient also has rheumatoid arthritis, and it is possible that this condition may have resulted in immune complex formation or platelet antibody formation, resulting in increased platelet destruction.

Quinine-quinidine purpura

Quinine purpura was first described in 1895 and that with quinidine in 1916. Ackroyd investigated sedormid (a hypnotic which was withdrawn from the market many years ago) purpura and postulated that a combination of the drug with the platelet surface gave a hapten antigen which stimulated antibody production. His classical studies in 1949 demonstrated that the antibody attack on the patients' platelets occurred only in the presence of the drug, which produced platelet agglutination, complement fixation and platelet lysis. The destruction of the platelet by the drug antibody was also demonstrated by its ability to inhibit clot retraction. Similar results were obtained with plasma from patients with quinine and quinidine thrombocytopenia, and Ackroyd postulated a similar mechanism to explain this form of drug induced purpura. Shulman (1958), however, demonstrated that the affinity of quinine and quinidine for the platelet membrane was too low to enable it to act as a hapten, and also showed that increasing concentrations of quinidine *in vitro* would not inhibit the binding of the drug to the platelet surface, such as would be expected in classical hapten theory if the drug was bound to a protein on the cell surface. He, therefore, postulated that the binding must be due to a drug antibody immune complex, subsequently binding to the cell's surface in an 'innocent bystander' like reaction. Kunicki and Aster (1978) have shown that Bernard–Soulier platelets do not react with most quinine–quinidine antibodies and that the membrane component, glycoprotein Ib, missing or abnormal in this disorder must be present for the immune complex to bind to the cell. The nature of the plasma component with which quinine is thought to act as a hapten to form the antibody and subsequent immune complex, is still unknown. Earlier work from our laboratory suggested that this was due to von Willebrand factor, but we have been unable to reproduce these results. Most quinine and quinidine antibodies are specific for the particular optical isomer although in some instances there is cross reaction, so that there is some antibody binding in the presence of the isomer. The drug to which the patient was exposed is always the more effective in *in vitro* demonstration of the antibody. The incidence of this antibody is relatively low and so far there has been no way of determining why certain individuals have this particular problem, although it seems to be more common in elderly people (but these drugs are more commonly given to elderly people), and in a number of our patients there have been some other auto-immune problems such as rheumatoid arthritis or discoid lupus. Most patients who have this problem and who for one reason or another are re-exposed to the drug, have a rapid recurrence of their acute thrombocytopenia. This is not invariably so, as is demonstrated by one of Shulman's patients who was re-challenged with quinidine some months after the initial episode of quinidine-induced purpura without effect. This seems to be very unusual, since most people have reported that even if patients are re-exposed to the drug 12 months later a rapid recurrence of thrombocytopenia ensues. Occasional patients have been reported in whom there is an associated neutropenia, and even less commonly an acute Coombs positive haemolytic anaemia. In the latter instances there are two different types of antibodies involved.

Heparin induced thrombocytopenia

The incidence of this problem appears to have increased greatly over the last 5 years. In part this may relate both to the more frequent use of heparin, in particular in low dose subcutaneous prophylaxis against thrombo-embolism, and the more frequent platelet counts being undertaken on patients in hospital. There are two mechanisms involved in the production of thrombocytopenia with heparin. One relates to an *in vitro* phenomenon of platelet agglutination by heparin, although the amounts required for this are usually quite high. This is a direct effect of the heparin which may be more marked in some people's platelet-rich plasma than in others. This phenomenon probably accounts for a very frequent form of transient thrombocytopenia which occurs early in the course of heparin treatment, and which produces no ill effect, the platelet count returning to normal despite continued heparin therapy. This often follows the very first injection of heparin.

With the other mechanism the thrombocytopenia is more severe and persists. It resembles the situation in quinidine or sedormid purpura since an antibody is in the plasma, usually IgG, but sometimes IgA, which requires the presence of heparin to cause platelet agglutination and fixation of complement. Studies have not yet revealed a specific platelet site against which this antibody is active. The clinical setting of this heparin dependent platelet antibody is that of a patient who has been receiving heparin either in treatment of a deep venous thrombosis or for a thrombo-embolic phenomenon such as pulmonary embolus, or a patient who is receiving prophylactic low dose heparin subcutaneously following a myocardial infarction or an operative procedure. The thrombocytopenia is usually not apparent until after 5 or 6 days of heparin therapy and commonly there are no bleeding manifestations. Indeed there is a striking incidence of further thrombo-embolic problems, and occasionally a resistance to heparin is noted where this is being given continuously intravenously and is being monitored by routine coagulation times. In some, but not all patients, evidence for disseminated intravascular coagulation accompanies the fall in platelet count, so that there may be elevated split products, but this is far from universal. The platelet count is often around $20-50 \times 10^9/l$. This type of picture has been seen with both bovine lung heparin and porcine mucosal heparin, although it may be more common with the bovine lung preparations. The resistance to the heparin when it develops has been attributed to the heparin damaging the platelets and releasing platelet factor 4, and perhaps also to the lowering of ATIII levels when disseminated intravascular coagulation occurs. Investigations reveal a high platelet associated IgG level and also an increased C3 level. Where platelet survival studies have been undertaken they have been reduced, and the bone marrow shows increased or normal numbers of megakaryocytes. The studies of the patients' platelet-rich plasma or of patient serum or immunoglobulin fractions against normal platelet-rich plasma, show a heparin dependent factor which binds complement to platelets and which causes their aggregation and serotonin release. This factor can be readily demonstrated using a standard aggregometer. Once identified, heparin should be stopped and reversed with protamine sulphate and the patient treated with dextran (500 ml of dextran 40 every 12 hours) and commenced on warfarin, because there is such a high incidence of thrombotic episodes in these patients, which are often arterial in nature. It has been postulated that these result from heparin induced platelet aggregation and damage with subsequent activation of the coagulation pathway. It is also thought that heparin may inhibit activation of the fibrinolytic pathway whilst not inhibiting coagulation due to the released platelet factor 4. The mortality of this problem in most series has been quite high but hopefully early recognition and the appropriate steps will reduce this. The overall incidence varies from series to series but judging from reports in our own hospital, it is unlikely to be much greater than 1% although in some series, up to 30% involvement has been noted. This latter figure is much higher than has been observed in Australia and perhaps results from the use of a different heparin preparation.

Other drugs which should be particularly sought and are reported frequently to cause a drug dependent platelet antibody interaction are listed in Table 8.5. Sedormid and ristocetin are both no longer available for patient use. The latter drug causes thrombocytopenia through its direct induction of platelet agglutination. A fuller list of drugs which have been reported to cause platelet damage can be found in Williams' or Wintrobe's textbooks of haematology.

Tests for detecting platelet–drug interaction are largely divided into (1) observation of the drug's effect on clot retraction, (2) the production of platelet agglutination using either washed platelets or normal platelet-rich plasma to which a heat inactivated sample of the patient's serum is added together with the appropriate concentrations of the drug, and observing platelet agglutination either on a plate or in an aggregometer, and (3) testing platelet factor 3 release with or without the presence of the drug and more recently, measuring binding of IgG and/or complement to normal platelets in their native platelet-rich plasma to which have been added heat inactivated patient's serum with and without the drug. The heparin type antibody cannot be studied using the platelet factor 3 test because this test is determined by a clotting end point which would be blocked by heparin.

Disseminated intravascular coagulation (DIC)

This condition is more fully discussed in Chapter 9, but since purpura and thrombocytopenia may be a striking feature of DIC, this diagnosis must always be excluded when a patient presents with thrombocytopenic purpura. It is often suggested by the presence of one of the conditions listed in Table 9.7, but a routine screen should always be undertaken. Management of this condition is outlined in Chapter 9.

Other causes of thrombocytopenia associated with thrombosis are the so-called Kasabach–Merrit syndrome in which giant congenital naevi or vascular malformations result in a condition of disseminated intravascular clotting occurring within the abnormality. Massive thrombosis where there is again a consumption of platelets may be difficult to distinguish from DIC because of accompanying FDPs, but in this instance the thrombocytopenia is transient and because of the size of the thrombosis required, there is clinically little difficulty in establishing the correct diagnosis.

Idiopathic thrombocytopenic purpura

Idiopathic thrombocytopenic purpura (ITP) is sometimes called auto-immune thrombocytopenia (ATP). This disorder remains a diagnosis by exclusion and must be distinguished from the other causes of thrombocytopenia listed in Tables 8.1, 8.2, 8.3 and 8.4. The aetiology of this disorder is still not known but may follow a viral infection, e.g. infective mononucleosis, or the child-hood exanthemata or present with other auto-immune diseases such as systemic lupus erythematosus (SLE), and sometimes ITP patients will develop florid features of SLE later. There is an increased incidence in diseases which have immune problems such as chronic lymphatic leukaemia, hereditary and acquired agammaglobulinaemia and IgA deficiency, more recently an increased incidence has been reported in homosexuals and a link suggested with acquired immune deficiency syndrome (AIDS). Harrington's classical studies in 1951 first demonstrated the presence in these patients' blood of a factor which, when injected into normal people, resulted in a dramatic fall in platelet count. He introduced an *in vitro* technique which detected the presence of platelet agglutinins in a high percentage, but later it was suggested that these agglutinins might be simply the generation of thrombin in the serum samples and thus be largely artifactual. Harrington demonstrated that the plasma factor causing a reduction in platelet counts following infusion into volunteers was present in the immunoglobulins and that it could be adsorbed out by passaging with normal platelets and this has been repeatedly confirmed. Harrington also postulated that the beneficial effect of splenectomy might be due to the removal of a site of antibody production as well as a mass of reticulo-endothelial cells removing platelets damaged by antibodies. He showed that splenectomized animals were more resistant to antibodies prepared against platelets than those that were not splenectomized. These concepts originally put forward by Harrington, have now been confirmed by work showing that splenic lymphocytes synthesize immunoglobulins which can be demonstrated to bind to platelets *in vitro*, and also histologic studies showing reticulo-endothelial cells of the spleen containing platelets in various stages of digestion. There is still debate as to whether the antibodies are specifically directed against a platelet antigen or are immune complexes binding at the platelet's Fc receptor or perhaps other sites to cause an 'innocent bystander' type reaction.

Most series report a 2–3:1 female to male incidence with a peak occurrence in the 2nd–4th decades, but it can appear at any time from early childhood to old age. The usual presenting features are bleeding and bruising which may or may not be spontaneous. The date of onset of the problem can often be ascertained in the woman from her menstrual history and in the man, from questioning about the effect of procedures such as teeth extraction, tonsillectomy and other operations. Increasing numbers of patients are being found who have extremely low platelet counts discovered by chance and who have not noted any susceptibility to bleeding or bruising. Sometimes the patient may present with anaemia due to occult blood loss and there may be accompanying features of iron deficiency such as koilonychia, glossitis, chelosis and sometimes, rarely, a history of difficulty in swallowing (the Plummer–Vinson or Patterson–Kelly syndrome). Haematuria may also occur, but is uncommon except in the acute onset of severe thrombocytopenia or when caused by viral disease such as infectious mononucleosis or chicken pox.

Physical examination often reveals a petechial rash which is most marked in the lower limbs and sometimes widespread purpura with ecchymosis. Mouth blood blisters may be evident and reflect very severe thrombocytopenia with an acute onset. Fundoscopic examination is usually normal, and when fundal haemorrhages are present other problems such as associated hypertension, systemic lupus erythematosus, leukaemia or aplasia should be sought. The presence of fundal haemorrhages and/or headache suggests the possibility of a cerebral haemorrhage and demands immediate treatment for the patient.

The remainder of the physical examination is usually remarkably negative, and in particular it is unusual to have splenomegaly or lymphadenopathy and their presence should make one seek other causes. Haemorrhoids should always be excluded by a rectal examination and occult bloods performed on the faeces. If the occult bloods are repeatedly positive a local lesion in the gastro-intestinal tract giving bleeding should be excluded. A micro urine should be undertaken to look for haematuria and to help exclude renal involvement e.g. casts.

A skin bleeding time is prolonged and the Hess test is positive unless the patient has received steroids which may rapidly (within 24 hours) convert the Hess test from positive to negative without necessarily altering the skin bleeding time or the platelet count. The peripheral blood film reveals thrombocytopenia, but the remainder of the film is quite normal, unless the patient has some underlying condition or associated iron deficiency. Bone marrow examination reveals a cellular marrow with normal red cell and white cell maturation, and normal to increased numbers of megakaryocytes with higher preponderance of Type I and II forms and this reflects increased platelet production and is probably analogous to the increase in erythropoiesis with a shift towards the more immature forms seen in haemolytic anaemia. An iron stain should always be done to assess the iron stores and the marrow examination is very useful in excluding many of the causes of thrombocytopenia (Tables 8.1 to 8.4).

Over the years there have been many tests introduced to detect platelet antibodies. Despite many papers on this subject, there is still no absolute test for detecting idiopathic thrombocytopenic purpura or excluding the diagnosis. It is true that an elevated platelet associated immunoglobulin (PA IgG) or the presence of immunoglobulin and complement on the platelet's surface, are both consistent with the diagnosis of ITP and it is uncommon for such tests to be negative when the patient is first seen. Tests which rely on platelet factor 3 activation, that is where the patient's serum is added to normal platelet-rich plasma and then the platelet procoagulant activity studied over a time period, have been claimed to yield a high percentage of positive results in some workers' hands, but not in others. In our own laboratory, positive platelet factor 3 antibody tests are only present in approximately 30% of our patients with ITP. This contrasts with platelet associated IgG (PA IgG) which is increased in approximately 80%. Different incidences have been reported from different centres and in one instance platelet associated IgM levels have been reported to be increased in a greater proportion than PA IgG. In more than 60% both PA IgG and PA IgM were elevated, perhaps suggesting the role of immune complexes. High PA IgG may be seen in septicaemia and in other auto-immune conditions such as lupus, rheumatoid arthritis, chronic active hepatitis with and without thrombocytopenia, and one report suggests that the PA IgG may increase in any circumstances where there is an increased production of platelets and another in any instance where the plasma IgG level is elevated.

Platelet survival studies employing platelets from normal donors with the same blood group are usually strikingly reduced so that a majority of patients with ITP have a platelet survival of less than 12 hours, compared with a normal survival of 10 days. A number of studies have claimed that surface scanning may help predict the outcome of splenectomy by showing increased accumulation in this organ in preference to other sites such as the liver or bone marrow. This has not been the case in our hands, nor in a number of other centres. This study may also be complicated by the presence of anti-HLA antibodies but it is particularly helpful if the survival is found to be normal or only slightly reduced, since this is against the diagnosis of ITP and would favour another cause such as hereditary thrombocytopenia or some factor reducing platelet production.

Other investigations are tests to exclude DIC and SLE. The prothrombin time, FDP and protamine precipitation tests as well as antinuclear factor and double stranded DNA should be negative. Immune complexes should also be undertaken as in some series these have been found in the majority of patients. This has not been our experience, but this may be for technical reasons in view of the different techniques for measuring immune complexes.

An increased incidence of thyroid disease, especially thyrotoxicosis and peptic ulcer, has been reported in ITP and attention should be given to these possibilities at the bedside. A number of instances have also been recorded of an identical picture to ITP being seen in the presence of cancer. This may be a chance association, but one has been struck over the years on a number of occasions, where cancer of the lung and hypernephroma have been associated with ITP without features of disseminated intravascular coagulation. This association should always be considered in the elderly patient presenting with ITP and a chest X-ray and micro urine and occult blood examinations of the faeces are useful screening tests.

Treatment of ITP

The overall mortality of patients with ITP is extremely low, < 1%, with modern therapy and the majority of deaths result from a cerebrovascular accident. The general principles of treatment are to prevent further bleeding, to arrest any that is currently taking place, to reduce the production or the effect of the antibody or the immune process underlying the disease either by inhibiting antibody production, reducing its effect on the cell or prohibiting the attacked cell's uptake by the reticulo-endothelial system. In the majority of instances, the patient presents during an acute phase, although there may not be a problem of active bleeding. Any bleeding sites should be attended to and all intramuscular injections should be avoided. In the case of women who are menstruating, an oral contraceptive should be commenced immediately and this usually is effective in reducing menstrual loss. If the patient's menstrual period has not yet commenced, she should still start on continuous oral contraceptives and if she is already taking these tablets, they should be continued until the platelet count has improved or returned to normal levels. If this is unsuccessful in arresting menstrual loss or if this loss is excessively heavy, ε-aminocaproic acid (EACA) or tranexamic acid should be commenced initially intravenously, and then orally and 10 units of platelets given together with prednisolone. Should measures have been taken prior to seeing the patient such as nasal packing, or even uterine packing, it is wise to leave these in place until the patient has had therapy such as prednisolone and/or oral contraceptives for 48 hours. Withdrawal of the packing should follow the administration of EACA or tranexamic acid either intravenously or orally as is clinically indicated in standard doses and a cover of 10 units of platelets, i.e. the equivalent of platelets from 5 litres of blood, given during the removal of the packing and another 10 units immediately after.

Drug therapy

The most commonly employed treatment has been prednisolone and its dramatic effect on the management of this disorder is illustrated by the disappearance of 'crash' splenectomies to control bleeding. A dose of 0.75 mg/kg of body weight daily is given (60 mg prednisolone daily is given to a person of average build). Some believe it is best given in divided doses of 15 mg q.i.d., but evidence is anecdotal. Steroids are believed to prolong the platelet survival by interfering with the phagocytic function of the reticulo-endothelial system and ultimately a reduction in antibody titre. Should the bleeding manifestations not be controlled in the first 24 to 48 hours, this dose may be doubled and the level maintained for approximately 2 weeks following which the dose is lowered. The rate at which the dose is lowered depends on the clinical response to treatment and the platelet count. In most instances it is perfectly safe to reduce the daily dose by 10 mg per week until a level of 10 mg daily is achieved. It is important not to maintain the patient on high dose steroids if no response to therapy is being obtained because of the increasing incidence of steroid side effects with time and the suppressant effect on the platelet count. It is particularly important to remember the unfortunate cosmetic effects of this drug since the patient is often a young woman. Fortunately the majority of patients respond to this form of treatment although in a proportion it is impossible to cease the drug without a return of thrombocytopenia and bruising. A complete remission following prednisolone therapy has been reported to be only 10–15% in some series, but up to 40% in another where 30% were still in remission 4 years later. Alternative treatment should be considered when steroid therapy has to be continued. Should longterm prednisolone be contemplated then alternate day therapy should be instituted since there is evidence that this reduces the risk of complications, i.e. if the patient requires 10 mg prednisolone daily, 20 mg may be given on alternate days. During the administration of the drug, steroid complications should be anticipated and the patient should have routine urine tests for sugar or random blood sugars as well as be questioned about back pain, muscle weakness and any mood abnormalities. One of the most distressing complications with this drug is the production of psychotic features and this demands its immediate reduction and possible withdrawal. Should glycosuria develop early in the course of steroid treatment it can be readily controlled by oral hypoglycaemic agents until the disease remits or alternative therapy instituted. Gastric upsets are usually controlled by standard antacid therapy.

Equivalent doses of hydrocortisone may be given intravenously if demanded by the clinical situation and some believe that this route may lessen gastric symptoms.

Splenectomy

Splenectomy is the treatment of choice in young patients who have chronic idiopathic or auto-immune thrombocytopenic purpura of sufficient severity to warrant treatment. Chronic is defined as a patient who has had documented auto-immune thrombocytopenia for a period of more than 3 months. Unfortunately, this is often not the case on presentation and as a result most patients coming to splenectomy are those who have had a trial of prednisolone therapy and have either failed to respond or have relapsed following withdrawal of the treatment. All patients should be immunized with antipneumoccocal vaccine prior to the operation in view of the reported increased incidence of pneumoccocal septicaemia in patients following splenectomy. Although severe coronary disease used to be regarded as a contraindication to splenectomy we have managed a couple of patients who had their splenectomy immediately prior to bypass surgery with an uneventful recovery. In most series there is an overall response rate of approximately 70% yielding a complete remission, and up to 95% having an improvement in the overall clinical situation of the patient with some increase in platelet count and a lessening in the bleeding tendency so that further medical treatment is not required. The mortality of an elective splenectomy for a patient with idiopathic thrombocytopenic purpura is extremely low, in the order of 0.1%. The risk of distressing complications by medical treatment is greater and the overall mortality probably the same. All these points should be fully discussed with the patient and if the patient is a woman she should be warned that her children may still have problems with neonatal thrombocytopenia, even if she is in complete clinical remission, since the autoantibody may persist without there being any clinical evidence of it (v. infra). Favourable results from splenectomy are said to be more common in patients who have had an initial response to steroid therapy, in patients where chromium survival studies have shown splenic sequestration, and where the operation is performed early in the course of the illness, but none of these are absolute. Some patients who have predominantly liver sequestration demonstrated by chromium survivals have responded well to splenectomy, and some patients with an initial response to steroid therapy have not responded to the operation. Following splenectomy the most common response is for the patient's platelet count to return rapidly to normal and frequently overshoot that level, so that a thrombocytosis of $700 \times 10^9/l$ to over $1000 \times 10^9/l$ is not uncommon by the 6th or 7th post-operative day. It is our policy to use low dose heparin (5000 units b.d.) in patients whose counts climb very rapidly to levels greater than $800 \times 10^9/l$ in the 1st week post-operatively since we have seen pulmonary embolism occurring in such patients. It is unusual for this to be required and it may be that antiplatelet agents may be equally effective. Even where the platelet response is greater than $1000 \times 10^9/l$, it does not necessarily mean that a prolonged remission will be obtained and some of these patients do relapse and return with thrombocytopenia, but more usually the platelet count falls back to normal levels and remains there. When thrombocytopenia recurs after an interval of a few months or more, the possibility of an accessory spleen should be considered. This problem has not been identified in our experience if the peripheral blood continues to show the features of post-splenectomy changes, but in view of a report to the contrary we always undertake nuclear scans in such patients using red cells labelled with technetium. Accessory spleens are routinely searched for at the time of operation. Another group of patients shows a significant increase in platelet count immediately post-splenectomy, but over the ensuing days the count drops back to the starting level. In a few instances the count may return to normal some weeks or months after the operation. Table 8.6 lists therapeutic measures which may be considered if treatment with steroids and/or splenectomy has been unsuccessful.

Table 8.6 Treatment of auto-immune thrombocytopenia refractory to steroids and splenectomy

Vincristine (VC) and vinblastine (VB)
  Standard
  VC or VB loaded platelets
Azathioprine
Danazol
Cyclophosphamide
IgG infusion
Plasmapheresis
Platelet transfusion

Vincristine and vinblastine

These agents have been used in two ways in the management of auto-immune thrombocytopenia. Introduced by Harrington in 1974, vincristine is given at weekly intervals at doses of 1.5-2 mg i.v. for up to 6 weeks provided complications such as peripheral neuropathy, recurrent laryngeal nerve palsy, etc. do not intervene. These are extremely uncommon and this agent is the most effective in its rapidity of reversing the thrombocytopenia, the platelet counts sometimes returning to normal within 1-2 weeks. Its side effects, and its possible mutagenic properties, makes it a worrying drug to use in the younger age groups. The drug's use is restricted in our clinic to patients who are past the reproductive age and who have failed to respond to other types of therapy. Most reports show that 50–60% of patients who have failed to respond to steroids and/or splenectomy, will remit with vincristine, or vinblastine used in a similar manner, but in doses of 10 mg i.v. This form of treatment may result in permanent remission in a significant proportion of patients.

Another technique has been used with vincristine or vinblastine by pre-incubation of the drug with normal platelets and then infusing the platelets into patients. This treatment has again been most commonly used in patients who have been refractory to other forms of treatment. The theory behind this approach is that the microtubules in the platelets will bind the vincristine or vinblastine and will carry it to the reticulo-endothelial cells which are removing the platelets from the circulation. After phagocytosis the platelets will release the vincristine which will then attack the phagocytic cell. Initial results reported almost 100% response in patients with refractory ITP, however studies from a number of other centres have not been able to reproduce this high therapeutic success rate. In our own hands this form of approach has frequently given an increase in the platelet count, but without long term response, and the patients have usually relapsed some months following treatment. The most prolonged remission has been 9 months, but the patients in whom we used this technique were all long standing refractory ITP who had unsuccessful splenectomy and courses of prednisolone, azathioprine, cyclophosphamide and in some instances i.v. vincristine as was the case in some of the patients in the initial series (Ahn *et al*, 1978). Currently this technique should be reserved for patients who have failed to respond to other forms of therapy and who have a sufficient bleeding manifestation to warrant therapy or who require a short term cover for operative procedures or teeth extractions.

Azathioprine

Depending on the size of the patient this is usually given in doses from 100 to 300 mg daily. The most common indication for this therapy is in patients who require high doses of steroids, 10 mg or more, to maintain their platelet count, in whom splenectomy has been refused or is unsuccessful and vincristine or vinblastine treatment is felt unsuitable. The drug must be continued for 3–4 months before reducing the glucocorticoid dosage. It is successful in approximately 20–50% of patients who have failed to respond to steroids and splenectomy. It is an immunosuppressant drug and has all the risks of such therapy as well as its bone marrow suppression action, and full blood counts should be performed at weekly intervals initially. Neutropenia is almost always reversible so that if there is a fall in white cell count, a simple reduction of the dose will usually suffice. Nonetheless, the possible risk of causing the patient to be more liable to other forms of malignancy and leukaemia make it a drug which one is reluctant to use in the long term, especially in the younger age group and in those patients of reproductive age. This form of therapy usually has to be maintained to ensure the response although it may enable the complete withdrawal of steroid therapy and after 6 months of further treatment attempts should be made to withdraw the azathioprine.

Danazol

This anabolic steroid has been reported by Ahn *et al* (1978) to be of value in patients with refractory ITP. The dose recommended is 400–800 mg/day and women should be carefully assessed for possible masculinizing effects and warned to report any side effects such as nightmares.

Cyclophosphamide

Cyclophosphamide is a very effective agent in the treatment of auto-immune thrombocytopenic purpura, but its possible side effects, which include sterility, cystitis, hair loss and subsequent development of malignancy of either the haematopoietic or other systems make it an unacceptable drug in the younger age group. We believe it should be reserved for patients who have failed to respond to all other forms of therapy and who are in an age group over 45. The dosage usually recommended is 200 mg or 2.5 mg/kg daily with a reduction in dose if the white cell count falls to 2.5×10^9/l, and high fluid intake is advised to reduce the possibility of haemorrhagic cystitis. The response to this agent in speed lies midway between that of vincristine and prednisolone, and therefore the treatment should be maintained for 2–3 months before abandoning it as being unsuccessful. This drug should be maintained for 2 weeks after a remission is achieved. Cyclophosphamide, vincristine and prednisolone given in doses employed in standard lymphoma treatment every 3 weeks depending on the full blood count, has been successful. The clinical indication for the use of cyclophosphamide in any form is extremely rare and this approach has not been used by the author for the past 10 years.

Gammaglobulin

Intravenous gammaglobulin therapy has recently been used successfully in the therapy of childhood thrombocytopenia and also in adults. Its greatest place probably lies in paediatrics since it is more common for it to result in a permanent cure, probably because such thrombocytopenias are usually of an evanescent nature. Most success has been reported with high doses namely 15 g per day for 4–5 days. The success rate in children is virtually 100% and a similar rate has been claimed in adult thrombocytopenic purpura. However, in the adult cases it appears to be short-lived since the platelet count usually has fallen back to its original levels after 10–14 days. Most of these cases were patients who had thrombocytopenia which failed to respond to all other forms of treatment, and it may offer an excellent method by which elective surgery or procedures such as tooth extraction could be covered with a minimum of morbidity to the patient. The type of intravenous gammaglobulin used may be important. Its mode of action may be to produce a reticulo-endothelial (RE) cell blockade so that platelets attacked by antibody are not removed by the RE system, perhaps due to the Fc receptor on the RE cells being occupied by the infused gamma globulin. Most studies have been reported with a Sandoz intravenous gammaglobulin preparation. Our own experience in refractory adult idiopathic thrombocytopenia has not been as encouraging as those reported from other countries, but this may reflect a difference in the gammaglobulin preparation employed.

Plasmapheresis

Most centres which have tried this technique have not been impressed with its value in auto-immune thrombocytopenia in contrast to thrombotic thrombocytopenic purpura (*v. infra*), although occasional remissions have been reported and plasma infusion *per se* is occasionally associated with a remission, but it is possible that these instances were in patients with Upshaw–Shulman syndrome or some related variant or possibly related to a similar effect seen with IgG infusions.

Platelet transfusion

Since the platelet survival time in most patients with ITP is frequently less than 6 hours, it would be anticipated that the usefulness of platelet transfusions would be limited. It is also difficult at times to know how much of a contribution this treatment has made. Platelet transfusions are recommended in ITP in patients who have retinal haemorrhages or when there is clinical suspicion that a cerebral haemorrhage may be imminent such as severe headache or hypertension and in patients who are actively bleeding, from sites such as the nose, peptic ulcer or the genito-urinary tract, when emergency surgery is required both at the time of operation and post-operatively or if a nasal or uterine pack is to be withdrawn. Where splenectomy has been undertaken for ITP the platelets should be given following the ligation of the splenic pedicle. The equivalent of 10 platelet packs are given as concentrates and the cells are infused rapidly, within 20–30 minutes. Since the introduction of platelet concentrates we have found platelet transfusion reactions to be extremely uncommon.

Refractory idiopathic thrombocytopenic purpura

Despite all the approaches that have been outlined above there remain a group of patients who fail to respond. Essentially these are people who have had a splenectomy and one or all of the regimes outlined above without permanent benefit although there is almost always some improvement in their clinical condition. The question must be asked as to how far one should go with these patients since although they may be considerably incommoded by their disease due to recurrent bruising, the majority may enjoy a normal lifespan with a relatively unimpaired life style. The question, therefore, of employing drugs which are possibly mutagenic must be considered extremely carefully and they are only justified where the degree of haemorrhage is extremely inconveniencing to the patient, or where there are associated medical problems such as hypertension which add to the risk of cerebral haemorrhage. Surgical procedures should not be denied these patients, as in the majority one technique or other can produce a significant improvement in the platelet count often to normal levels and normal haemostasis for an operative procedure, and so surgical remedies for disorders such as a chronic peptic ulcer can usually be implemented. In our own clinic it is this group of patients in which the use of platelets incubated with vinblastine has been most valuable but this approach may now be replaced by IgG infusion.

Whether this group with thrombocytopenic purpura has a different pathogenesis is unknown, but there is evidence in some of our patients at least, that this may be so since some have normal platelet associated IgG levels.

ITP and pregnancy

ITP is not a contraindication to pregnancy, but such women of childbearing age should be fully informed of the problems which may occur, and the precautions which should be taken should they wish to have children. There is currently no satisfactory way or formula for predicting the outcome of such a pregnancy either in regard to recurrence of the ITP should the patient be in remission, or progression of the disorder should the patient already have ITP. It is better to manage a patient who presents with ITP and who is pregnant with cortico-steroid therapy, rather than to undertake splenectomy for fear of inducing an abortion, and in one series a 30% fetal mortality resulted. Most physicians prefer to manage the patient with steroid therapy until after delivery. Steroid therapy does increase the incidence of pre-eclampsia, and there is always the worry of adrenal suppression developing in the fetus plus all the other side effects of steroids to both the mother and fetus, but there are rarely major problems and pre-eclampsia can be avoided by careful observation. The evidence that splenectomy causes problems is not well documented, and some believe that if the thrombocytopenia is not easily controlled by steroids in the first trimester, splenectomy should be performed under cover of platelet transfusions.

Idiopathic thrombocytopenic purpura may be exacerbated by pregnancy and may reappear in patients in remission, but maternal morbidity is extremely low and there has been no reported maternal death with ITP since 1950.

Spontaneous abortion has been reported to be between 10 and 30% compared with the normal population of 10–15%, and perinatal mortality of the fetus has been also reported to be as high as 20% in contrast to normal infants which is 1.5%. Vaginal delivery is probably the best from the mother's point of view since post-partum haemorrhage is usually not a problem due to uterine contraction, but the fetal mortality and also the risk of an intracranial bleed resulting in mental retardation if the baby survives per vaginal delivery, have prompted many to advocate caesarian section prior to the onset of labour.

A number of attempts have been made to predict which infants will be thrombocytopenic. In one series the mothers were divided into two groups, one in whom the platelet count at the time of delivery was less than $100 \times 10^9/l$ and 79% of infants in this group were found to be thrombocytopenic, whilst in the other group with counts greater than $100 \times 10^9/l$ thrombocytopenia was present in 27%. From these observations it was recommended that caesarian sections should be undertaken in all mothers in whom the platelet count was less than $100 \times 10^9/l$ and vaginal delivery in those with counts greater than $100 \times 10^9/l$. This still leaves a number of babies at risk and other series have shown no relation between the maternal and neonatal platelet counts. Nor does the level of PA IgG in mothers necessarily identify neonates at risk. It has been claimed that the level of circulating antiplatelet antibody in the plasma rather than PA IgG is correlated with the presence and degree of neonatal thrombocytopenia. This would seem to be logical, since the mechanism of neonatal thrombocytopenia is presumably due to the transplacental passage of the mother's immunoglobulin which is directed against platelets and which would be expected to cause the fetus' platelet count to be reduced unless its platelets were unreactive to the antibody. Further reports on this technique will have to be awaited to see whether it is reliable. Studies by Karpatkin et al (1981) have shown that administration of steroids prior to delivery will elevate the neonate's platelet count compared with those that are not so treated, and they have advocated the use of 10–20 mg prednisolone daily for 2 weeks prior to delivery in mothers who are in remission with ITP. Another approach has been the use of fetal scalp vein sampling and it has been suggested that should the scalp vein platelet count be below $50 \times 10^9/l$, then a caesarian section should be undertaken, whereas if the count is above this level, the baby may be delivered safely per vaginum. It is very important to emphasize that patients who have had a splenectomy and in whom the platelet count may be perfectly normal may still deliver a child who is quite severely thrombocytopenic. Our current practice is to recommend that all patients who have had ITP should be commenced on 10 mg prednisolone 2 weeks prior to delivery, and that a scalp vein sample should be undertaken as recommended. If the latter procedure is not possible a caesarian section should be undertaken until a definite method is developed to predict the infant's platelet count, perhaps by the detection of circulating platelet antibodies in the mother's plasma.

Neonatal thrombocytopenia can be managed by platelet transfusion and the administration of steroids. The lowest count usually occurs around the 6th postnatal day and often recovers rapidly, although it may persist for some weeks or even months. Although an exchange transfusion will remedy the situation, the risks and complications of this procedure rarely warrant its use. Another approach which may be worthy of consideration is the use of high dose γ-globulin infusions into the mother in the anticipation that the γ-globulin would be transferred across the placenta and perhaps blockade the RE system in the infant in the same way as it has been reported in other patients with thrombocytopenia.

Platelet autoantibodies due to secondary causes

Table 8.4 lists secondary causes of autoantibodies.

Chronic lymphatic leukaemia is a disorder in which there is almost total immune paresis due to abnormal B cell function in the majority of instances. Chronic lymphatic leukaemia is associated with thrombocytopenia in two forms. One of these is auto-immune with elevated platelet associated immuno-globulins, a diminished platelet lifespan and increased megakaryocytes in the bone marrow, providing quite a dramatic appearance of megakaryocytes laid out on a carpet of small lymphocytes. The other form of thrombocytopenia is secondary to bone marrow replacement by the leukaemic cells. When the thrombocytopenia is auto-immune in type it frequently responds well to standard glucocorticoid therapy, but may require splenectomy. The diagnosis is usually simple since the peripheral blood shows a preponderance of lympho-cytes with elevated total white cell count and the patient has lymphadenopathy and splenomegaly. Lymphocyte typing, bone marrow, platelet IgG levels and, if necessary, a platelet survival confirm the diagnosis. The incidence of secondary ITP in chronic lymphatic leukaemia is between 5 and 10%.

ITP syndrome is also seen in patients with non-Hodgkin and Hodgkin lymphoma as well as in various other forms of malignancy. Some series of ITP have reported high incidence of malignancy, that of DiFino et al (1980), being approximately 20%. Whilst we have not encountered as frequent an asso-ciation as this, malignancy should always be thought of when ITP presents in a patient over 40 years. Apart from lymphoma, there seems to be no particular cancer involved although we have seen it most commonly with bronchial carcinoma. Removal of the tumour does not influence the course of the disease.

Systemic lupus erythematosus and other collagen disorders rarely present with thrombocytopenic purpura, although this may complicate the course of the illness. In some instances, in SLE in particular, the patient may first present with isolated idiopathic thrombocytopenic purpura without any other clinical or laboratory features of the disease and only develop the full blown picture some months or years later. One should always ask patients whether they have suffered recently from recurrent mouth ulcers or Raynaud phenomenon, have had any photosensitive skin rashes, spot alopecia or joint manifestations, and if the answer is in the affirmative, a more diligent search for possible lupus erythematosus should be undertaken. Splenomegaly is usually, but not always, present and apart from an antinuclear factor, double stranded DNA and immune complexes, a skin biopsy from an unexposed area of skin and examination with immune fluorescent labelled antibodies to immunoglobulins may show the changes of lupus. Fundal haemorrhages are more common with lupus erythematosus because of the associated vasculitis. The basic management of the condition remains the same as that for ITP and in particular splenectomy should be undertaken if clinically indicated, since an early report, that this might exacerbate the lupus erythematosus, has not been substantiated.

Drugs producing auto-immune antibodies have been poorly identified, but aldomet is a possibility since it has been reported to cause destructive thrombocytopenia and it has a well known association with inducing Coombs positive red cells and sometimes auto-immune haemolysis, so that a similar mechanism for thrombocytopenia is likely.

Evan syndrome

Evan syndrome is the association of auto-immune haemolytic anaemia (Coombs positive) and idiopathic thrombocytopenic purpura. The description of this syndrome first suggested to Harrington and Moore that idiopathic thrombocytopenic purpura might be an auto-immune phenomenom due to platelet antibodies, analogous to the red cell autoantibodies in Coombs positive haemolytic anaemia, and led to their experiments infusing plasma from patients with ITP into normal volunteer recipients. Both the haemolytic anaemia and the thrombocytopenia in these patients usually respond to prednisolone therapy. This particular association is also seen in chronic lymphatic leukaemia.

Other forms of antibodies which can develop are the result of platelet antigens. The commonest situation where one sees this form of thrombocytopenia is in the newborn where the mother has an unusual platelet group such as Pl^A1-ve and the child is Pl^A1+ve. It may also occur following blood transfusion. The patient is usually a woman who has had one or more pregnancies, and the antibody is most commonly directed against Pl^A+ve platelets although the patient is Pl^A-ve, so that the reason it attacks Pl^A-ve platelets is difficult to understand but may relate to the platelets' ability to take up blood group and HLA antigens (*see* Chapter 3). The thrombocytopenia may persist for some months and initially bleeding manifestations may be difficult to manage since it often arises after surgery. Exchange transfusion may be dramatically effective and prednisolone is often given but has no proven value. Platelet transfusions are contra-indicated since severe febrile reactions may occur.

Thrombotic thrombocytopenic purpura (Moschowitz syndrome)

This condition often presents in a very acute and dramatic fashion although more rarely it can pursue a less acute and even chronic course, but it is unusual not to cause death within 6–12 months unless recognized and treated. It is characterized by the pentad of pyrexia, haemolytic anaemia, changing neurological symptoms and signs, thrombocytopenic purpura and renal dysfunction. There may be a prodromal period with a variety of manifestations which may extend from 2 months or rarely to years. These may include features such as recurrent fever, anaemia, proteinuria, bleeding manifestations, joint problems and even transient pareses. The onset of the final stage of the disease is often explosive with pyrexia and varying states of consciousness with changing neurological signs, such as cranial nerve palsies and even hemiparesis with a marked microangiopathic anaemia with raised reticulocyte count and thrombocytopenia which may be extreme and associated with widespread purpura. There is often gross proteinuria and biochemical changes of renal failure with raised creatinine and urea; there may also be haematuria. Diagnosis is confirmed by biopsy of vessels either from the gingival margin or sometimes from bone marrow biopsy showing occlusive subintimal deposits of PAS + ve material in the terminal arterioles and capillary junctions. These can be shown to consist of fibrin and fibrinogen and are thought to result from platelet thrombi.

The peripheral blood shows the classical changes of microangiopathic anaemia with helmet cells, schistocytes, polychromatic macrocytes and triangular shaped cells as well as a striking reduction in platelets. It is important to realize that the syndrome may not present with every feature of the pentad, and often the patient will complain of increasing weakness with nausea and such symptoms as occipital headaches with diarrhoea and vomiting. Pancreatic involvement may give abdominal pain. The reasons for these protean manifestations are the widespread nature of the small vessels that are involved since no organ in the body is exempt. The neurological signs may be quite bizarre with the patient becoming incoherent and complaining of paraesthesia which come and go and may initially be mistaken for hysteria. Abdominal pain and nausea and vomiting are common and although virtually all patients are thrombocytopenic on presentation, not all have haemorrhagic manifestations. Many of the patients are clinically jaundiced and hepatosplenomegaly occurs in approximately one quarter of the patients. Although most patients are between the ages of 10 and 40 years, it can occur at any age group, the peak incidence being in the 3rd decade, and females more frequently affected than males with a 3:2 ratio. Investigations usually show haematuria, marked proteinuria and occasionally some granular and hyaline casts. Coagulation and clotting screens are usually normal, and evidence of disseminated intravascular coagulation is very uncommon and if present should make one reconsider the diagnosis or suspect an associated disorder such as SLE. The remaining haematological findings are an anaemia with a reticulocytosis often greater than 10%, a platelet count which is usually lower than $100 \times 10^9/l$ and frequently a leukocytosis. Bone marrow usually shows a moderately hypercellular marrow with increased megakaryocytes and some normoblastic hyperplasia consistent with haemolysis. A trephine may show occlusions of small arterioles. Other biochemical findings relate to renal malfunction and include a raised urea and creatinine, and there may be non-specific changes in liver function consistent with widespread arteriolar thrombosis and hyperbilirubinaemia is very common. The aetiology and pathogenesis of this disorder remain unknown and it may be that there is more than one way in which this disorder may be precipitated. Studies of the lesion may show, in some instances, the presence of IgM and complement as well as fibrin and fibrinogen, but these findings have not been universal. Similarly, a number of papers have reported circulating immune complexes to be present whilst others have not found this to be the case. A very similar syndrome to thrombotic thrombocytopenic purpura (TTP) has been reported in infective endocarditis and here immune complexes were demonstrated. Possibly immune complexes account for its occurrence in a small percentage of patients with lupus erythematosus. Lian and co-workers have reported a high incidence of a platelet aggregating factor in plasmas of patients with TTP, but other classical examples have been found in which a platelet aggregating factor has not been discovered. Some workers have demonstrated a cytotoxic anti-endothelial cell antibody in the patient's serum, but again this has not been found in all instances. Currently the diagnosis must rest on the characteristic clinical features as well as the histological features in the small vessels.

Another suggestion has been that there is a plasma factor lacking that normally stimulates vascular synthesis of prostacyclin (PGI_2) and that this deficiency may be present in relatives of these patients, although in a much less pronounced form and therefore these people are asymptomatic. There has been a report of a patient with thrombotic thrombocytopenic purpura who had initially low levels of circulating 6-keto PGF_1 which is the stable end product of PGI_2 and these levels returned to normal after the patient had had a remission induced by plasma exchange.

When the diagnosis is made, treatment must be commenced as a matter of urgency. It is our policy to give the patient a bolus dose of hydrocortisone 200 mg and cyclophosphamide 150 mg i.v. then oral steriods at 60–120 mg daily and to undertake immediate plasmapheresis removing at least 3 litres of plasma and replacing them with fresh frozen plasma. Plasmapheresis should be continued on a daily basis together with heparin 30 000 units daily and dipyridamole 300–400 mg daily. The patient's progress should be monitored by the neurological features, the blood count and bleeding time. Should there be no improvement in these parameters, then splenectomy should be undertaken. In a recent report one patient who failed to respond to standard treatment with steriods, antiplatelet drugs, plasma infusion and plasmapheresis, was given an intravenous infusion of PGI_2 over a 72 hour period with an improvement in his mental condition, and a further continuous infusion of prostacyclin over a number of days, resulted in a complete remission. One feature of this patient was a high urinary excretion of thromboxane B_2 despite high aspirin dosage. This was reduced dramatically following PGI_2 infusion. The platelet aggregating factor described by Lian and colleagues is not inhibited by prostacyclin which may explain why many patients do not respond to therapy with antiplatelet drugs. That in some patients at least there may *not* be a factor in the blood causing TTP is suggested by two reports where the blood from the patient was transfused into normal recipients without untoward effects. It is still difficult to assess the overall success rate in this disorder, but it appears from reports in the World literature, that with vigorous management, the recovery rate in this disorder should now be greater than 70%, in striking contrast to the prognosis a few years ago where the mortality was close to 100%.

Another related condition, but strikingly different in its natural history, is that of chronic relapsing thrombotic thrombocytopenic purpura (also called the Upshaw–Shulman syndrome) (*v. supra*).

Haemolytic–uraemic syndrome (Gasser syndrome)

This is primarily a disorder of children which has at times been reported in epidemics and is often preceded by a brief febrile illness. This may be bacterial or viral in nature and it has been reported following immunization against diphtheria, tetanus, polio, measles and smallpox. Numerous instances have been reported following Shigella infections and a gastroenteritis type picture is a common clinical presentation. It is quite common in South Africa in children who have recently migrated to that country. Sporadic cases have been described in teenagers and young adults and also in women during pregnancy, but most commonly post-partum, and also in women taking the contraceptive pill. The patient may present febrile with vomiting, diarrhoea, abdominal pain and oliguria. On examination patients might be slightly jaundiced, have purpuric eruptions and moderate hepatomegaly but splenomegaly is rare. Kidneys may be palpable and tender and in some instances rebound tenderness is seen. The neurological features may include drowsiness, convulsions and sometimes transient paresis, although these features are usually not as prominent as in thrombotic thrombocytopenic purpura. Examination of the blood often shows a severe anaemia with marked thrombocytopenia (but this is not invariable) and leukocytosis. The blood film shows many fragmented cells and a picture typical of micoangiopathic haemolytic anaemia with poly-chromasia and a reticulocytosis. Haemoglobin may be detected in the plasma and noted on naked eye examination and methaemalbumin is usually present. Haptoglobins are low and bilirubin is usually mildly elevated. The urine may contain haemoglobin, haemosiderin and protein, and on microscopic exami-nation red cells and casts may be seen. Coagulation findings suggestive of DIC are occasionally found, but usually the coagulation screen is normal although high levels of fibrin breakdown products have been reported in the urine. Renal biopsy has shown IgM, C_3 and fibrin in the glomerular deposits. Circu-lating endotoxin was reported in 50% of patients who had associated HUS following shigellosis, but only in 5% of patients who had uncomplicated shigella diarrhoea. Immune complexes have also been frequently reported. In children the prognosis is usually good with a mortality rate under 5%.

The pathogenesis of this syndrome remains unclear, although its striking similarity to thrombotic thrombocytopenic purpura has led to suggestions that there may be a lack in a plasma factor which normally stimulates PGI_2 production by endothelial cells, and this explains the beneficial effects of plasma exchange reported in this disorder, although this may also relate to removal of immune complexes. One intriguing study revealed that two patients with this disorder had the Thomsen–Friedenreich (T–F) antigen exposed on the erythrocytes and the glomeruli. It was suggested that this resulted from attack of the cells by neuraminidase from bacteria, in this instance pneumoccocus, resulting in the exposure of this normally hidden antigen. The exposed antigen was postulated to interact with anti-T-FIgM antibody in plasma to produce the lesions of haemolysis and thrombosis in the renal glomeruli. Unlike thrombotic thrombocytopenic purpura, the vascul-ature involved is primarily that of the glomerulus.

The therapy of this condition remains controversial, but most people approach the problem conservatively using packed cell transfusion to control the anaemia keeping a careful monitor on fluid and electrolyte balance and urine output. The most important aspect of the management appears to be that of the renal problems and should simple restriction of fluid intake and control of blood pressure not be adequate, then peritoneal or haemodialysis may be required. Debate continues as to the role of antiplatelet agents, antico-agulants such as heparin and fibrinolytic agents. Most favour the use of anti-platelet agents, possibly combined with infusions of fresh plasma or plasma exchange.

Acquired biochemical defects

Acquired biochemical defects of the platelets resulting in increased destruction have not yet been clearly defined, although they may play a part in some forms of thrombocytopenia associated with severe metabolic problems in the body such as uraemia or hepatic failure.

Thrombocytosis

Thrombocytosis may be defined as a condition where the patient's platelet count is consistently in excess of $450 \times 10^9/l$. Its causes are listed in Table 8.7. Most of the conditions listed in this table cause a thrombocytosis which is usually less than $1000 \times 10^9/l$. The main exceptions to this are chronic blood loss, especially where this is associated with an inflammatory bowel disorder such as ulcerative colitis, immediately post splenectomy particularly where there is an underlying condition which has an increased platelet production such as the myeloproliferative disorders or idiopathic thrombocytopenic purpura and the myeloproliferative condition alone, e.g. myelofibrosis and essential thrombocythaemia. Virtually the only situations where the thrombocytosis causes clinical problems are post splenectomy or with essential thrombocythaemia, myelofibrosis or polycythaemia vera.

In the myeloproliferative disorders a syndrome of microvascular insufficiency may develop where, despite normal peripheral pulses, the patient may have painful feet associated with a patchy or general peripheral cyanosis and sometimes small infarcts. These may be associated with clinical symptoms of pain on walking and if unattended, go on to produce areas of gangrene, not dissimilar to that seen in diabetic microvascular disease. Less commonly there may be deep venous thrombosis and/or thrombophlebitis and more rarely still, transient ischaemic attacks and amaurosis fugax. Pulmonary emboli usually occur only after operative procedures and splenectomy in patients with these disorders appears to be especially dangerous, probably because of a frequently associated rapid increase in platelet count as well as the local pain, making physiotherapy and breathing more difficult, and splenectomy should be avoided unless specifically indicated. Usually the micro-circulatory problems can be readily controlled by the introduction of aspirin 300 mg daily and dipyridamole 200–400 mg t.i.d. or q.i.d. where tolerated, and in the case of polycythaemia vera the initiation of a venesection programme. Should the use of antiplatelet agents fail to control the symptoms and signs of microvasculature problems, consideration should then be given to other forms of treatment which may control the thrombocytosis by reducing platelet production. In the case of polycythaemia and myelofibrosis, the two most commonly employed manoeuvres are to use myleran or ^{32}P. The latter is preferred if the patient is felt to be at all unreliable or lives in a part of the country where routine blood tests cannot be obtained. If for some reason it is desirable to rapidly reduce the platelet count, consideration can be given to the use of plateletpheresis or drugs such as nitrogen mustard or hydroxyurea. Myleran is usually used in a dosage of 6 mg daily with weekly blood counts, reducing the dosage appropriately as the counts come under control and then ceasing it when they are at the desired level. Radioactive phosphorus (^{32}P) is most commonly used in patients with polycythaemia who are difficult to control with venesection or in whom the platelet count has increased following the venesection and

Table 8.7 Thrombocytosis

Chronic blood loss and iron deficiency

Infections
    Pneumonia – usually chronic rather than acute

Inflammation
    Rheumatoid arthritis
    Bowel disease
    Crohn
    Ulcerative colitis
    Lupus

Neoplasia

Lymphoma
    Hodgkin

Myeloproliferative disorders
    Chronic myeloid leukaemia
    Polycythaemia rubra vera
    Myelofibrosis
    Essential thrombocythaemia
    Acute leukaemia
    Refractory anaemia with excess blasts. 5q anomaly

Asplenia or splenectomy

Drugs
    Vincristine
    6-Mercaptopurine

Rebound

symptoms are not controllable by the use of antiplatelet drugs. In these circumstances ^{32}P is given intravenously in doses of 3–4 mCi, depending on the size of the patient, and the platelet count is checked in 3 months. Should there be no change in the count, the same dose is administered again. Should the count return to normal the patient is followed at 3 monthly intervals. Should the count be only partially restored to normal, then an appropriately reduced amount of ^{32}P is given and the patient is rechecked in 3 months. It has been most people's experience that patients with polycythaemia and leukocytosis usually require more ^{32}P to bring them under control than those with a normal white cell count.

    Essential thrombocythaemia is a rare disorder which may present in younger age groups and appears to be more frequent in women than men. The patient may present with microvascular problems or more frequently is discovered by chance to have splenomegaly, and an investigation of the blood film reveals thrombocytosis without other changes. A bone marrow in these circumstances shows a striking increase in megakaryocytes, but the remainder of the marrow is normal and the chromosome studies are also normal. This disorder may pursue an extremely benign and lengthy course and require little or no treatment. Indeed most of the patients who have run into problems that we are acquainted with have been those who have received aggressive chemo-therapy or have had splenectomy undertaken. One paradoxical feature of these extreme forms of thrombocytosis where the count may exceed $2000-5000 \times 10^9/l$ is an associated bruising and bleeding tendency which may be the reason why therapy has to be instituted since only the reduction of the overall platelet count will restore haemostasis to normal.

In general terms thrombocytosis should be managed conservatively, and many books state that post-operative thrombocytosis may exceed $800-1000 \times 10^9/l$ and have little or no incidence of thrombotic complications. This has not been our experience following splenectomy for haematological problems such as myeloproliferative disorders or ITP, so that our own policy is to use prophylaxis routinely post-splenectomy, should there be a rapid rise of the platelet count in the first few days.

The basic cause of the increased platelet count in the disorders listed in Table 8.7 is poorly understood. It is thought that the situation of chronic blood loss may be the result of an overall increase in bone marrow stimulation resulting in thrombocytosis, but the factors involved in situations of infections, inflammation, neoplasia and lymphoma are unknown. In the case of myeloproliferative disorders, there is an increased mass of megakaryocytes producing platelets. Chronic myeloid leukaemia frequently has a platelet count between 700 and $1000 \times 10^9/l$ but may have normal or reduced numbers and still be Philadelphia positive and have all the other classical features.

There is one type of refractory anaemia with excess blasts, namely the 5q anomaly in which there is an increased number of megakaryocytes whose nuclei do not show the normal lobulation seen in mature megakaryocytes, and characteristically has an associated thrombocytosis. In all of the situations of the myeloproliferative disorders where platelet survival studies have been undertaken, they have been found to be perfectly normal.

The most common cause of asplenia causing thrombocytosis is splen-ectomy. As outlined earlier, the normal spleen contains 20% of the body's total platelet mass, however post-splenectomy for whatever cause, it is not unusual to find the platelet count rise above $1000 \times 10^9/l$, and although in most patients in the following weeks the count returns to normal, there are others in whom this increased count persists for no apparent reason. This persistence of thrombocytosis is more common in patients who have their spleens removed for haemolytic anaemia such as pyruvate kinase deficiency, where although there is clinical improvement and the haemoglobin may rise, the anaemia is not completely corrected. In these patients it is believed that the thrombocytosis is a reflection of an overall increase in bone marrow mass attempting to compen-sate for the continuing anaemia. Other conditions of asplenia with thrombo-cytosis are coeliac disease, sickle cell anaemia and dermatitis herpetiformis, and more rarely congenital absence. This is diagnosed by the red cell changes of Howell–Jolly bodies, target cells and crenated cells which are seen following a total splenectomy in the peripheral blood, and is confirmed by radio-isotope scan showing faulty or absent splenic reticulo-endothelial cell function. This type of thrombocytosis rarely requires any therapy.

Drugs

Vincristine has been shown to increase platelet counts in approximately 30% of patients with lymphoma treated with this drug alone. This increase in count is not necessarily accompanied by resolution of the tumours and appears to be a direct effect since reproducible increases in platelet counts following vincristine can be induced in animals. Its mode of action is unknown.

6-Mercaptopurine increases platelet counts in some patients with chronic myeloid leukaemia, and may be a useful agent to employ in patients with this disorder who present with a low platelet count.

Rebound

This term describes the 'overshoot' of platelet count that may follow acutely induced thrombocytopenia either secondary to drug administration or associated with cyclical or intermittent thrombocytopenia. This form of thrombocytosis rarely exceeds $1000 \times 10^9/l$.

References

ACKROYD J.F. (1949). The pathogenesis of thrombocytopenic purpura due to hypersensitivity to sedormid. *Clin. Sci.*, **7**, 249

AHN, Y.S., BYRNES, J.J., HARRINGTON, W.J., CAYER, M.L., SMITH, D.S., BRUNSKILL, D.E. and PALL, L.M. (1978). The treatment of idiopathic thrombocytopenia with vinblastine-loaded platelets. *N. Engl. J. Med.*, **298**, 1101

CARLOSS, H.W., McMILLAN, R. and CROSBY, W.H. (1980). Management of pregnancy in women with immune thrombocytopenic purpura. *J. Am. Med. Assoc.*, **244**, 2756

CLANCY, R., JENKINS, E. and FIRKIN, B. (1971). Platelet defect of infectious mononucleosis. *Br. Med. J.*, **4**, 646

COHEN, P., and GARDNER, F.H. (1961). The thrombocytopenic effect of sustained high-dosage prednisone therapy in thrombocytopenic purpura. *N. Engl. J. Med.*, **265**, 611

DIFINO, S.M., LACHANT, N.A., KIRSHNER, J.J. and GOTTLIEB, A.J. (1980). Adult idiopathic thrombocytopenic purpura. Clinical findings and response to therapy. *Am. J. Med.*, **69**, 430

GROTTUM, K.A., HOVIG, T., HOLMSEN, H., ABRAHAMSEN, A.F., JEREMIC, M., and SEIP, M. (1969). Wiskott–Aldrich syndrome: Qualitative platelet defects and short platelet survival. *Br. J. Haematol.*, **17**, 373

HALSTEAD, S.B. (1980). Dengue haemorrhagic fever – a public health problem and a field for research. *Bull. WHO*, **58**, 1

HARRINGTON, W.J., HOLLINGSWORTH, J.W., MINNICH, V. and MOORE, C.V. (1951). Demonstration of a thrombocytopenic factor in the blood of patients with thrombocytopenic purpura *J. Lab. Clin. Med.*, **38**, 1

KARPATKIN, M., PORGES, R.F. and KARPATKIN, S. (1981). Platelet counts in infants of women with autoimmune thrombocytopenia. *N. Engl. J. Med.*, **305**, 936

KUNICKI, T.J., JOHNSON, M.M. and ASTER, R.H. (1978). Absence of the platelet receptor for drug dependant antibodies in the Bernard-Soulier syndrome *J. Clin. Invest.*, **62**, 716

LACEY, J. V. and PENNER, J. A. (1977). Management of idiopathic thrombocytopenic purpura in the adult. *Semin. Thromb. Hemostas.*, **3**, 160

LIAN, E. C.-Y., HARKNESS, D. R., BYRNES, J. J., WALLACH, H., NUNEZ, R. (1979). Concise report: presence of a platelet aggregating factor in the plasma of patients with thrombotic thrombocytopenic purpura (TTP) and its inhibition by normal plasma, *Blood*, **53**, 333

ONDER, O., WEINSTEIN, A. and HOYER, L. W. (1980). Pseudothrombocytopenia caused by platelet agglutinins that are reactive in blood anticoagulated with chelating agents. *Blood*, **56**, 177

MURPHY, S. (1972). Heriditary thrombocytopenia. *Clin. Haematol.*, **1**, 359

NEAME, P. B., KELTON, J. G., WALKER, I. R., STEWARD, I. D., NOSSEL, H. L. and HIRSH, J. (1980). Thrombocytopenia in septicaemia: The role of disseminated intravascular coagulation. *Blood*, **56**, 88

NEL, J. D., STEVENS, K., MOUTON, A. and PRETORIUS, F. J. (1983). Platelet-bound IgM in autoimmune thrombocytopenia. *Blood*, **61**, 119

NELSON, E. R., BIERMAN, H. R. and CHULAJATA, R. (1964). Hematologic findings in the 1960 hemorrhagic fever epidemic (Dengue) in Thailand. *Am. J. Trop. Med.*, **13**, 642

SCHULMAN, N. R. (1958). Immunoreactions involving platelets I. A steric and kinetic model for formation of a complex from a human antibody, quinidine as a haptenic and platelets: and for fixation of complement by the complex. *J. Exp. Med.*, **107**, 665

9
Involvement of platelets in non-haematological disorders and thrombosis

The human disorders in which the platelet has been identified as playing a role are listed in Table 9.1. The precise involvement is often hard to define, since in most instances it may represent subtle interactions between the blood vessels' blood clotting components, and depend on physical elements such as viscosity and blood stream jetting with secondary eddy pool formation which could initiate platelet activation and form platelet aggregates.

Table 9.1 Disorders in which platelets play a role

(1)	Raynaud syndrome
(2)	Migraine
(3)	Coronary disease Angina Myocardial infarction Sudden death
(4)	Cerebrovascular disease Transient ischaemic attacks Stroke
(5)	Amaurosis fugax
(6)	Peripheral vascular disease
(7)	Diabetes
(8)	Respiratory disorders
(9)	Glomerulonephritis
(10)	Thrombosis

Raynaud syndrome

Raynaud syndrome is a condition where exposure to cold results in a series of colour changes in the patients' extremities, the fingers first becoming pale and then blue and painful, so that the patients warm their hands in warm water for relief. Most commonly it occurs in the hands alone, but the feet may also be involved. It is usually bilateral and if unilateral some local pathology such as a cervical rib or other cause of thoracic outlet compression should be considered. The most common precipitating cause is exposure to cold, but emotion may also be a trigger. Table 9.2 lists the medical problems which may cause Raynaud syndrome, which is therefore an important clinical signpost. In large series, approximately one quarter of the patients are idiopathic, but since most of this data is published from centres interested either in connective tissue diseases or in vascular problems, the almost equally high incidence of scleroderma and collagen disorders may be due to the interests of the clinic involved. In clinical practice, mild Raynaud phenomenon in young women is extremely common and is usually unrelated to any sinister process, but the development of Raynaud phenomenon after the age of 25 should always be regarded seriously and the conditions listed in Table 9.2 excluded.

The pathogenesis is unknown and evidence for and against a hyper-viscosity state at low temperatures in idiopathic Raynaud syndrome has been reported. Claims for increased levels of catecholamines and the precipitation of attacks by serotonin have also been made and disputed. The association of red blood cell sludging in patients with cold agglutinins and Raynaud phenomenon does suggest an obvious mechanism in these circumstances, and the presence of cryoglobulins would also lend credence to a cold hyperviscosity state, but how this could induce digital artery spasm by cold or emotion in the idiopathic cases is uncertain, perhaps by platelet activation and release of thromboxane A_2 and serotonin or other vasospastic agents (*v. infra*). Why Raynaud syndrome is not more commonly seen in other hyperviscosity states, such as polycythaemia primary or secondary, in macroglobulinaemia

Table 9.2 Possible causes of Raynaud syndrome

(1)	Idiopathic	(6)	Occupation
(2)	Scleroderma		Trauma and especially use of vibrating machinery or tools
(3)	Immune complex		Exposure to vinyl chloride
	Systemic lupus	(7)	Drugs
	Rheumatoid arthritis		Beta blockers
	Polyarteritis		Oral contraceptives
	Hepatitis B antigen		Chemotherapy
	Drug induced		Ergot
(4)	Cryoglobulinaemia	(8)	Neurological causes
	Essential	(9)	Cold injury
	Mixed		
(5)	Obstructive vascular disease	(10)	Cold agglutinins
	Atherosclerosis		
	Buerger disease	(11)	Chronic renal failure
	Cervical rib or thoracic outlet syndrome	(12)	Occult neoplasm

(without cryoglobulinaemia) and other paraproteinaemias is difficult to explain if viscosity is a major pathogenetic factor. That platelet activation may occur is suggested by the increased plasma levels of β-thromboglobulin (BTG) and platelet factor 4 in patients in whom an attack has been induced. A high plasma von Willebrand factor level has been reported and this increases when the patient is exposed to cold. The increase in this protein could be either the result of release from platelets or from endothelial cells, and this remains a subject for further study. The improvement of some patients treated with reserpine suggests some role for serotonin, and since such treatment lowers platelet serotonin levels it could support the hypothesis of serotonin release from platelets as a trigger for an attack. The role of the platelet is also supported by the increased levels of plasma BTG and hyperaggregability of the patient's platelets to ADP which were restored to normal following repeated plasmapheresis. This was accompanied by clinical improvement.

Migraine

Migraine is another episodic disease believed to be due to an initial vasospasm resulting in slowing of the cerebral circulation followed by vasodilatation and headache. The trigger for these attacks is unknown, but there is evidence for platelet aggregation and activation of the platelet release reaction, and a serotonin releasing factor has been demonstrated in blood during the attack. There are increases in plasma BTG as well but no change in TXB_2, the stable end product of TXA_2. Platelets can release a number of vasoconstrictive substances, in particular thromboxane A_2 and 5-hydroxytryptamine (serotonin), as well as ADP and ATP which display both excitatory and inhibitory effects on vascular smooth muscle cells. The platelet serotonin concentration actually increases during the prodrome and then falls during the headache phase perhaps due to serotonin release, and it has been postulated that the platelet serotonin acts with bradykinin to produce the vascular pain. Platelet function anomalies can be produced by stress with a loss of second phase aggregation to adrenalin, and release of serotonin and platelet factor 4 is also diminished. This could be explained by platelet activation producing a type of acquired storage pool defect, and the release induced by stress initiates the vasospasm of an attack. The role of platelets may explain the effectiveness in some patients of anti-inflammatory agents which block prostaglandin receptors, such as tolfenamic acid which has been reported to be as effective as ergotamine tartrate in relieving a migraine attack. Aspirin is less effective, but is superior to placebo. Agents which are effective in reducing the frequency and severity of the attacks are propanolol, a β-adrenergic blocker, and pizotifen, which is an anti-histamine and a serotonin blocking agent, and these could both act through their respective effects on platelets.

Coronary disease

Platelets may contribute to vascular disease and result in problems in two major ways. One is in the development of atherosclerosis and atheromatous lesions which are so commonly associated with myocardial, cerebrovascular and peripheral vascular disease, and the other is in the acute event which precipitates medical emergencies such as coronary occlusion, stroke or peripheral artery occlusion.

One of the most popular hypotheses at present invokes the 'wear and tear' concept of induction of vascular wall damage by the adherence of platelets to the subendothelial tissues exposed by the removal of endothelial cells following damage, with consequent platelet aggregation and release reaction. This is followed by a migration of smooth muscle cells, perhaps as a response to chemotactic substances, into the intima of the vessel through gaps in the internal elastic lamina, with consequent proliferation, which is proposed to result from stimulation by the platelet mitogenic factor, of smooth muscle cells, but which has no effect on other cells, e.g. endothelial cells. This has also been called the platelet derived growth factor (PDGF), and is a cationic protein with a molecular weight of between 10 000 and 30 000 whose amino acid sequence is remarkably similar to a simian oncogene virus causing a sarcoma. PDGF is active in cell culture at levels of 100 ng/ml. The smooth muscle proliferation and formation of new connective tissue is followed by lipid deposition in animals with a high plasma cholesterol. Baboons in whom a chronic state of homocystinaemia was induced had a 50% decrease in platelet survival, at autopsy 10% of the endothelium of the thoracic and abdominal aorta was missing, and if the homocystinaemia was maintained not only did the platelet survival remain decreased, but there was marked intimal smooth muscle proliferation at the sites of missing endothelium. Treatment of the animals with dipyridamole restored the platelet lifespan to normal, but did not reduce the amount of endothelium that disappeared although there was now no intimal smooth muscle proliferation. Chronic hypercholesteraemic states have also been shown to cause a loss of endothelium in the major vessels. In another investigation, matched groups of swine were rendered hypercholesteraemic by appropriate diets. One group was homozygous for von Willebrand disease and therefore their platelets would be less able to adhere to damaged vessels. Extensive atherosclerotic lesions were seen in the normal swine but virtually none in those with von Willebrand disease. In man the effect of smoking, diet and disorders such as diabetes has been extensively studied over the past few years with regard to a number of aspects of platelet function including lifespan. Unfortunately, not all these results have been reproduced in all laboratories, for example the platelet lifespan in patients with homocystinaemia, was reported to have been very significantly reduced by one group, but in a similar group of patients studied by others, it was normal. There are numerous reports of patients with diabetes having platelets which were hyperaggregable, whilst other workers have found them to be normal. Most reported studies in patients with diabetes, particularly those with micro-vascular disease, have shown that the platelets are hyperaggregable and the platelets' lifespan reduced, supporting the concept of a 'wear and tear' hypothesis in atheroma formation. One has the uncomfortable feeling that there may be a number of instances where studies are not reported simply because the results are negative. This is highlighted by a letter in the *Lancet* from J. R. O'Brien who reported the inability of his own laboratory to repeat findings reported 4 years earlier on the effect of diet on platelet function. They were also unable to detect platelet aggregates in patients in the first week following myocardial infarction which has been reported by a number of laboratories including our own, and which in our study correlated well with a reduction in platelet survival. Presumably these differences result from different populations of patients studied, or differences in techniques employed in the particular laboratories concerned. The majority of studies on groups of patients with coronary artery disease in a stable condition have normal platelet aggregation results and do not show any increase in platelet aggregates; however in situations such as unstable angina, or acute myocardial infarction the platelet aggregates have been increased. Most reported platelet survival studies show a reduced platelet survival in patients with coronary disease, although in our hands, this is seen in the acute post-infarct phase and patients studied when their condition is stable some months after the infarct and without any recent acute episodes of ischaemia have normal platelet lifespans. There are now a number of papers in the literature reporting increased levels of β-thromboglobulin (BTG) and platelet factor 4 in exercise-induced myocardial ischaemia, and also in patients with unstable angina immediately after an attack. Raised levels of platelet factor 4 and β-thrombo-globulin have been reported up to 4 hours following such episodes, and throm-boxane B_2, the stable end product of the platelet derived thromboxane A_2, was also elevated during these forms of chest pain. There is much experimental animal work showing that the induction of platelet aggregation in coronary vessels will result in cardiac ischaemia and infarction. Prinzmetal angina, which results from coronary artery spasm, may be initiated by platelet activation and release of thromboxane A_2, due to platelet activation by exercise. Drugs which are useful in promoting coronary vasodilatation, such as glycerin trinitrate and calcium channel blocking agents as well as dipyridamole, have antiplatelet effects. These drugs may relieve angina and reduce its incidence but there is little evidence that they prevent infarction or improve lifespan, although a series of patients with unstable angina treated with 324 mg of aspirin daily showed a reduction in non-fatal myocardial infarction and possibly deaths compared to placebo.

One of the major unanswered questions in medicine today is what actually precipitates the onset of coronary thrombosis. Why is it that a person who has lived for years with either recurrent episodes of angina or even in apparently good health, suddenly, without any obvious precipitating cause, has an acute myocardial infarction? This question is even more difficult to answer when one looks at autopsies of patients past their 80s who die of pneumonia or some other non-vascular cause who have vessels which are extraordinarily distorted or obstructed with atheroma or thrombus, and yet apparently have had no symptoms. A popular theory currently is that the episode is initiated by platelet activation either by platelets adhering to some damaged part of the vessel wall, e.g. exposed atheromatous plaque, or aggregation triggered by some physical whirlpool effect resulting from jetting with the initiation of platelet clumps. This is supported by rheological models. Perhaps here the phenomenon of spontaneous platelet aggregation demonstrated *ex vivo* (*see* Table 9.5) may be of importance. Stress may play a role in a synergistic fashion since minimal doses of adrenalin, which do not induce platelet aggregation, will make them much more susceptible to aggregation with other agents, but although acute stress is often being claimed as a cause of myocardial infarction, the only proven relationship has been in groups of patients who have been depressed or who have recently lost a dearly loved one. The correlation of myocardial infarction with acute anxiety states is poor, but such emotional events may well trigger an attack of angina, and so different mechanisms may be involved although such an attack of angina may proceed to myocardial infarction as is illustrated in medical history by John Hunter's death. Another trigger could be immune complexes which might bind to the platelet and cause aggregation or induce the release reaction, or both. If the platelet is the trigger for the events of myocardial infarction, one would expect antiplatelet agents to reduce the incidence of this phenomenon. So far studies have largely been confined to the use of aspirin which has not been strikingly effective, although one study reported an overall reduction, but this was confined to non-fatal infarcts. Perhaps the right combination of agents is necessary to prevent a particular initiating step, and the size of the infarct or indeed whether or not the infarct will occur at all may be determined by other factors in the blood, such as anti-thrombin levels and/or protein C, plasma coagulant activities and/or the vessel wall's capacity to produce prostacyclin as well as fibrinolytic activity.

The syndrome of sudden death has attracted considerable attention over the past 4–5 years. In most instances it is thought that these deaths result from ventricular fibrillation and may occur without actual coronary thrombosis, but a number of studies have shown platelet aggregates in the myocardial micro-vasculature. Others have suggested that the onset of ventricular fibrillation may be precipitated by platelet aggregates causing intermittent disturbances during their passage through the coronary vasculature and breaking up to be undetectable in histological preparations. In a recent study in dogs employing glass bead embolization as a technique to induce myocardial infarction, it was found that sudden death could be reduced by previously treating the animals with carbenicillin at a dosage which induced platelet functional changes, and that this reduction in this model was not seen when anti-arrhythmic agents such as quinidine or lidnocaine were employed. The actual myocardial infarction was not altered by the treatment with carbenicillin, but the mortality was reduced, and it was postulated that carbenicillin reduced platelet aggregation and distal embolization thereby preventing ischaemia in the microvasculature distal to the occluded vessel. This type of phenomenon might explain the lack of a coronary thrombosis in patients who die suddenly with ventricular fibrillation since the obstruction in the distal microvasculature might result in an electro-excitable focus due to the resultant ischaemia and cause the arrhythmia. Aspirin was not effective in reducing sudden death in this animal model. Carbenicillin may be more effective than aspirin because it reduces platelet adhesion to collagen as well as inhibiting primary platelet aggregation, whereas aspirin only acts on blocking the release reaction and the secondary phase of aggregation (*v. infra*).

Cerebrovascular disease

The possibility of antiplatelet agents being an effective measure in reducing transient ischaemic attacks and stroke is being investigated in many centres. Similar pathogenetic mechanisms have been postulated in these disorders as for coronary artery disease, and a number of studies have been encouraging in the use of antiplatelet agents to prevent stroke. The most widely quoted is the Canadian stroke study, which showed a significant reduction in stroke in male but not female patients who were treated prophylactically with 1.2 g aspirin daily. The sex difference in this study is surprising and difficult to understand, although some work has shown differences between female and male platelets, e.g. the number of Fc receptors is higher in female platelets than in male. Such differences could account for the more ready response of platelets to immune complexes, resulting in platelet aggregation and thrombosis. Others have reported, both in animal and human studies, that females have a lower skin bleeding time following aspirin ingestion than males, and there may be a sex difference in the pharmacokinetics of the drug. Platelet function studies (*see* Table 9.5) of groups of patients with cerebrovascular disease have shown similar findings to those in myocardial infarction. These include an increased incidence of platelet aggregates, shortened platelet lifespan, increased levels of factor VIII, and in particular a decreased ratio of VIII antigen to VIII:C, higher platelet factor 3 availability and a shortened platelet cyclo-oxygenase regeneration time, supporting an increased platelet production and a reduced platelet survival and an increased release of ADP on platelet exposure to collagen.

Amaurosis fugax

This disorder is characterized by intermittent visual loss, and has been documented to be due to circulating platelet aggregates or cholesterol fragments which can be visualized in the retinal vessels by examination with the ophthalmoscope. It is thought that the platelet aggregates originate from 'jetting' on carotid artery stenotic lesions or following their activation by atheromatous plaques. There have been a number of studies in animals showing that experimental platelet aggregation producing platelet aggregates in the cerebral circulation can be prohibited by treating the animal with antiplatelet agents such as dipyridamole. It has been shown that in some clinical studies the symptoms of amaurosis fugax can be controlled with the administration of aspirin and dipyridamole.

Peripheral vascular disease

The use of antiplatelet agents has had a limited role in peripheral vascular disease, but the pathogenesis of this condition is thought to be similar to coronary and cerebrovascular disease. One circumstance where we have found antiplatelet agents to be helpful clinically, has been in patients who have increased platelet 'aggregates' associated with thrombocytosis and who often have symptomatology which would be compatible with platelet blockage of the micro-circulation resulting in paraesthesia and other uncomfortable symptoms including pain in the periphery. Following the use of aspirin the platelet aggregate ratio returned to normal and the symptoms disappeared. It seems here, as perhaps in coronary disease, that platelet aggregates could be important in causing obstruction in the micro-circulation, and hence transient ischaemic events which may be readily controlled. It may be that this type of approach will be helpful in reducing the incidence of gangrene in selected patients with diabetes. All patients with extensive vascular disease have a variable increase in acute phase reactants such as fibrinogen, haptoglobulin and Factor VIII:Ag, an increased incidence of platelet 'aggregates' and a diminished platelet lifespan, as well as increased levels of plasma PF4 and BTG. There is considerable variation in the findings of individual patients, and in some groups where the extent of the vascular disease may be less widespread, such as recovered myocardial infarcts, there seems more disagreement. This may be largely due to patient selection or the techniques employed.

Diabetes

Much investigation has been carried out on the role of the platelet in the pathogenesis of the vascular complications of this disease. The increased incidence of coronary occlusion and arterial occlusion in peripheral vascular disorders has been documented, but no increase found in cerebral thrombosis. Although there have been some contradictory findings, most studies have reported abnormalities in platelet function in diabetics, especially in those with microvascular changes of the juvenile diabetic type. Reports in this group of patients have shown increased platelet adhesiveness, the presence of circulating platelet 'aggregates' in a high proportion of patients, increased sensitivity to aggregating agents such as ADP and collagen, and increased BTG levels, as well as diminished platelet lifespan.

One report has suggested that the increased sensitivity of the platelet to aggregating agents may relate to increased prostaglandin pathway activity, with a heightened production of thromboxane A_2 and other metabolites. Other studies report that platelets from diabetics yield more fibrinogen binding sites on stimulation than do cells from normals. The platelet abnormalities have been attributed to plasma factor anomalies such as disturbed fatty acids and increased cholesterol and triglyceride levels which change the composition of the platelet membrane, and which may lead to increased prostaglandin synthesis or an intrinsic abnormality in the platelet itself, such as the increased number of fibrinogen binding sites. Depression of prostacyclin synthesis by the endothelial cells in diabetics has been reported. A reduced fibrinogen survival time in diabetes was corrected with better metabolic control of the patients. The oral hypoglycaemic gliclazide, a sulphonyl urea derivative, corrected the hyperaggregability and increased adhesiveness seen in patients with diabetes, but this appears to be due to some effect of the drug itself since control of the disease (reduction in blood sugar) occurred before the improvement in platelet function. Gliclazide has an *in vitro* action by stimulating adenylate cyclase and increasing the platelet's level of cAMP which inhibits platelet release reaction induced by thrombin and collagen. This does not explain the *in vivo* effect which takes time to develop. Perhaps it is related to some subtle alteration in fatty acids in the blood. Increased VIII:C, VIII:RAg and VIII:RCoF have been reported in diabetes, but this is probably linked directly to the presence of vascular disease, since patients with atherosclerosis from other causes have similar elevations.

Respiratory disorders

Suggestions that platelets may be involved in the pathogenesis of respiratory disorders have gained momentum since it has been appreciated that many patients with acute respiratory failure have a mild thrombocytopenia of around $100 \times 10^9/l$. Furthermore, diminished platelet aggregation to adrenalin and collagen in particular has been demonstrated in asthmatics whose attacks are induced by allergic stimulants such as pollens, and these platelet abnormalities have been shown to be more common and more marked when the patient is examined during the pollen season. Similar results have been obtained in patients with nasal allergy. These patients had elevated levels of IgE and pollen specific radio-allergosorbent binding (RAST). The abnormal adrenalin and collagen induced aggregation returned to almost normal levels some months after the pollen season had ended. IgE molecules have been observed to bind to platelets, and on ferritin labelled studies with the electron microscope form patches on the platelet membrane, and this might account for the aggregation findings. Further evidence for possible platelet involvement is that of increased levels of platelet factor 4 in plasma following antigen-induced airway reactions in asthmatic subjects. This is thought to arise by the release of platelet activating factor (PAF) (*see* Chapter 4) from basophils in the lung which are sensitized to the antigen, although the PAF could be released from endothelial cells in vessels. Uptake of serotonin (5 HT) by platelets from the migrainous patients and those with asthma is different from normals (*v. supra*). There has been a recent description of striking changes in the factor VIII molecule during severe acute respiratory failure. In this report factor VIII antigen was found to be disproportionately elevated compared to VIII procoagulant activity and VIII:RCoF activity. In the most severe group there was a striking right shift on the crossed immunoelectrophoresis consistent with an increase of low molecular weight forms of factor VIII, and it was postulated that these may have been derived from damaged endothelium which is known to occur in this syndrome. Other investigators have reported that endothelial cells primarily synthesize the high molecular weight form of factor VIII polymers, and it would therefore be necessary to postulate a second step to convert these to the lower molecular weight polymers found in the circulation. This type of picture is similar to that seen in patients with von Willebrand Type IIB or pseudo von Willebrand disease, described earlier. What alterations these dramatic changes have on the micro-circulation or platelet function is as yet unclear, but the occurrence of thrombocytopenia in patients with pseudo von Willebrand disease and the similar degree of thrombocytopenia frequently seen in acute respiratory failure, pose intriguing questions.

Glomerulonephritis

Kincaid-Smith has championed the concept that activation of the haemostatic mechanism may be of considerable pathogenetic importance in some forms of glomerulonephritis, and in an uncontrolled trial showed benefit in these patients with the administration of dipyridamole. Subsequent trials in glomerulonephritis have yielded conflicting results. Investigations have shown reduced platelet survival and morphologic evidence of platelet clumps in patients with glomerulonephritis, and also the involvement of platelets in the production of experimental glomerulonephritis, e.g. produced by the Habu snake venom. BTG levels have been increased, but this is difficult to interpret since they may be elevated in renal failure without implying increased platelet turnover. Serotonin levels in platelets have been found to be significantly lower in patients who have progressive glomerulonephritis, and the serum serotonin levels have been found to be higher in these circumstances. The latter finding may represent platelet activation and release resulting in platelets with an acquired storage pool defect. Activation of platelets in these circumstances can be readily envisaged in view of the damaged endothelium and also the frequent presence of immune complexes which might in their own right, induce platelet aggregation in the micro-circulation and then induce glomerular damage. Although increased circulating platelet 'aggregates' have been reported, subsequent studies from the same laboratory have failed to confirm this finding.

Thrombosis

Thrombosis is usually regarded as having a Yin–Yang relationship with haemostasis and to represent an over-reaction of the haemostatic system, in contrast to bleeding disorders being due to an under-reaction. Unlike the bleeding disorders where an identifiable defect or number of defects is usually now possible, in the case of thrombosis the recognition of one or even two identifiable causes is unusual. The exceptions to this are the rare hereditary conditions of homocystinuria, some hereditary dysfibrinogenaemias, antithrombin III deficiency, protein C deficiency and some vascular anomalies, namely the Hughes–Stovin syndrome (pulmonary artery aneurysms with pulmonary emboli associated with peripheral venous thromboses usually presenting in young males) and the Kasabach–Merrit syndrome (giant capillary haemangioma with thrombocytopenia secondary to disseminated intravascular coagulation). Hereditary 'hypercoagulability' is far more rare than hereditary hypocoagulability. There are no tests which can predict that a patient will definitely have thrombotic problems, nor are there any laboratory blood tests which will firmly make the diagnosis of the occurrence of thrombosis with the exception of disseminated intravascular coagulation. Table 9.5 lists a series of investigations which we employ in our own laboratory as a 'thrombosis screen' but although these tests may frequently be positive in groups of patients who have an increased tendency to thrombosis, they will in no way predict that the event will actually occur even if the patient is subjected to a defined trauma such as surgery of the hip. Positive results are often obtained in one or other of these tests but their significance is uncertain, e.g. the presence of spontaneous aggregation in the patient who has recently had a superficial thrombophlebitis. On the other hand, the presence of a shortening of the PTTK on mixing suggesting the presence of a clotting activator, and when prolonged with the classical findings of a 'lupus inhibitor' may be related to thrombotic events. Similarly, reduced ATIII levels, provided there is no ready explanation such as heparin therapy, are usually of significance especially where there is a family history. Protein C deficiency has now been reported in a number of families with striking histories of venous and/or arterial thromboses. Much more difficult to interpret are findings such as spontaneous aggregation, or hyperaggregability, or the presence of a lowered platelet aggregate ratio suggesting circulating platelet 'aggregates'. These must be interpreted in the clinical context (see p. 187).

Table 9.3 sets out some of the associations which are recognized to predispose to thrombosis. Clinically, problems with thrombosis may be divided into deep venous thrombosis, arterial thrombosis, embolism and disseminated

Table 9.3 Factors predisposing to thrombosis

Stasis
    Prolonged bed rest
    Splinting
    Paralysis of a limb
    Congestive cardiac failure
    Arm hanging over a chair or out of a car window

Operative procedure
    Any operative procedure requiring subsequent bed rest
    Specific surgery
        Hip surgery
    Splenectomy

Specific disorders
    Hereditary
        Vascular abnormalities
        Varicose veins
        Cavernous vein haemangioma
        Hughes–Stovin syndrome
        Anti-thrombin III (ATIII) deficiency
        Protein C deficiency
        Abnormal fibrinogen
        Polycythaemia
        Homocystinuria
        Hypercholesterolaemia

Genetic
    Race
    Blood group

Acquired disorders
    Collagen disorders, SLE
    Neoplasia
    Alcoholism
    Hormonal
        Pregnancy
        Oral contraceptive
    Metabolic
        Diabetes
    Varicose veins
    Haematological disorders
        Polycythaemia
        Myelofibrosis
        Essential thrombocythaemia
        Secondary thrombocytosis
        Acute myeloid leukaemia
        Chronic myeloid leukaemia
        Paroxysmal nocturnal haemoglobinuria (PNH)
    Nephrotic syndrome
        Low AT III
        VIII:CAF
    Cardiovascular
        Cardiac arrhythmia
        Mitral stenosis
        Artificial cardiac valve prothesis
        Coronary graft

intravascular coagulation, although the latter often presents as a bleeding problem rather than one of thrombosis and will be dealt with separately. There is a histological difference between the architecture of a venous thrombosis and one in an artery. A section of a venous thrombosis is not dissimilar to that seen in a clot in a test tube with platelets and white cells being scattered evenly on a carpet of fibrin with red cells in the interspaces. Arterial thrombosis on the other hand has clumps of platelets encircled by neutrophils surrounded by fibrin and red cells. Identical appearances can be obtained *in vitro* by applying different rheological forces to blood whilst it is clotting. The differences, therefore, probably relate to the differences in viscosity and rate of flow, even if initiating factors and subsequent biochemical events are similar. Everyone, during their lifetime, has several instances of venous thrombosis which pass unnoticed, as judged by the frequency of calcified phleboliths seen in pelvic veins on radiological examination, and by the presence of small thrombi in venous valves in leg veins dissected at autopsy. Using modern investigative techniques such as venography, ^{125}I fibrinogen with subsequent scanning and impedance plethysmography, it has become recognized that venous thrombosis is extremely common in medical situations – following stroke where it has been reported to occur in 50% of patients, and in myocardial infarction where reports range from 10 to 40%, the higher percentage probably reflects the number of patients with congestive cardiac failure as well as the degree of patient mobilization. In surgery, post-operative deep venous thrombosis is related to the site of surgery and also the extent and length of the operation. Total hip replacement has a particularly high incidence – approximately 50%, and appears to be additionally dangerous because of the frequent involvement of the femoral vein, pulmonary embolism has been reported in as many as 10%. In other forms of surgery, the deep venous thrombosis usually occurs more peripherally and is accordingly felt to be less dangerous, and certainly has a lower incidence of pulmonary embolism. Low dose heparin is of no value in prophylaxis following total hip replacement and most centres employ either higher dose heparin prophylaxis or warfarin. Very high incidences of deep venous thromboses are also found in knee surgery and following tibial fractures, the overall incidence is also being approximately 50%, but here low dose heparin prophylaxis is satisfactory. Urological and gynaecological procedures are operations which have high rates of DVTs with incidences ranging from 20 to 50% in patients with open prostatectomy, compared with only 10% in patients who have transurethral resections. Standard abdominal operations appear to have incidences of 15–30% perhaps influenced by the extent of the operation and its length. The cause of this high incidence of thrombosis probably relates to stasis, tissue trauma and the post-operative upsurge of acute reacting proteins which include fibrinogen and factor VIII. This is associated with increased platelet adhesiveness which is usually most obvious on the second post-operative day. That stasis is an important factor is suggested by the effectiveness of employing intermittent pneumatic compression of the calves during and after the operation, and also the use of dihydroergotamine which increases venous tone, and thereby is thought to reduce stasis. Amongst other factors which may be important is the fall in antithrombin III after surgery. A recent study of changes preceding deep venous thrombosis after spinal cord injury showed that the thrombotic event was preceded by a marked increase in VIII:Ag and VIII:RCoF (?vWf) and an increased aggregability of the platelets to collagen. Interestingly, VIII:C clotting was only slightly increased and the platelet aggregate ratio was normal until after the thrombosis had occurred when it dropped, indicating platelet activation. It was theorized that the increase in factor VIII was secondary to endothelial damage, and the increase in VIII:RCoF would enhance the platelets' adhesion to the damaged subendothelium which would in turn activate the platelets' procoagulant properties.

The very low incidence of deep venous thrombosis in patients undergoing similar surgery in Singapore and Hong Kong has drawn attention to racial differences. The incidence of deep venous thromboses detected by ^{125}I-labelled fibrinogen tests in Chinese patients following a stroke was approximately 20% compared with the 50% in Europeans. Similarly, low incidences were reported in Chinese patients post-operatively, again using techniques of ^{125}I-labelled fibrinogen, only 2.6% occurring after major operative procedures. One postulate is that this difference relates to the lack of reduction of ATIII levels in Chinese after surgery. That genetic factors are important is supported by the statistically higher incidence of deep venous thrombosis post-operatively in patients who are blood group A.

The above figures referred to studies searching for deep venous thrombosis by sophisticated techniques. They have established accurately the frequency of this problem and have shown that it is rare for peripherally placed thrombi to cause pulmonary embolism in patients, unless the thrombus is extending or is associated with thrombus in the ilio–femoral regions. These studies have highlighted the difficulty in correctly diagnosing a deep venous thrombosis clinically and show that it is essential to undertake venography, or, if available, impedance plethysmography combined with ^{125}I fibrinogen scanning to establish the diagnosis. It should be remembered that even what appears to be an obvious peripheral venous thrombosis, as judged by distension of the peripheral veins, swelling and calf tenderness, may be the result of other causes ranging from myositis, panniculitis, bone disease or even a ruptured Baker cyst to a syndrome of pseudo thrombophlebitis whose aetiology is unknown. Young women on the pill or pregnant can also develop unilateral symptoms and signs which are identical to that of a DVT, and which are thought to relate to the dilatation and stasis of the veins secondary to hormonal influences since venography in these patients shows no thrombus. Apart from the deep venous thrombosis the conditions listed in Table 9.3 may predispose to superficial thrombophlebitis. This is a condition where the superficial veins in the arms or legs become tender, reddened and inflamed, and may thrombose to form a tender, thickened cord. Whereas most people would treat deep venous thrombosis with anticoagulants these are unnecessary for this condition which usually responds well to anti-inflammatory drugs such as aspirin, indomethacin or, if these fail, butazolidine. Whilst one always worries about the possibility of underlying disorders, in particular lupus erythematosus and malignancy in the older age group, the vast majority of these patients have no identifiable cause, but occasionally have troublesome recurrences. In this event, agents which stimulate the fibrinolytic pathway may be valuable, such as phenformin and danazol. These drugs should be continued for 6 months following the recurrent episode, before withdrawal.

Embolism

Pulmonary embolism is one of the most worrying and feared of surgical and medical complications. In medical situations it has been termed the great mimicker because it may present in a number of ways clinically, e.g. recurrent episodes of wheezing, when it may be mistaken for asthma, with fever and chest signs and radiological features of pneumonia, and even as a pyrexia of unknown origin with relatively little clinical respiratory manifestations, as well as the classical pleuritic chest pain post-operatively with haemoptysis and a mild to moderate pyrexia. It can be particularly difficult to diagnose if it occurs in someone who has already established chronic obstructive airways disease and who presents with increasing breathlessness. Clinically, DVTs in the legs are often not detectable but venography may reveal a thrombosis. Particularly valuable are ventilation and perfusion scans which when taken together with the clinical situation, the chest X-ray and venous venography, give a 95% guarantee of a correct diagnosis. There are still some investigators who believe that the diagnosis can only be substantiated by undertaking pulmonary angiography. Even then, the diagnosis may be missed, only to be found at autopsy. So far other investigations, such as measuring fibrin breakdown products and platelet release factors, e.g. BTG, only offer circumstantial evidence. At present a minimum of perfusion and ventilation scan, venography of the legs and a chest X-ray should be undertaken since the diagnosis automatically labels the patient as having a very serious problem which will require intensive medical therapy. Any recurrence of chest pain will often lead to the assumption that another infarct has occurred. There have been many instances of people misdiagnosed as having pulmonary embolism who have been subjected to recurrent anticoagulation and subsequent maintenance on warfarin for years. This is dangerous and expensive therapy associated with considerable mortality and morbidity. Whilst blood gases may be of value in the immediate workup of the patient, once a diagnosis is established they are rarely indicated in view of the risks involved in arterial puncture in patients who are fully anticoagulated.

Anticoagulant therapy

Once a diagnosis has been established, it is essential to have a prothrombin time, a PTTK and a platelet count prior to the instigation of therapy. There is considerable debate and controversy about the best way to administer heparin. Provided there is no contra-indication to the use of anticoagulants our own policy is to give an immediate push dose of 7500 units i.v. to a small to medium sized individual, increasing to 10 000 units in a person weighing 85 kg or more, following this with continuous infusion heparin at a rate to deliver 25 000 units in the next 12 hours and another 25 000 units in the following 12 hours, giving a total of 60 000 units in the first 24 hours. At the end of that time a repeat PTTK and/or whole blood clotting time, is undertaken, and the dose adjusted up or down if the clotting time is not in the therapeutic range of $2-2\frac{1}{2}$ times normal. We adjust the dosage of heparin depending on the platelet count so that if the platelet count were high, $600 \times 10^9/l$, we would tend to give an extra 10–20 000 units i.v. of heparin in 24 hours and if low, that is, less than $150 \times 10^9/l$, we would reduce the dose. It is the usual mistake to give too little rather than too much heparin in the first 48 hours, and it is very uncommon for anyone to have a bleeding problem from heparin in the first 48 hours, unless there is some underlying problem such as peptic ulcer, hypertension, thrombocytopenia or trauma. Following the first 48 hours where an overall dose of between 100 000 and 120 000 units i.v. heparin is often necessary, it is usual to find that the dosage required drops to around 25 000–30 000 units daily. The dose is adjusted according to the coagulation studies which are undertaken every 24 hours. On the seventh day following the embolus, warfarin therapy is commenced, undertaking a prothrombin time which is usually around 16 seconds with a control of 12 seconds in a patient who is fully heparinized. Warfarin is commenced at a dosage commensurate with the patient's size and with regard to the presence of other drugs listed in Table 9.4 which may increase or decrease the warfarin requirements. A small woman would be started on a daily dose of 5 mg, an average sized person 8 mg and a large person 10 mg, the dosage adjusted up and down if drugs listed in Table 9.4 have to remain in use. This is maintained for 3 days, and then the prothrombin time is performed. If this is in the therapeutic range of $1\frac{1}{2}$–2 times the control one-stage Quick prothrombin time, heparin is ceased. If not, we continue the heparin in the current dosage and increase the warfarin by 2 mg daily. One should never hurry or be concerned to take a little longer to get the prothrombin time at therapeutic levels by this technique, and should resist the temptation to attain so called therapeutic range by using loading dose methods. The reasons for this are that the ultimate management of the patient is much smoother and less hazardous. It should be remembered that the ease of control of warfarin is directly related to the numbers of other tablets the patient is on, and drugs listed in Table 9.4 should be avoided unless essential. Useful drugs to remember are chlorthiazide, which

Table 9.4 Drugs which interact with warfarin

Enhance action	
Acetyl salicylic acid	Oral hypoglycaemics
Phenylbutazone	Mefenamic acid
Sulphinpyrazone	Oral antibiotics
Metronidazole	Nortriptyline
Trimethoprim-sulphamethazole	Quinidine
Clofibrate	Allopurinol
Heparin	Phenyramidol
Diphenylhydantoin	Benziodarone

Reduce action
Barbiturates
Diuretics
Cholestyramine (may enhance if vitamin K reserves are depleted)
Rifampicin
Glutethimide
Dichloralphenazone
Griseofulvin

does not affect warfarin and is a useful diuretic, diazepam and thiodiazepam may be used as hypnotics or sedatives and paracetamol for headache. After a major thrombotic episode such as a pulmonary embolus, oral anticoagulants should be continued for at least 3 months, and if control is well maintained and there is no other factor of concern, e.g. dyspepsia, it is our policy to continue for 6 months. Elastic stockings are routinely ordered to support the patient's legs. If there is a recurrent episode the patient is again anticoagulated for 6 months and then commenced on aspirin 300–600 mg daily and dipyridamole 200–400 mg daily, depending on tolerance, for another 12 months.

A major problem with warfarin therapy is the numerous drugs which interact with it, either enhancing or reducing its activity. In general terms the drugs may act by diminishing or improving the availability of vitamin K from the diet, diminishing or increasing the rate of absorption of warfarin from the gastro-intestinal tract, increasing or reducing the breakdown of the active warfarin metabolites and increasing coagulation factor turnover, enabling warfarin to act more rapidly and increasing the rate of synthesis of vitamin K clotting factors sometimes seen with oestrogen administration. Liver disease may enhance the effect of a drug, both by reducing synthesis of clotting factors and also by producing a vitamin K deficiency state due to abnormalities in the biliary tract or even outright biliary tract obstruction. Vitamin K may also be diminished by poor dietary intake combined with bowel disorders and/or oral antibiotics reducing the bacterial flora producing vitamin K, the latter being a particularly important source in patients who are receiving intravenous therapy only. Increased sensitivity to warfarin is also seen in febrile patients as well as patients with thyrotoxicosis, and reduced effects may be seen in patients with hereditary resistance and also in some patients with renal failure. It should be noted that there are certain drugs which in some instances appear to increase the anticoagulant effect and in others to decrease it. Examples of this are cholestyramine which usually decreases the response to warfarin, but may enhance it where vitamin K reserves are depleted. Phenytoin is another drug which may either enhance or reduce the effect of warfarin. Long term warfarin therapy should always be avoided in patients who are unreliable such as alcoholics or the elderly, unless there is someone who can administer the drug. An alcoholic binge may also precipitate bleeding due to its acute toxic effects on liver. Finally, any drugs which affect haemostatic mechanism, in particular those drugs which affect platelet functions should also be avoided (*see* Table 7.4 and 7.5). Should serious haemorrhage result from the use of these drugs, reversion may be obtained rapidly by the infusion of 4–6 units of fresh frozen plasma or 4 units of a suitable plasma concentrate of K-dependent factors such as prothrombinex (CSL). Vitamin K should also be given (50 mg i.v.) if the haemorrhage be profuse or in dangerous sites such as the central nervous system or pericardium. Vitamin K should not be used for minor bleeding episodes where warfarin needs to be continued, such as in patients with valvular prostheses, since control with warfarin will be difficult for some time following the use of vitamin K.

Other clinical situations which may be associated with emboli are the recent onset of atrial fibrillation, particularly if associated with mitral stenosis, thyrotoxicosis if the patient is in cardiac failure and patients with valve prostheses. All of these patients require longterm anticoagulation with the exception of thyrotoxicosis where the anticoagulants may be ceased following correction of the cardiac failure and control of the thyrotoxicosis.

Other embolic phenomena occur in patients who have transient ischaemic attacks which may be based on atheromatous carotid or basilar vessels. The emboli in these instances may be either atheromatous plaques or cholesterol or platelet emboli. If a stenosed and atheromatous vessel can be identified which correlates anatomically with the clinical symptoms then surgical excision should be undertaken. In current knowledge, antiplatelet drugs such as aspirin and dipyridamole should then be employed. If nausea or headache prohibits the latter, then it should be substituted with sulphinpyrazone.

More controversial areas include crescendo angina without a completed infarct in which the patient is having recurrent chest pain with ischaemic electrocardiograph changes but without evidence of a completed infarct by E.C.G. or examination of serial cardiac enzymes. This has been fiercely debated over the years, and studies for and against the the use of anti-coagulants litter the literature and textbooks. If pain cannot be controlled in 24 hours by current standard anti-anginal treatment, such as calcium channel blockers, nitroglycerin infusions etc., then it would be our policy to anticoagulate the patient with heparin and if coronary graft surgery is not possible, commence him on warfarin for the period of 12 months to 2 years.

Complications of anticoagulant therapy

The major complication of anticoagulant therapy is bleeding, and usually absolute contra-indications are diabetic retinopathy, uncontrolled hypertension and active peptic ulcer. In these instances, consideration should be given to surgical intervention, such as inferior vena caval plication in patients with pulmonary embolism secondary to deep venous thrombosis. In life-threatening situations anticoagulant therapy may still have to be introduced together with aggressive medical therapy for the hypertension or peptic ulcer, and careful monitoring by fundoscopic examination be undertaken in patients with diabetic retinopathy. In prolonged oral anticoagulation therapy in outpatients, the incidence of bleeding complications has been reported as ranging from 5 to 48% when minor bleeding episodes are included such as epistaxis, mild haematuria and minor bruising. Major haemorrhages are usually defined as life-threatening episodes or bleeding which leads to hospital admission and/or interrupts the patient's usual activities such as work. These include cerebral haemorrhage, haematemesis or melaena, retroperitoneal haematomas, severe haematuria, retinal haemorrhage, menorrhagia, extensive ecchymoses, haemarthroses, haemoptysis and nerve entrapment syndromes. Most would accept that there is an incidence of these major episodes of about 4% per treatment year. This emphasizes the dangers of anticoagulant therapy and the importance of close monitoring and careful patient instruction of situations which might influence the level of anticoagulation, e.g. gastro-intestinal upsets, the introduction of drugs listed in Table 9.4 and patient compliance. Common contributing factors to haemorrhage are the introduction or withdrawal of drugs, error in dosage either by the patient or the doctor and alcohol. One of the most commonly reported drugs causing haemorrhage with anticoagulants is aspirin. Two syndromes which the clinician must be alert to, enabling early diagnosis, are epidural haematoma and intramural bleeding in the bowel. The latter may present with non-specific symptoms which are gradual in onset and most frequently consist of recurrent abdominal cramping pain and distension, ultimately going on to vomiting. Often the patient has other signs of haemorrhage and in some instances an associated rectus abdominus haematoma. The prothrombin time is usually greatly prolonged and barium studies may show segments of small bowel with thickened mucosal folds giving appearances which have been variously described as the 'coiled spring' sign or the 'picket fence' sign. The other syndrome is that of epidural haematoma which is a medical emergency since it is potentially curable if it is diagnosed early enough, but which can go on to quadriplegia if missed. There is severe persistent back pain which may radiate in a root distribution. This should be treated immediately by reversing the anticoagulants and if necessary undertaking neurological investigation.

A particularly difficult situation arises when anticoagulants have to be given during pregnancy. Oral anticoagulants cross the placenta and cause fetal abnormalities which during the first trimester have been termed warfarin embryopathy and include nasal hypoplasia, eye abnormalities, asplenia, stippled epiphyses, hypoplastic digits and mental retardation. In the second trimester, optical atrophy, abnormal brain growth and developmental retardation have been reported. Use of these drugs in the third trimester can cause fetal haemorrhage, either before, during or after delivery and there is also an increased risk of haemorrhagic placental detachment. If coumarin drugs are used in pregnancy, approximately 16% will result in an abnormal live born child and 16% will have an abortion or still birth. Oral anticoagulants are secreted in only very small amounts in milk and so these drugs can be safely commenced after the birth of the child. Most obstetricians advocate the use of heparin if anticoagulation is necessary during pregnancy since its high molecular weight prevents it crossing the placenta, but heparin too is associated with increased fetal wastage and maternal deaths, although rare, have occurred. Unless there is a serious problem such as a pulmonary embolus which would require normal clinical dosage of heparin intravenously, the common dose of heparin advocated is 5000 IU 12 hourly throughout the pregnancy, ceasing when labour begins but recommencing 8 hours post partum and continuing for 6 weeks, although oral anticoagulants could be introduced earlier if long term anticoagulation is necessary.

Apart from bleeding complications, heparin has been associated with alopecia and osteoporosis. These complications are rare in the short term use of heparin.

The current upsurge of coronary bypass surgery has led to a considerable endeavour to ensure that the newly installed grafts do not block, and this complication can be reduced by the use of antiplatelet agents such as aspirin and dipyridamole. One is hopeful that the many new drugs that are appearing on the scene will be even more effective. The role of anticoagulation and antiplatelet drugs in the prevention of coronary disease and in the prophylaxis of recurrence remains uncertain. It does seem, in some very rigidly controlled trials in Holland, that there is benefit in long term anticoagulation using warfarin following an infarct, but many countries do not have the same excellent centralized monitoring system, and unless patients can be allocated to such a clinic, then the dangers of the treatment may outweigh its benefits. Whether antiplatelet drugs will be of value or not is as yet unknown. It is interesting that there are some reports that the β-adrenergic blockers at therapeutic concentrations reduce platelet 'aggregates', and this could be one explanation for their apparently beneficial effect following an infarct. It seems possible that micro-aggregates of platelets, rather than the main thrombus in the case of coronary vessel disease and perhaps also in stroke, will determine the extent and therefore the outcome for the patient, if not cause the initial attack. It is in these areas that one hopes advances will come in the not too distant future.

Table 9.5 Thrombosis screen

(1)	Full blood count, film and ESR
(2)	Prothrombin time, thrombin time, partial thromboplastin time with *kaolin* (PTTK) *or:* activated partial thromboplastin time (APTT) and mixing 1:1 with normal control
(3)	Fibrinogen level, protamine sulphate precipitation and fibrinogen split products (FDP)
(4)	Platelet aggregate ratio
(5)	Platelet hyperaggregability Collagen $5\,\mu g/ml$, $0.5\,\mu g/ml$ ADP $5 \times 10^{-6}\,mol/l$, $5 \times 10^{-7}\,mol/l$, $5 \times 10^{-8}\,mol/l$ Adrenalin $1.5 \times 10^{-7}\,mol/l$, $1.5 \times 10^{-8}\,mol/l$ Spontaneous aggregation
(6)	Plasminogen assay and euglobulin lysis with and without exercise
(7)	VIII:Ag, VIII:RCoF, VIII:C, DIEP VIII:FMP
(8)	ATIII Biological Immunological
(9)	Protein C Biological Immunological
(10)	Platelet lifespan
(11)	Elevated platelet release product β-Thromboglobulin (βTG) Platelet factor 4 (PF4) Thromboxane B_2 (stable breakdown product of TXA_2 (TXB_2)) Thrombospondin
(12)	6-Keto $PGF_{1\alpha}$ (derived from PGI_2)

The hypercoagulable or pre-thrombotic state

Table 9.5 sets out the current techniques available for investigating a thrombotic tendency in a patient. Spontaneous aggregation refers to the clumping of platelets in platelet-rich plasma stirred in a cuvette prior to the addition of any agonist such as ADP, collagen, etc. We have observed this phenomenon in people who are otherwise quite normal, and would be loath to attribute any significance to it in individual patients unless it occurred regularly and correction (with aspirin for example) led to improvement in clinical symptoms which could be attributable to platelet activation. Hypersensitivity to aggregation agents may be of more significance, since one can readily establish normal ranges for matched controls. Whether such findings indicate patients who are developing atheroma or who are more likely to have a thrombotic event, either *de novo* or secondary to some other precipitating cause such as surgery, is uncertain. The demonstration of platelet 'aggregates' in the blood by the platelet aggregate ratio is most commonly undertaken by the technique of Wu and Hoak in which two samples of blood are collected

Table 9.6 Common anti-platelet agents used therapeutically

Drug	Dosage
Acetyl salicylic acid	300 mg daily 1.2 g daily in divided doses
Sulphinpyrazone	600–800 mg daily in divided doses
Dipyridamole	100–400 mg daily in divided doses

from the patient, one into a standard anticoagulant mixture and the other into a syringe containing both the anticoagulant mixture and formalin. The principle of the test is that the formalin will preserve the platelet aggregates and, therefore, the platelet count in this tube will be lower than that collected in the syringe containing EDTA which will disrupt the aggregates. One problem with this test is that venous blood is employed, and our own attempts to obtain arterial blood at coronary artery catheterization, etc. have not given reproducible results. With venous blood samples the test has been reproducible in our hands, although it is critical that the blood be collected without a tourniquet and through a butterfly cannula of fixed length. It is possible that the aggregates form during collection rather than being present in the circulation, but nonetheless would represent platelets which are more readily activated than normal and therefore be of clinical relevance. We repeat it on two occasions before accepting a reduced ratio as being abnormal. Platelet lifespan is discussed elsewhere (Chapter 10). Specific components of the platelet such as BTG and platelet factor 4 are being increasingly used as guides to platelet activation *in vivo* but their clinical relevance remains unclear.

Role of antiplatelet drugs in thrombotic problems

In view of the role of the platelet postulated in the many situations described in this chapter, it is hardly surprising that there has been much attention in recent years to the possible advantages of drugs which impair platelet function in their treatment and control. Table 9.6 lists the three most commonly employed agents in this regard and the doses used. Not in this list are a number of drugs which affect the platelet's qualitative function (*see* Chapter 7) either because these drugs have been shown to be ineffective or have not been thoroughly evaluated. There are also a great number of new drugs which are currently being developed having an antiplatelet effect which may prove superior to those currently available. Whilst the drugs listed in Table 9.6 have all been shown to be beneficial in experimental animal situations, their results in man have been somewhat disappointing; most of the trials which have not been subject to debate and controversy have not shown any benefit statistically in the important situations such as the prevention of recurrent infarction and death following a myocardial infarct. In the Canadian Stroke trial, using aspirin alone at a dosage of 1.2 g daily, there was a statistically beneficial effect in male patients who had transient ischaemic attacks in preventing the occurrence of stroke. A number of authorities have also pointed to the fact that the 'trends' in all of these trials are in favour of the antiplatelet drugs although they do not reach significant levels, but to the sceptical outsider one must take the view of the Scottish verdict – not proven. The exceptions to this are the prevention of occlusion after coronary artery graft surgery where aspirin and dipyridamole treatment in combination reduces the re-occlusion of the grafts, and in situations where there is a thrombocytosis with secondary symptoms in the micro-circulation where in all instances so far reported, aspirin has been successful in correcting the symptomatology. Aspirin on its own has had no effect in preventing deep venous thrombosis, but there is evidence that in combination with dipyridamole it is effective in reducing thrombotic episodes in valve prostheses, in abolishing the problem of amaurosis fugax and in some studies reducing post-operative venous thrombosis. Dipyridamole has a high incidence of causing headaches and abdominal discomfort at doses higher than 200 mg daily, although these are sometimes controlled by the concurrent administration of aspirin. Whilst so far the use of these drugs has been relatively unrewarding it must be remembered that this may relate to the dosage and schedules thus far employed. For example, low dose aspirin could be expected to inhibit the platelet production of thromboxane A_2 and not inhibit prostacyclin production, whereas high dose aspirin might inhibit both, combinations such as aspirin and dipyridamole would be expected to be more effective because of dipyridamole's effects on increasing platelet cAMP and also stimulating prostacyclin production in the endothelial cells. This is supported by a recent report showing that aspirin doses of 80 mg daily were effective in inhibiting platelet function, and unlike higher doses, did not affect prostacyclin production in vessels. So far therefore, antiplatelet agents, apart from the areas indicated, have been relatively disappointing. One reason for this may be individual patient variations in response to the drugs. In one of the earlier studies on aspirin in man, Miekle *et al* (1969) showed that at doses of 900 mg daily approximately half of the healthy volunteers showed no alterations in the skin bleeding time, whereas the remainder had significant prolongation. The dose used would be expected to induce qualitative platelet aggregation defects in all the recipients. This would imply responders and nonresponders to aspirin in a significant number of normal people and could well affect the therapeutic usefulness of this drug in individual patients.

Disseminated intravascular coagulation (DIC)

Disseminated intravascular coagulation most commonly presents with a bleeding manifestation such as purpura or mucosal bleeding. More rarely it may occur in association with a deep venous thrombosis and/or embolic problems. It may also be diagnosed when a routine coagulation screen shows abnormalities which on further investigation prove to be due to this phenomenon. Table 9.7 lists some of the causes of disseminated intravascular coagulation. In most descriptions the trigger for this event is stated to be the release intravascularly, or perhaps extravascularly, of some procoagulant substance such as thromboplastin, endotoxin or collagen, or tissue damage which activates the clotting pathway and which at the same time may activate other pathways through the contact system such as fibrinolysis and complement and bradykinin. More rarely it may follow the administration of activated clotting factors given therapeutically in patients with liver disease or following snake bite. The LeVeen shunt, in which ascitic fluid is transported from the peritoneal cavity to the superior vena cava by a plastic tube implanted subcutaneously, is a very effective measure for controlling refractory ascites, but in our hospital is invariably accompanied by DIC. The evidence for the triggering events of DIC is usually circumstantial and may vary considerably in each clinical circumstance. In the case of the LeVeen shunt ascitic fluid contains little 'thromboplastic' activity, but has a considerable concentration of soluble collagen which when infused into animals, produces disseminated intravascular clotting, and which Salem et al (1981) postulated to be the cause of DIC seen in patients with LeVeen shunts in whom the ascitic fluid is perfused unfiltered back into the patient's venous system. This concept is supported by the reduction of the incidence and degree of DIC in these patients

Table 9.7 Causes of DIC

(1)	Obstetrical complications
(2)	Infections
(3)	Neoplasms

(4)	Haematological disorders
	    Promyelocytic leukaemia
	    Intravascular haemolysis

(5)	Vascular disorders
	    Hereditary
	      giant haemangioma
	    Acquired
	      aneurysm
	      grafts
	      lupus and other vasculitides

(6)	Shock

(7)	Miscellaneous
	    Purpura fulminans
	    LeVeen shunts
	    Heat stroke
	    Graft vs. host
	    Snake bite
	    Pancreatitis
	    Drugs
	    Lactic acidosis

if they are concurrently given aspirin. Likewise, although amniotic fluid embolism has been regarded for years as being due to thromboplastin present in the amniotic fluid, analysis of amniotic fluid has shown that there is a significant amount of collagen present and that this may, in part at least, account for this syndrome by activation of platelets and the clotting mechanisms. If the concept of there being a variety of precipitating factors is correct it may explain the very wide variation that is seen in the various patients studied with this disorder. One's attitudes are also coloured by clinical experience since physicians most commonly see this problem associated with septicaemia and neoplasia, whereas surgeons see it in association with trauma and shock. Particularly notable in the latter is its incidence following gunshot wounds to the head, where its onset is abrupt, but almost always circumscribed and lasting only 24–48 hours. Post-operative shock is the other common situation seen by surgeons. There are the very well known associations with pregnancy where the best form of therapy is to clear the uterus either of the dead fetus, the pregnancy or the placenta.

The diagnosis of the condition depends on the clinical situation, a peripheral film and platelet count, a protamine precipitation test which detects circulating fibrin monomers, fibrin degradation products (FDP) which usually detect the D and E fragments, the fibrinogen level and a prothrombin and thrombin time. In DIC, one would expect a reduced platelet count, prolonged prothrombin and thrombin times, significantly increased fibrin split products and a reduced fibrinogen level. Care must be exerted in interpreting this since

Table 9.8   Elevated fibrin degradation products (FDPs)

Chronic renal disease and uraemia
Pulmonary embolism
Retro-peritoneal bleed or large thrombus after trauma
Cirrhosis
Haemolytic uraemic syndrome
DIC

many patients have started with an elevated fibrinogen, and therefore a normal level may really be a significant reduction. The presence of fibrin monomers by protamine precipitation must be carefully interpreted since this test is often falsely positive. FDPs may be elevated in other conditions without active DIC (Table 9.8). Other clotting parameters which are sometimes quoted include a reduced ATIII level, reduced factor V and factor VIII levels and an incongruously shortened partial thromboplastin time with kaolin which is believed to be due to circulating activated clotting factors. Since the fibrinolytic system is usually activated there is often a reduced plasminogen level and evidence of fibrinolysis as demonstrated by a shortened euglobulin lysis time. These latter tests, however, rarely are helpful in coming to a decision concerning the diagnosis.

Table 9.9 Differential diagnosis of DIC

Fibrinogenolysis or fibrinolysis
    Rare condition
    Fragmented red cells *not* seen in peripheral film   }   Except when other pathology
    Protamine sulphate precipitation negative   }   is present
    Platelet count normal
    Clot lysis present, euglobulin lysis time markedly
    shortened
    FDPs are increased
    Prothrombin time, thrombin time, APTT are
    abnormal
    Factors V and VIII may be decreased

Liver disease
    Cirrhosis often has ↑ FDPs with *fibrinolysis*,
    also can occur with thrombocytopenia and
    clotting abnormalities making absolute diagnosis
    impossible
    Factor VIII levels often increased   }   In contra-distinction to DIC
    Factor VII and IX often decreased)

Microangiopathic haemolytic anaemia
    Peripheral film change and ↑ reticulocytes and other signs of haemolysis
    FDPs *normal* or slightly elevated unless there is co-existent renal failure
    No significant clotting factor deficiency

Post extra-corporeal circulatory operation
    Exclude heparin
    Thrombocytopenia + heparin 'rebound' – pseudo DIC

'Heparin' thrombocytopenia
See Chapter 8

In summary, the most helpful are the platelet count, fibrin degradation products, thrombin time and protamine precipitated monomers. The differential diagnosis of DIC is listed in Table 9.9 and the method of differentiation is shown in this table. It can be seen from this that liver disease with fibrinolysis may not be distinguishable from DIC, and note post-cardiac surgery where thrombocytopenia may result from the use of the pump, and heparin rebound occur, resulting in a situation which resembles DIC but which can be readily distinguished by the use of protamine to neutralize the heparin in the clotting studies.

Specific indications for treatment in DIC are as follows:

(1) Heparin should be given if there is an associated venous thrombosis or thrombo-embolism.
(2) It should also be given where there are ischaemic changes in the limbs or where the patient has purpura fulminans. The latter is a rare and very dramatic condition where the patient presents with haemorrhagic lesions especially marked in the upper and lower limbs with patches of purpura and necrosis with peripheral gangrene following unless treated promptly. Laboratory findings are severe thrombocytopenia with

disseminated intravascular clotting. The only effective treatment is immediate heparinization, failure to do so results in further bleeding and development of areas of gangrene together with sloughing and bleeding from the gastro-intestinal tract and death.

(3) Less specific indications are the use of heparin to control the bleeding in the patient prior to labour with a retained dead fetus.

(4) Heparin is probably also indicated in DIC which is associated with large venous anomalies such as in the Kassabach–Merrit syndrome, and it has also been advocated as a prophylactic measure during the treatment of promyelocytic leukaemia although this has been debated.

Replacement therapy employing cryoprecipitate and platelets should be considered if surgery is indicated, if bleeding is excessive and the diagnosis uncertain, such as may be the case in liver disease, and in abruptio placentae immediately prior to the evacuation of the uterus. One of the worries one always has in replacement therapy is the possibility that one may be 'adding fuel to the fire', and some consideration should always be given to the possible associated use of heparin in these circumstances. There is little need to add heparin in abruptio placentae, for example where the uterus can be readily evacuated. When looking through the reports of this disorder and in reviewing one's own experience, it is rare that replacement therapy causes problems. The overall outcome of the patient with disseminated intravascular coagulation rests entirely on the underlying condition causing the disorder, as is shown by the mortality associated with abruptio placentae being less than 1%, whereas the overall deaths from these conditions *in toto* listed in Table 9.7 is 50–80%. The use of anti-fibrinolytic agents such as ϵ-aminocaproic acid and tranexamic acid is absolutely contra-indicated since the inhibition of the fibrinolytic system in the acute stage of this condition could result in massive thrombosis, and the use of activated clotting factor preparations, e.g. prothrombinex, CSL (Commonwealth Serum Laboratories) are probably also contra-indicated.

References

ABRAHAMSEN, A.F. (1968). Platelet survival studies in man with special reference to thrombosis and atherosclerosis. *Scand. J. Haematol.*, (Suppl.), No. 3

ARKEL, Y.S., HAFT, J.I., KREUTNER, W., SHERWOOD, J. and WILLIAMS, R. (1977). Alteration in second phase platelet aggregation with emotionally stressful activity. *Thromb. Haemost.* (Stuttgart), **3**, 552

BLUNT, R.J. and PORTER, J.M. (1981). Raynaud Syndrome. *Semin. Arth. and Rheum.*, **10**, 282

CHESEBRO, J.H., CLEMENTS, I.P., FOSTER, V., ELVEBACK, L.R., SMITH, H.C., BARDSLEY, W.T., FRYE, R.L., HOLMES, D.R., VLIETSTRA, R.E., PLUTH, J.R., WALLACE, R.B., PUGA, F.J., ORSZULAK, T.R., PIEHLER, J.H., SCHAFF, H.V. and DANIELSON, G.K. (1982). A platelet-inhibitor-drug trial in coronary-artery bypass operations. Benefit of peri-operative dipyridamole and aspirin therapy in early postoperative vein–graft patency. *N. Engl. J. Med.*, **307**, 73

GREEN, D., ROSSI, E.C. and HARING, O. (1982). The B-blocker heart attack trial: Studies of platelets and factor VIII. *Thrombos. Res.*, **28**, 261

KINCAID-SMITH, P.S., LAVERN, M., FAIRLEY, K.F. and MATHEWS, D.C. (1979). Dipyridamole and anticoagulants in renal disease due to glomerular and vascular lesions. A new approach to therapy. *Med. J. Aust.*, **1**, 145

LANCE, J.W. (1981). Headache. *Ann. Neurol.*, **10**, 1

LEWIS, H.D. Jr., DAVIS, J.W., ARCHIBALD, D.G., STEINKE, W.E., SMITHERMAN, T.C., DOHERTY, J.E., SCHNAPER, H.W., Le WINTER, M.M., LINARES, E., POUGET, J.M., SABHARWAL, S.C., CHESLER, E. and De MOTS, H. (1983). Protective effects of aspirin against acute myocardial infarction and death in men with unstable angina. *N. Engl. J. Med.*, **309**, 396

MIELKE, C.H., KANESHIRO, M.M., MAHER, I.A., WEINER, J.M., and RAPAPORT, S.I. (1969). The standardised normal Ivy bleeding time and its prolongation by aspirin. *Blood*, **34**, 204

O'BRIEN, J.R. (1980). *Lancet*, (letter) 1, 981

ROSS, R. (1979). The arterial wall and atherosclerosis. *Ann. Rev. Med.*, **30**, 1

SALEM, H.H., KOUTTS, J. and FIRKIN, B.G. (1980). Circulating platelet aggregates in ischaemic heart disease and their correlation to platelet lifespan. *Thrombos. Res.*, **17**, 707

SALEM, H.H., KOUTTS, J., HANDLEY, C., VAN DER WEYDEN, M.B., DUDLEY, F.J. and FIRKIN, B.G. (1981). The aggregation of human platelets by ascitic fluid: A possible mechanism for disseminated intravascular coagulation complicating LeVeen shunts. *Am. J. Haematol.*, **11**, 153

The Canadian Co-operative Study Group. (1978). A randomised trial of aspirin and sulfinpyrazone in threatened stroke. *N. Engl. J. Med.*, **299**, 53

WEKSLER, B.B., PETT, S.B., ALONSO, D., RICHTER, R.C., STELZER, P., SUBRAMANIAN, V., TACK-GOLDMAN, K. and GAY, W.A. Jr. (1983). Differential inhibition by aspirin of vascular and platelet prostaglandin synthesis in atherosclerotic patients. *N. Engl. J. Med.*, **308**, 800

WU, K.K. and HOAK, J.C. (1974). A new method for the quantitative detection of platelet aggregates in patients with arterial insufficiency. *Lancet;* **2**, 924

10
A clinician's approach to the investigation of a patient with a bleeding diathesis

Accurate diagnosis rests on a thorough history of the patient's problems, and adequate physical examination combined with the knowledge of the physiology and pathology of haemostasis. Patients usually present with a history of easy bruising, epistaxis, excessive menstrual loss, bleeding from minor operative procedures such as teeth extractions. Anaemia may be the mode of presentation with bleeding from the gastro-intestinal tract or with menstrual loss. Occasionally haemostatic mechanisms have been found to be abnormal when tests have been conducted before an operation or during the course of an investigation of another illness. The latter are most commonly either thrombocytopenia or some abnormality of one of the more routine clotting tests, e.g. prolonged prothrombin time or a prolonged partial thromboplastin time with kaolin.

It is important to pinpoint the date of onset since this may determine whether the problem is familial or acquired. A careful family history should be taken, since in mild bleeding disorders there may be another member of the family more severely affected in whom the diagnosis may be more readily identified; this applies especially to von Willebrand disease and platelet release problems. It is not enough to ask the patients whether they have any relatives who have bleeding problems, but one must ensure identification of each particular close relative, mother, father, siblings, uncles, aunts and ask whether they have had any epistaxis, bleeding after minor operations such as dental extractions or tonsillectomy, menstrual abnormalities, blood transfusions etc. If the parents are available they should be asked whether there was any problem at childbirth of bleeding from the umbilicus, or, in a male, whether circumcision caused any bleeding problems. In the female, a careful menstrual history should always be taken and specific questions asked as follows:

(1)   Are your periods ever so heavy that you are socially embarrassed by them and have to stay at home?

(2)   Do you ever have to wear towelling rather than the standard tampon or pad?

(3)   Do you have to wear a pad as well as a tampon?

(4)   Do you ever have to wear two pads at once?

(5)   Do you ever soak through the tampon or the pad?

(6)   Has the blood loss increased with menstruation? When did you first notice this increase?

A positive reply to any of these questions may indicate that the patient has excessive menstrual loss, although the only absolute way of being certain in this regard would be to measure the amount lost using chromium labelled red cells. A change in the character of menstrual loss is also important, since in an acquired situation such as idiopathic thrombocytopenic purpura the woman's periods may be relatively light, only to become excessive when she develops the thrombocytopenia.

Questioning should then be directed towards minor operative procedures such as teeth extractions or other operative procedures, e.g. tonsillectomy. Any patient who has had a tonsillectomy without bleeding problems or blood transfusions, is very unlikely to have had a clinically significant bleeding diathesis at the time of operation. With a mild to moderate bleeding diathesis, bleeding after a tooth extraction may continue for 2 or more days and require a return to the dentist for attention. One should always ascertain the effects of trauma and whether or not bruising has occurred spontaneously. Has the patient ever had problems with playing active sports such as football, baseball, cricket, hockey or basketball?

The type and site of bleeding should be sought. Spontaneous bruising is only seen in serious bleeding defects and usually results in obvious laboratory abnormalities. Should spontaneous bruising not be associated with abnormal tests, the possibility of factitious purpura should be considered (v. infra). The site of the bleeding may suggest a purely local vascular lesion or trauma such as epistaxis, however if such bleeding is associated with other bruising or petechial eruptions, then consideration of other haemostatic factors is required. The history of blood on the toothbrush may reflect peridontal problems or result from a bleeding diathesis.

The bleeding is often episodic and in these instances special attention should be paid to the possibility of exposure to toxins, for example, alcohol or drugs, and laboratory investigations should be done at a time when the patient has his/her haemostatic problems. Some years ago the term cocktail purpura was introduced to describe the association of sensitization to quinine present in tonic water resulting in acute episodes of thrombocytopenia and purpura following the intake of this popular drink. Quinine has been used as a bitter ingredient in food flavouring, but this usage has not been reported to cause problems. The vast majority of patients with cocktail purpura referred to the author have bleeding problems as a direct result of their alcohol intake and not due to quinine sensitivity! It is often forgotten that alcohol is a potent depressant of bone marrow activity and can cause an acute destructive effect on platelets in certain patients.

The drugs reported to cause haemostatic problems are legion, and it is unwise to ignore the possibility that any drug may be capable of producing such problems. The ones to enquire particularly about are:

(1) The anticoagulants, remembering that there has been an increasing incidence of thrombocytopenia reported with heparin preparations over the past 5 years.

(2) The penicillins, especially carbenicillin, which in therapeutic doses causes qualitative platelet abnormalities, and therefore when being used in extremely sick patients may contribute to a bleeding diathesis.

(3) Penicillamine and gold salts.

(4) The thiazide diuretics.

(5) Chlorpromazine (in high doses there is a high incidence of a lupus-like anticoagulant but *without* bleeding (*v. infra*)).

(6) Aspirin will produce abnormal platelet function studies and may confuse the diagnostic picture and more rarely may cause hypoprothrombinaemia. In addition, aspirin has its local gastric effects, producing erosions and bleeding, and the non-steroidal anti-inflammatory drugs, e.g. indomethacin have similar properties.

(7) Quinine, which is most commonly found to cause thrombocytopenia when used by the elderly for night cramps, and quinidine, still one of the more popular cardiac anti-arrhythmics, may cause identical problems.

(8) Radiotherapy and cytotoxic agents.

(*see* also Tables 7.5, 8.3 and 8.5).

Enquiries should be made concerning wound healing, either following trauma or operative procedures. Abnormal wound healing has been reported with factor XIII deficiency, afribrinogenaemia, some of the congenital dysfibrinogenaemias, and with Ehler-Danlos syndrome where it may be due to an abnormality in fibronectin and/or collagen.

In children and young adults the acute exanthemata and infectious mononucleosis must be considered, and the typical features of these conditions sought.

Renal failure may be associated with a bleeding diathesis, and usually the patients are anaemic with rather a muddy complexion, and half and half fingernails, and may be found to be hypertensive. This presentation is now uncommon except where the renal failure is associated with some other medical condition such as myeloma, and here the bleeding diathesis is more commonly secondary to underlying disorders.

Scurvy is a rare cause of purpura in the Western societies, however instances of babies being fed food sterilized by over-zealous mothers thus destroying the heat labile vitamin C continue, as does its occasional appearance in patients who are 'down and out'. By far the most common vitamin deficiency causing either clinical problems or abnormal laboratory tests is that of vitamin K deficiency. This can be either due to malabsorption of vitamin K in such conditions as coeliac disease and steatorrhoea, or obstruction of the common bile duct or cholestatic liver disease. Synthesis of vitamin K dependent clotting factors may be abnormal in liver disease or during the intake of drugs such as warfarin. Only patients with liver disease or hereditary coagulation defects will not respond to vitamin K. A past history of recurrent acute abdominal pain together with a high alcohol intake may alert one to the possibility of pancreatitis causing steatorrhoea, as may bulky offensive stools which fail to flush readily in the toilet.

Recent descriptions of laboratory abnormalities induced by eating Chinese food (Schezwanese purpura) where the active ingredient is believed to be the Chinese fungus Mo-Er, and the description of Eskimos and volunteers receiving high amounts of salmon oil leading to prolonged skin bleeding time as well as other minor abnormalities in the platelet function profile, alert one to the possibility that dietary eccentricities may precipitate a mild bleeding diathesis (Chapter 7).

The remainder of the interview should be directed towards other areas of haematological significance such as the history of any past episodes of anaemia, any recent or recurrent infections, and the state of the health in general, appetite, weight stability, etc. Some enquiry should also be made concerning the non-haematological disorders which may classically involve the haemostatic mechanisms, some of which have already been alluded to, such as liver disease and steatorrhoea, but one group in particular which should always be remembered, are the collagen diseases. Questions should be directed towards past history of joint problems, pleurisy, recurrent mouth ulceration, patchy alopecia and Raynaud phenomenon, especially if this has been of recent onset. Apart from the direct involvement of the haemostatic mechanism, e.g. thrombocytopenia, these disorders are also characterized by a frequent relationship with vasculitis due to circulating immune complexes which may mimic the purpuric manifestations of thrombocytopenia. Much more rarely they may be associated with circulating anticoagulants directed against VIII:C resulting in severe haemostatic abnormalities. The most common circulating anticoagulant detected in the laboratory in patients with lupus erythematosus has little or no haemostatic effects, but may be associated with an increased incidence of thrombosis and recurrent spontaneous abortions in females.

Having completed the history, a careful physical examination should be undertaken. The distribution and extent of the bruising and purpuric eruptions should be noted and a search conducted for telangiectasia. If the patient has been ambulant, petechial eruptions secondary to thrombocytopenia are usually most marked in the lower limbs, and in mild cases may only be observed there. Petechial eruptions are small pin point areas, red in colour and having the appearance of a flea bite without the associated urticarial reaction. In the case of scurvy these eruptions are localized to the follicular region and are associated with changes in hair growth, which instead of being straight becomes corkscrew in appearance. If the thrombocytopenia is more severe, the petechiae will be more generalized and may appear on the thorax and abdomen as well as the back and upper limbs. In severe thrombocytopenia these become confluent and will form ecchymoses 1–4 cm in diameter or larger, while in very severe instances spontaneous deep ecchymoses and bruising occur.

In infectious mononucleosis even without thrombocytopenia, petechiae are often noted over the soft palate. The appearance of large blood blisters in the mouth appears to relate to the severity of the thrombocytopenia and may be seen in any situations where the platelet count suddenly drops, e.g. with drugs or in infectious disorders such as Onylai seen in South Africa. The lips, tongue, mouth and nose should be examined for spider naevi which may be associated with Osler disease or hereditary telangiectasia. The tongue may show atrophy of the filiform papillae which may be seen in iron deficiency, folate or B_{12} deficiency, and the gums and teeth margins may be hypertrophied and bleeding in acute monocytic leukaemia, but also in other forms of leukaemia. Mouth ulcerations may occur in a number of situations including lupus erythematosus and leukaemia.

The distribution of the bruises is particularly helpful. Superficial bruising often associated with pigmentation is frequently seen on the forearms and backs of hands in senile purpura. An identical form of purpura is seen in patients who are receiving high doses of prednisolone or who have Cushing syndrome. There are often associated skin changes which are frequently seen in elderly people, namely transverse linear white scars (cigarette paper skin), and an apparent loss of skin elasticity and turgor. Usually such changes are of no special significance, but they may be exaggerated when they are accompanied by any form of bleeding diathesis.

Waldenstrom hypergammaglobulinaemic purpura is characterized by recurrent episodes of purpuric eruptions, usually localized to the lower limbs leaving areas of pigmentation due to haemosiderin deposition and is associated with high ESR and increased globulin levels.

Vasculitic lesions associated with systemic lupus are characteristically seen in the periungual regions of the nail fold or as small infarcts on the fingertips and sometimes a splinter haemorrhage in the nail itself. They may be accompanied by vasculitic skin lesions in the periphery which are similar to those seen in any form of immune complex including mixed cryoglobulins related to underlying inflammatory conditions or to cryoglobulinaemia and paraprotein-aemias. These may vary from haemorrhagic eruptions to circumscribed punched out areas of necrosis. Henoch–Schonlein purpura has a characteristic distribution usually involving the extensor surfaces of the knee and often appearing over the buttocks, but it may be very diffuse and involve most of the extremities. Sometimes urticaria is a striking feature. It most commonly occurs in children and young adults and frequently is accompanied by poly-arthralgia, recurrent abdominal pain and haematuria.

Amyloid disease may have a very characteristic appearance with two black eyes due to ecchymosis around the upper and lower eyelids without a history of trauma. Other features of the disease may be present such as scalloping of the edges of the tongue or a very firm infiltrated and painful tongue. This condition is curious because of the sometimes quite dramatic association of pinch purpura in which the pinching of a fold of the skin on the neck or other areas of the body may result in the rapid appearance of a bruise. Amyloid should be excluded in any patient who presents with isolated factor X deficiency, since the amyloid fibrils have the property of absorbing this factor and may shorten its life span sufficiently to cause factor X deficiency.

Hyperelasticity of the skin, particularly around the neck, and hyper-extensibility of the joints may alert the physician to consider Ehlers-Danlos syndrome where the poor support given to the blood vessels may result in bruising occurring after very minor trauma, the condition may be associated with factor VII deficiency. One family has been reported with abnormal platelet aggregation which was corrected by the addition of fibronectin, and some workers have reported that surface bound platelet fibronectin is the membrane receptor on the platelet for collagen, although this has been disputed.

Bruising which is unusual in nature and distribution such as that confined to the breast, that which has abnormal shapes, lesions which are uniformly symmetrical and which only appear in places which the patient can reach all should raise the question of the possibility that this is artifactual (*v. infra*).

Pseudo xanthoma elasticum with the characteristic 'chicken skin' appear-ance and angioid streaks in the fundus may present with gastro-intestinal bleeding. Angiodysplasia is another situation which may result in severe blood loss in the gastro-intestinal tract, and is a vascular malformation usually confined to the large bowel especially on the right side. It has been reported associated with vWd (*see* Chapter 6), and with aortic valve lesions and mitral valve prolapse (Barlow syndrome) as well as appearing spontaneously.

Racial background and bleeding problems have been associated, and factor XI deficiency is the best documented being uncommon in people without Jewish ancestory.

Following the assessment of the patient's blood pressure, a Hess test should be performed. It is undertaken by placing the blood pressure cuff in the usual position and inflating it to 100 mmHg, checking that this does not obliterate the radial arterial pulse. Prior to inflation the arm should be carefully examined and any petechiae or telangiectasia noted. Following inflation the arm should be observed and the cuff maintained at 100 mmHg for 5 minutes unless the patient complains or a shower of petechial eruptions appear when the cuff should be deflated. Following the 5 minutes the cuff is deflated and the arm is observed over the next 2–3 minutes. Should ten or more petechiae develop, the test is positive. A heavy shower of petechiae strongly supports the possibility that the patient has thrombocytopenia and should be confirmed by undertaking a skin bleeding time (*v. infra*).

The patient's fundus should be examined after dilating the patient's pupils. The occurrence of retinal haemorrhages constitutes a medical emergency since the patient is at risk of visual loss, hence a diagnosis must be reached rapidly and appropriate measures instituted. It is very important to observe any other changes which may have occurred in the retina, especially engorgement of the veins with segmentation (cattle trucking) which is the characteristic appearance of the hyperviscosity syndrome seen in macroglobulinaemia and other paraproteinaemias. It should be emphasized that fundal haemorrhages rarely, if ever, occur in situations of chronic idiopathic thrombocytopenic purpura, and their appearance immediately alerts one to the possibility that the patient has an underlying disease process such as leukaemia, aplastic anaemia, lupus erythematosus or one of the paraproteinaemias. Rarer causes include pernicious anaemia and folic acid deficiency where they may result from a combination of qualitative platelet defects as well as a usually mild degree of thrombocytopenia and severe anaemia.

Next the examination should concentrate on the haematopoietic system. Pallor is assessed by examining the hands and palmar creases, the conjunctival and the oral mucosa. The presence of bone pain is sought by pressure over the sternum, pelvis or ribs. The presence of an enlarged spleen or liver should be noted, and a careful examination performed of the inguinal axillary and cervical regions for lymphadenopathy as well as looking in sites such as the epitrochlear nodes and the lingual and pharyngeal tonsils. A complete physical examination should then be conducted, remembering that conditions such as disseminated intravascular coagulation can be associated with many disorders such as cancer, septicaemia, subacute bacterial endocarditis and liver disease. Late systolic mitral bruits characteristic of prolapsed mitral valves have been reported to be associated with von Willebrand disease. Hypertension may increase the risk of an intracranial bleed and diabetes may be accentuated by steroid therapy. The presence of scoliosis should be noted since a mild platelet defect has been reported in this condition.

INVESTIGATIVE TESTS FOR HAEMOSTASIS

Platelet disorders

The following investigations should be undertaken on patients with a haemo-

Table 10.1   Tests to be undertaken in haemostatic disorders due to platelet abnormalities

Hess test
Skin bleeding time
Urine
Peripheral blood film
Full blood count and ESR
* Bone marrow aspirate and trephine
Coagulation screen (Table 10.2)
* Glass bead adhesiveness
* Prothrombin consumption test
Platelet factor 3 release
* Platelet associated immunoglobulin
* Platelet surface associated immunoglobulin
Platelet aggregation studies
* Platelet lifespan

*tests which need to be undertaken when dictated by clinical circumstances

static disorder due to platelet abnormalities (Table 10.1). Asterisks indicate tests which need to be undertaken when dictated by clinical circumstances. The remainder constitute an initial routine screen for a patient in whom a platelet abnormality is suspected.

At the bedside, one should always examine the urine for the presence of blood and also send off a sample of urine for microscopic examination. Skin bleeding time should be performed by either the Duke or the Ivy method. In the former, the earlobe is lanced by a stylet used for obtaining peripheral blood from the finger, and every 30 seconds the blood is removed by a filter paper, taking care not to touch the lacerated area. The normal range for a Duke bleeding time is $3\frac{1}{2}$–$4\frac{1}{2}$ minutes. The other bedside technique is the Ivy technique in which a blood pressure cuff is applied to the arm and set at 40 mmHg. Three lacerations are made on the volar surface of the forearm, being careful to avoid superficial veins, using the same kind of stylet as indicated before. Filter paper is again used to remove the blood every 30 seconds, once more taking care not to touch the site of laceration. The average of the time for the three bleeding sites to stop is made, and this is 2–7 minutes. More accurate assessments of skin bleeding time can be made using specially prepared templates to standardize the depth and diameter of the cut.

The Hess test is a very rough test but can be helpful in distinguishing clotting from platelet abnormalities. A positive Hess test indicates either that the platelet count is low, there is a qualitative platelet defect such as Glanzmann disease, or that some disorder is present which is affecting the capillaries, making them less effective in haemostasis, such as scurvy. A faintly positive test, e.g. ten petechiae, can be seen in normal people, and one must carefully inspect the skin to exclude previously present small microhaemangioma which bleed following this procedure resulting in an appearance resembling a petechial eruption.

A peripheral blood count should be undertaken and a blood film examination together with an erythrocyte sedimentation rate (ESR). If the peripheral film is obtained by a needle-prick platelet clumps may be observed making aggregation platelet defects less likely, and the morphology of the platelet may be helpful in unusual problems such as the Bernard–Soulier syndrome or the Gray platelet syndrome. Giant platelets and circulating megakaryocytic fragments may also be seen in a number of the myeloproliferative disorders and a population of large platelets is often seen in a regenerative thrombocytopenia, e.g. ITP. The remainder of the peripheral film may give a clue as to the underlying haematological condition causing a disturbance in platelet count or platelet function.

If the platelet count is increased, then features may be seen in the peripheral film which may help make the diagnosis, such as the presence of polychromasia and hypochromia in chronic blood loss, tear drop red cells in a patient with myelofibrosis, etc. Similarly, when the platelet count is decreased, the peripheral film may be very helpful, e.g. the lymphopenia associated with either a collagen disorder such as lupus erythematosus or uraemia, the presence of blasts in a patient with acute leukaemia, or the presence of hypersegmentation of white cells together with oval macrocytosis suggesting B_{12} or folic acid deficiency.

The ESR is useful, since it may support the possibility of some underlying inflammatory state or may point to the suggestion of an abnormal protein or circulating immune complexes. More information can be obtained if the ESR is performed at 4 °C as well as at room temperature, 25 °C, since cold agglutinins will cause a higher sedimentation and cryoglobulins a lower one at 4 °C.

If the platelet count is abnormal a bone marrow aspirate and trephine should be performed with stains for iron and collagen tissue in the marrow, and should there be signs of dyshaematopoiesis in the peripheral blood, chromosomal analysis also undertaken. A standard coagulation screen (Table 10.2) is obtained, and this consists of a whole blood clotting time with assessment of clot retraction by eye at $\frac{1}{2}$ hour, 1 hour and 2 hours. Should it be required, a semi-quantitative method of clot retraction can be undertaken using either whole blood or recalcified platelet-rich plasma in graduated test tubes, into which a corkscrew type rod is suspended and at the end of an appropriate time interval, say 2 hours, is removed, and with it the attached clot. One can then measure the remaining fluid volumetrically. The less clot retraction, the less fluid left. A Quick one-stage prothrombin time, a partial

Table 10.2 Standard coagulation screen

Whole blood clotting time
Prothrombin time
Partial thromboplastin time with kaolin (PTTK)
Thrombin time
Fibrinogen
Clot stability to 5 mol/l urea (screen for factor XIII deficiency)

thromboplastin time with kaolin, a thrombin time and if the platelet count is diminished, a fibrin degradation products assay should all be employed. If the PTTK is prolonged a mixing test with normal plasma will exclude an anticoagulant as a cause.

Apart from being an important screen to ensure that the bleeding diathesis, if present, is not due to coincidental clotting problems, these tests may give a lead as to the underlying cause of platelet problems. For example, a patient with liver disease might have a slightly prolonged prothrombin time, normal PTTK and a thrombin time of 22 seconds against a normal of 12 seconds, and negative fibrin degradation products. The likely cause of a mild thrombocytopenia here would be secondary splenomegaly due to liver disease. The presence of a slightly prolonged or normal prothrombin time with a normal thrombin time and a prolonged PTTK which does not correct on 1:1 mixing with normal plasma, indicates the presence of an anticoagulant, and if the platelet count is reduced could indicate lupus erythematosus.

Glass bead adhesiveness should not be requested unless the laboratory concerned is particularly interested in bleeding diatheses and prepared to monitor this particular test very closely. It is a 'finicky' test and from a routine laboratory's point of view is largely covered by other investigations which can be more readily quantitated, such as ristocetin-induced platelet aggregation.

The prothrombin consumption test (PCT) or serum prothrombin time is also a test which would not be recommended for routine laboratories unless they had a special interest in haemostatic disorders. This test may be an important part of the documentation of unusual disorders such as Bernard–Soulier syndrome, Heckathorn disease and isolated families with a moderate bleeding diathesis in whom the only consistently abnormal haemostatic test is the PCT.

Platelet factor 3 activation or release tests consist of recalcifying platelet-rich plasma and sub-sampling at time intervals of 10–15 seconds, then adding 0.1 ml of the sub-sample together with stypven and calcium, and observing the clotting time. Over 20 minutes there is a progressive decrease of more than 10 seconds, in our laboratory, by from 45 to 33 s. Lesser drops will be seen in patients with thrombocytopenia, some qualitative platelet defects such as storage pool disorders, Bernard–Soulier syndrome and Glanzmann disease, as well as patients who are on drugs which inhibit release, such as aspirin. This type of test is also applied when one is seeking platelet antibodies to drugs and is, therefore, a valuable test at present to have in the routine laboratory.

Platelet antibody tests still represent an area of controversy since although a plethora of such tests have evolved over the past 3–4 years, it still must remain largely in the hands of the individual laboratory concerned as to which particular investigative procedure should be undertaken from the viewpoint of reliability, cost and expertise available. We continue to use one antibody test based on the platelet factor 3 reaction which is a minor modification of the test first proposed by Horowitz. Although this test is not uniformly positive in patients with auto-immune thrombocytopenia, it gives consistently positive results in situations of some drug-induced purpuras such as quinine and quinidine, and in transfusion purpura seen with PlA1 deficiency as well as HLA antibodies. In our hands it does not correlate with platelet associated immunoglobulin IgG levels in ITP. Platelet associated IgG levels are elevated in 80–90% of patients when they first appear with auto-immune thrombocytopenic purpura. Where this test falls down is that there are a number of other circumstances in which the platelet associated immuno-globulin levels may be elevated, such as in patients with inflammatory states, infections or cancer. Whether the measurement of immune IgG attached to the platelet membrane, Surface Platelet Immunoglobulin, or a ratio of this to total platelet IgG levels will be more valuable is yet to be elucidated. It does seem likely, however, from results in many different laboratories, that one should measure both platelet IgG, IgA and IgM levels as well as C3. Techniques for this are now available but are yet to be fully evaluated. The combination of Platelet Associated Immunoglobulin level (total Platelet Immunoglobulin levels or PAIg) together with Surface Associated Immunoglobulin, SAIg, i.e. those immunoglobulins detected on the cell's surface appears to be useful in both drug induced and auto-immune thrombocytopenia.

Platelet aggregation studies are undertaken in a nepthelometer and are currently one of the more important tests for detecting qualitative platelet defects. The platelet count in this test should be kept at a constant level, and the following agonists are added to the platelet-rich plasma in the cuvette:

(1) Collagen
(2) Adrenalin,
(3) Adenosine diphosphate
(4) Ristocetin 0.25 mg/ml, 1 mg/ml, 1.5 mg/ml, 2 mg/ml,
(5) Thrombin,
(6) Arachidonic acid
(7) Ionophore – calcium ionophore

The ADP concentration selected relates to whether one is looking for hyperaggregability, such as may be seen in some disorders such as diabetes, in which case the lower concentrations are included for ADP, adrenalin and thrombin. Low concentrations of ristocetin are added to detect one of the variants of von Willebrand disease which aggregates at concentrations of ristocetin far below that required for normal platelet-rich plasma to aggregate. The ionophore study is done not only to see whether or not it will induce aggregation, by examining the cell's ability to mobilize Ca^{2+} but also as a safety measure to exclude aspirin type defects, since patients who have taken aspirin or who have cyclo-oxygenase defects will respond to these agents. Such patients should be re-checked at a later date and warned not to take any drugs 10 days prior to the investigation.

Platelet lifespan and platelet survival studies

This investigation can be very helpful clinically in deciding whether a patient has acquired immune thrombocytopenia.

Table 10.3 Available techniques for performing platelet survival studies in humans

Technique	Method	Advantages	Disadvantages
Duke (1911)	Platelet transfusion. Daily platelet counts	Minimal handling of platelets. No isotopes required	Can be used only when recipient has low platelet count and platelets are always homologous
^{32}DFP	Inject ^{32}DFP intramuscularly. Collect samples daily	No handling of platelets during labelling procedure. Probably no re-utilization	Megakaryocytes labelled as well as platelets, and so survival is prolonged. All cells in peripheral blood are labelled as well as the plasma proteins. Because of the 'platelet atmosphere', probably impossible to wash platelets free of all contamination. Cannot employ surface counting technique
^{32}P	Platelets isolated from patient treated with ^{32}P, and transfused into recipient. Collect daily samples	Minimal handling of platelets	Re-utilization. ^{32}P is incorporated into nucleotides, proteins and phospholipids which are undergoing metabolic turnover, and may be exchanged with plasma. Platelets always homologous and perhaps abnormal. Cannot employ surface counting technique
^{51}Cr	Platelet isolated, incubated with ^{51}Cr and re-infused into recipient. Collect samples daily and surface scan	Readily available isotope, which can be measured in similar well-scintillation counter used in red cell survival. External surface scanning may be performed	Must handle platelets to label. Can use autologous platelets only when count is greater than 100×10^9/l

Table 10.3 *cont'd*

Technique	Method	Advantages	Disadvantages
[^{14}C] Serotonin	Incubate platelets with ^{14}C-serotonin and then infuse. The [^{14}C] serotonin may be given intravenously to the patient. Collect daily samples	Can employ autologous platelets at times. Can avoid handling of platelets	Specialized isotope equipment necessary. Cannot employ surface counting techniques. Risk of re-utilization and/or exchange with body pools
[^{75}Se]Methionine	Inject [^{75}Se] methionine intravenously. Collect samples daily	No handling of platelets for labelling	Re-utilization of isotope and other cell plasma proteins are also labelled
Aspirin	600 mg taken orally after 48 hours, daily samples taken and malondialdehyde production following thrombin stimulation of platelet-rich plasma measured by fluorometry until it returns to pre-aspirin levels	No handling of platelets to label	Not suitable in thrombocytopenia since it could aggravate bleeding
Indium	Platelets isolated but smaller volumes are required compared with ^{51}Cr technique. ^{111}In oxine is incubated, washed and infused into recipient. Daily samples and surface scanning	Best isotope for surface scan studies since high γ-emitter	Very short lifespan of indium requiring cyclotron in vicinity

Platelet lifespan studies have aided the classification of thrombocyto-penia and have been exploited to demonstrate shortened platelet survival in disorders involving the vasculature as well as blood, e.g. diabetes, athero-sclerosis, myocardial infarction, etc. They have also been used as a yard stick to measure the effectiveness of drugs in correcting a shortened platelet life-span.

The most commonly employed technique is chromium (^{51}Cr) although indium offers advantages and may be more commonly employed in the future. The latter isotope is impractical at present in Australia since it requires a cyclotron for its production and has a half life of only 2.8 days. Table 10.3 lists techniques which have been employed to estimate the lifespan of platelets in man and indicates their advantages and disadvantages. The ideal label would be one which could be injected intravenously into the patient, would

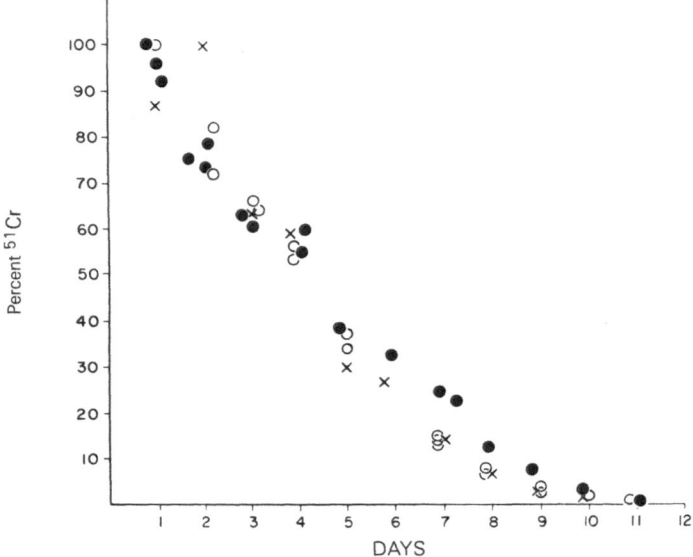

Figure 10.1 Platelet survival studies in three subjects using ^{51}Cr with frequent sampling to illustrate the reproducability of the technique. (From *J. Lab. Clin. Med.*, **64**, 195, reproduced by permission of the Editor)

specifically label platelets, enable surface counting and not be re-utilized. Although this ideal will be hard to achieve, a recent development in this direction has been the use of aspirin which binds irreversibly to the enzyme cyclo-oxygenase in platelets results in the inhibition of prostaglandin pathway and, therefore, malondialdehyde formation following thrombin stimulation. The patient is given one dose of aspirin and samples taken at daily or more frequent intervals; platelet malondialdehyde function following thrombin is measured, and the platelet survival estimated by the gradual restoration of production to normal. Its successful use in performing platelet lifespan studies in large groups of patients encourages the belief that better techniques may be developed in the future.

Figure 10.1 is a typical example of a normal platelet lifespan using ^{51}Cr-labelled platelets in three patients. Using ^{51}Cr the major portion of the graph is linear, and in our laboratory the T$\frac{1}{2}$ is 4.8 ± 0.42 days with a total lifespan of 9.2 ± 0.8 days. Another piece of information which may be obtained from this study is the platelet recovery or yield which is calculated by the following:

recovery % = platelet c.p.m./ml of blood × blood volume × $\dfrac{100}{\text{cpm/ml}}$ of infusion × volume infused.

Normally in our laboratory this is between 65% and 85%. The commonest cause of diminished recovery is splenomegaly secondary to cirrhosis.

It will be noted that the platelets' radioactivity is expressed as a percentage, 100% being taken as the highest activity recovered from the peripheral blood (Figure 10.1). If the time taken in the labelling procedure is prolonged, as is often the case when a technician is using the technique for the first few times, the 100% recovery often occurs 24 hours after the injection, and presumably represents the sequestering of mildly damaged platelets in areas of the body such as the spleen and then their re-entry and normal survival. Whether this is simply a case of the damaged platelets being metabolically reconstituted or secondary to the excessive handling resulting in them being more sticky with resolution after the first day or so in the body is not known. This phenomenon can be seen in patients after splenectomy, and then probably represents a pool of platelets in some other tissues in the body such as the lungs.

Coagulation disorders

Table 10.2 lists the coagulation tests which our laboratory employs as an initial screening procedure to investigate a patient with a bleeding problem; however a more common practice is to employ the prothrombin time, thrombin time and the partial thromboplastin time with kaolin (or activated partial thrombo-plastin time), all of which can be readily automated.

Table 10.4 Prothrombin time prolonged, thrombin time normal, PTTK (APTT) normal or prolonged

Causes
> Vitamin K deficiency
>> Malabsorption
>> Obstructed bile duct
>> Poor diet, and antibiotic or cholestyramine
>
> Liver disease
>
> Oral anticoagulants
>
> Spontaneous anticoagulant (e.g. anti-V)
>
> Hereditary causes

Action
> Depends on clinical situation. If urgent correction is needed, give fresh frozen plasma or appropriate blood products, but *always* store pre-infusion blood sample so subsequent assays may be performed if necessary.
> If non-urgent and not contra-indicated (e.g. wish to continue patient on oral anti-coagulants), give vitamin K

Tables 10.4–10.7 inclusive demonstrate the common finding with various coagulation abnormalities employing these three tests.

Table 10.4 sets out the situation when the predominant abnormality is an increased prothrombin time. If the thrombin time and the PTTK are both normal, this would imply that only factor VII deficiency was present (*see* Chapter 3). There may be deficiencies in other liver produced coagulation

Table 10.5 Prothrombin time normal, thrombin time normal, APTT/PTTK prolonged but returned to normal with 1:1 mix with normal plasma

---

Causes

Abnormality in contact system XI, XII, prekallikrein (Fletcher factor) high molecular weight kininogen (Fitzgerald, Williams, Flaujeac trait)

IX and VIII deficiency (haemophilia)

Possovoy defect

Miscellaneous

Action

Sample pre-treatment
If clinically indicated, fresh frozen plasma and/or cryoprecipitate

Appropriate factor assays

---

factors which are insufficient to prolong the PTTK, but significant deficiencies in factors X, V and prothrombin would increase the PTTK. In the case of liver disease a thrombin time would also often be prolonged since when the liver is sufficiently damaged it produces an abnormal fibrinogen which has more sialic acid than usual. Oral anticoagulants, when in therapeutic ranges, have an increase in the PTTK as well as the PT but only the PT may be prolonged where an inadequate dose has been given. A spontaneous anticoagulant would show poor correction on mixing of both the PTTK and the prothrombin time. If desirable, individual factor assays can be performed using the appropriate deficient substrates.

Table 10.5 outlines deficiencies associated with a prolonged PTTK which is returned to normal on mixing with normal plasma. If the PTTK is markedly prolonged and there is little or no history of a bleeding diathesis, then some abnormality in the contact system should be suspected and appropriate assays undertaken. If there is a story of bleeding, then it is likely that this patient will have either factor IX, factor VIII or perhaps factor XI deficiency which can be determined by the appropriate assays (*see* Chapter 3). The Passovoy deficiency refers to a mild to moderate bleeding disorder with an autosomal dominant inheritance which is categorized by menorrhagia in the female, bleeding after teeth extractions or surgery and some increased bruising on trauma, but rarely spontaneous bruising or haemarthroses. The defect remains present after lengthy incubation of kaolin with PTTK unlike some contact factor defects, and does not appear to be vitamin K dependent. The PTTK is only slightly prolonged, being only a few seconds above the control range, all the other coagulation tests are normal including the thromboplastin generation time using either diluted or undiluted components with normal plasma as a substrate. Correction occurs with mixing of normal plasma, but no correction occurs between patients. A number of these patients had been previously diagnosed as having factor XI deficiency. So far this factor has only been clearly identified from one laboratory, but it may be the cause of numerous descriptions of minor prolongations of the PTTK times of other laboratories.

Table 10.6 Prothrombin time normal or prolonged, thrombin time prolonged APTT/PTTK normal or prolonged

Causes
    Low fibrinogen
        Liver disease
        Disseminated intravascular coagulation
        Hereditary

    Abnormal fibrinogen
        Liver disease
        Hereditary

    Fibrin breakdown products
        DIC

Action
    Store sample

    If clinically indicated, give fresh plasma, fibrinogen or cryoprecipitate

    Other investigations to establish cause

There also appears to be a miscellaneous group with a mildly prolonged PTTK without any bleeding history and who can undergo surgery without any problems. In one survey examining all patients who passed through a routine laboratory and had a prolonged PTTK, some 10% lay in this group. Of the remainder, 10% were laboratory error and the others were associated with problems such as liver disease, etc. which were known to prolong the PTTK.

Table 10.6 shows situations where all three tests may be prolonged in which case the abnormality is related to fibrinogen.

Table 10.7 in which the PTTK solely is prolonged, but where there is no correction when mixing with normal plasma, suggests the presence of an anticoagulant. This is further confirmed by showing that reducing the ratio of the

Table 10.7 Prothrombin time normal, thrombin time normal, APTT/PTTK prolonged – 1:1 mix with normal plasma no correction

Causes
    Anticoagulant
        Lupus inhibitor
        VIII:C inhibitor
        Others – IX inhibitor

Action
    Store sample

    If clinically indicated, steroids and/or blood products

    Establish cause by appropriate investigations

patients' plasma to normal plasma, so that one part of the patient's plasma is mixed with nine of normal, and the test is still prolonged, strongly indicates that this is a result of the presence of an anticoagulant. This can then be further identified by individual factor assays or by isolation of IgG from the plasma by appropriate techniques, and then showing that the activity resides in the immunoglobulin fraction. Most of these anticoagulants are IgGs, but some have been reported in other immunoglobulins especially IgM. A common laboratory error in this regard is to forget to exclude the possibility that the patient has received heparin or that heparin has contaminated some of the collecting apparatus but then the thrombin time should be prolonged. This can be checked by using protamine sulphate to neutralize the heparin, or by obtaining another sample from the patient. One anticoagulant which is being increasingly recognized is the so-called 'lupus inhibitor'. This parti-cular inhibitor was first observed in patients with lupus erythematosus. Unlike VIII:C inhibitors, this anticoagulant is immediate in its effect and its presence can be confirmed by undertaking a prothrombin time using increas-ingly dilute amounts of substitute brain extract (the Simplastin dilution test). The majority of patients have an abnormal Simplastin dilution test and usually a prolonged PTTK, but in some instances only one of these tests is abnormal, and there is some evidence which suggests there may be more than one type of lupus inhibitor. In this test using the dilute phospholipid reagent, there is an increasing prolongation of the prothrombin time compared with normal on increasing dilution of the reagent. Occasionally the prothrombin time will be prolonged initially. Another test we have found useful is to delibe-rately activate platelets by preincubating with ADP or washing or freeze/ thawing them and adding to a PTTK. In the case of the lupus inhibitor, the PTTK will usually be corrected. Clinically these inhibitors occur in approx-imately 10–30% of patients with active lupus or following the exposure to certain drugs, most commonly chlorpromazine and in otherwise normal individuals, for no apparent reason.

Unlike the lupus inhibitor, the VIII:C inhibitor usually causes quite dramatic haemostatic problems with spontaneous bruising and severe bleeding episodes. This inhibitor can arise spontaneously in elderly people, pregnant women and very rarely in patients with lupus erythematosus. Its commonest occurrence is in patients with haemophilia who are receiving replacement therapy. Unlike the lupus inhibitor, this inhibitor may increase its effect on the PTTK on longer incubation. The specific nature of this inhibitor can be confirmed by factor VIII assays.

Inhibitors to other clotting factors have also been reported, most commonly directed against factors V, X and IX, but these are rare in comparison with the ones previously mentioned. Inhibitors directed to factors V and X have strikingly prolonged prothrombin times as well as prolonged PTTKs. Apart from auto-immune diseases, the patient should be investigated for paraproteinaemias.

If the screening tests are normal, further investigations depend largely on the clinical findings in the patient. If one is satisfied that there is a moderate to severe bleeding diathesis, then one should proceed to introduce other tests to exclude more unusual problems, such as factor XIII deficiency or abnormalities in the fibrinolytic pathway, and in such situations one may also consider the use of more complicated two stage tests, both as screening tests, e.g. the thromboplastin generation test or the thrombin generation test (*see* Chapter 3), or as individual tests to exclude individual clotting factor deficiencies as outlined in Chapter 3.

In particular clinical situations, artifactual or self-inflicted purpura should be considered. This is especially the case where the distribution and the nature of the purpura is unusual and artificial in appearance, or where it is very symmetrical and is in unusual sites such as the breasts, or where the only sites of the purpura are areas to which the patient would have ready access. This type of diathesis is most commonly seen in patients who are in the medical profession or have an occupation closely related to it, such as nursing, medical technicians, etc. There is sometimes a history of a previous accident in which there have been haematomas or even a genuine disorder such as thrombocytopenic purpura which has responded to treatment. The patient is most commonly female and may be highly intelligent. Whilst one always should suspect this condition where the haemostatic tests are normal, one should remember that such patients are quite capable of inducing abnormal tests by taking drugs, in particular warfarin and/or aspirin. An appropriate blood or urine drug screen may be helpful in determining this. Sometimes the diagnosis can be extremely difficult to sustain, but a useful trick in this regard is to modify the test used for auto-erythrocyte sensitization purpura. In this test the patient's own red cells are taken and washed and injected intradermally at spaced intervals in the forearm. Two different syringes are employed and the patient is allowed to learn that the doctor expects one of the injections to bruise and the other not to because of special treatment of the red cells. One then vacates the room for a few hours, or asks the patient to return the next day. A positive test is where one site has no more than the usual deposit of red cells under it and the other has marked bruising. Another technique which has been employed has been to encase an area in which bruising has occurred in a plaster, and in the case of self-inflicted problems, no fresh bruising will occur. Regardless of approach, the problem of discussing this with the patient is extremely difficult. In the author's experience there are basically two groups of patients involved, one in whom the artifactual bruising is done for some form of deliberate gain, e.g. to avoid school or work, or to prevent the discovery of an extra-marital relationship. These instances may be related to some form of hysteria, in others there appears to be a much deeper psychological disturbance which at times may be masochistic or even schizophrenic. In any event it is important in such circumstances, if the diagnosis is substantiated, to obtain expert psychiatric help and to involve one's psychiatric colleague in

Table 10.8 Post-operative bleeding

Unsecured bleeding point

Disseminated intravascular coagulation (DIC)
    Shock
    Sepsis
    Incompatible transfusion

Massive transfusion
    Deficent coagulation factors fibrinogen, V, VIII
    Thrombocytopenia
    Incompatible transfusion
    Citrate toxicity

Liver disease

Renal disease

Drugs
    Heparin
    Antibiotics

---

discussion with the patient and subsequent management.

Auto-erythrocyte sensitization is a bleeding disorder which may be a form of psychogenic purpura in most instances. These people are often patients who have been involved in previous trauma and later spontaneous bruising develops. Intradermal injection of the patient's own red cells may lead to severe bruising and hence the term auto-erythrocyte sensitization. For further information of this syndrome and psychogenic purpura the reader should consult the excellent review by Ratnoff.

One of the difficult areas of diagnosis in bleeding diatheses which may trouble the clinician is where the causes can be multi-factorial. Post-operative bleeding is of particular importance in this regard. Table 10.8 outlines some of the problems which may be encountered post-operatively. In this instance quick decisions have to be made as the patient is often desperately ill, and whilst it is only human to attribute continued bleeding to some fault in the haemostatic mechanism, it must be realized that the most common cause of this problem is some unsecured bleeding point. This must always be given the first consideration, even when some bleeding defect has been demonstrated, either before or after the surgery, and especially so if the haemostatic screening of clotting (Table 10.2), DIC (Chapter 9) and platelets (Table 10.1) are normal. Often, however, one is confronted with a desperately ill patient who has oozing from his surgical incisions and also bleeding around intravenous injection sites and lines, sometimes accompanied by spontaneous purpura and ecchymoses. There is no simple rule of thumb in this situation, however, all the points listed in Table 10.8 should be considered. Disseminated intravascular coagulation can rapidly be diagnosed using tests discussed in Chapter 9. If this diagnosis is sustained, it is essential to detect and reverse the trigger, and the three things to be thought of in this regard are shock, sepsis and incompatible blood transfusion. The latter is particularly important to remember and to exclude by undertaking tests for intravascular haemolysis such as a Shumm test for methaemalbumin, and checking that there is no haemoglobinuria. It is essential in these circumstances to do all in one's power to maintain renal function and urinary output by the appropriate use of volume expanders and osmotic agents such as mannitol and diuretics. Although the theoretical risk of transfusion of platelets and plasma coagulation factors has often been advanced as sustaining disseminated intravascular coagulation, it should be appreciated that deaths from this type of treatment have been rarely reported, and that the major aim and treatment of the disorder should be correction of the underlying cause, and that probably little harm results from using judicious replacement therapy with platelet infusions and fresh frozen plasma.

Post-operative bleeding following massive transfusion was first documented in the mid-1950s, and was reported in situations where patients had received between 5 and 20 litres of blood. This problem is particularly likely to arise where stored whole blood has been used in the post-surgical transfusions, and can be largely avoided by the use of packed cells, fresh frozen plasma and platelet packs, or by adopting some fixed policy such as giving one unit of fresh frozen plasma and two units of platelets for every five units of stored blood. The reasons for this are that the major deficiencies in stored blood are due to factors V and VIII and platelets. As a result most investigations of patients who have received massive amounts of stored blood without the precautions outlined above, have shown a prolonged prothrombin time and partial thromboplastin time with kaolin due to factor V and VIII deficiencies, as well as a thrombocytopenia of varying degrees. It should be emphasized that in the post-operative situation it is not safe to adopt any magic figure for platelet count if a patient is bleeding, and that any degree of thrombocytopenia in this circumstance should be regarded as a possible cause and treated with platelet packs of 6–8 units. It is also wise to add 2 units of cryoprecipitate to such a regime, since this is a good source of fibrinogen as well as factor VIII, and has the added advantage of possibly correcting platelet release abnormalities. The question of fibrinolysis as a cause of bleeding in this situation has often been raised and occasionally the use of anti-fibrinolytic agents such as tranexamic acid and ϵ-aminocaproic acid is advocated. Fibrinolysis as a cause of bleeding in man has rarely been documented and when present is usually a secondary phenomenon associated with disseminated intravascular coagulation. In most circumstances it is dangerous to use these agents in post-operative bleeding unless primary fibrinolysis has been established and disseminated intravascular clotting excluded. The introduction of specific peptide substrates for assaying plasmin and plasminogen activator may help in this problem. The only circumstance where fibrinolysis appears to be established as a cause of bleeding problems is in cyanotic heart disease, although even here the documentation is not absolute.

The problem of citrate toxicity has been widely debated over the years,

Table 10.9   Liver disease

---

(1)   Synthesis of coagulation factors prothrombin, fibrinogen, factors V, VII, IX and X.
High molecular weight kininogen.
Prekallikrein, ATIII, Protein C.
Vitamin K dependent.
Factors II, VII, IX, X.
Protein C.

> Reduced in amount
> Product is abnormal

(2)   Clearance of factors by RES

> Activated coagulation factors IXa, Xa, etc.
> FDPs and fibrin monomers
> Activated plasminogen.

(3)   Increased protein loss or catabolism

> ? Turnover of clotting factors
> ? Loss into ascitic fluid
> Protein losing enteropathy (PLE)

(4)   Thrombocytopenia

> Pooling
> Alcohol
> Folic acid deficiency
> DIC

(5)   Qualitative platelet defect

---

and there has been considerable controversy as to whether such toxicity can cause bleeding problems secondary to hypocalcaemia. It has been argued on theoretical grounds that the patient would die of cardiac arrest before citrate levels could reduce the ionized calcium to a level sufficient to interfere with blood coagulation. It has also been debated whether the administration of calcium chloride is of value in preventing such toxicity, although many people advocate using 2 ml of 10% calcium chloride to be administered with every unit of whole blood. Certainly anyone receiving massive amounts of citrated blood should have electrolyte monitoring, including calcium, and any abnormality corrected appropriately.

All of the above problems are compounded if the patient has abnormal liver or renal function. Table 10.9 lists the problems that may arise with the haemostatic mechanisms in liver disease; as the prime source of synthesis of most coagulation proteins any disorder of this organ can result in either reduced synthesis or the synthesis of abnormal coagulation factors. Not only does it synthesize the majority of the proteins concerned with the production of fibrin, but it also produces proteins which may be important in modulating coagulation and in preventing thrombosis such as anti-thrombin III (*see* Chapter 3) and the vitamin K-dependent protein, Protein C. Furthermore, the liver plays an important role, because of the concentration of reticulo-endo-

Table 10.10   Renal disease

Qualitative platelet defect
Thrombocytopenia due to suppressed bone marrow function
Abnormal factor VIII
Low von Willebrand factor activity

thelial cells in this organ, in removing activated coagulation factors and thus diminishing the risk of thrombosis, as well as removing fibrin degradation products and fibrin monomers which might inhibit the clotting process. There may also be an increased loss or turnover of coagulation factors, and thrombocytopenia may be produced in a number of ways as indicated in Table 10.9. More recently a qualitative platelet defect has been described in patients with liver disease. Table 10.10 outlines the problems seen in renal disease, which primarily are believed to be secondary to a qualitative platelet defect and/or a factor VIII anomaly (*see* Chapter 7).

Finally, drugs that are being administered, or have been administered to the patient should always be examined. The most frequent drug involved is heparin, especially after open heart surgery where normally adequate amounts of protamine have been administered, but for reasons which are not understood this has been insufficient to neutralize the heparin, and so-called rebound occurs. This is readily detected in a coagulation laboratory and corrected by the use of further protamine. Antibiotics and other drugs causing problems with the haemostatic mechanism have already been discussed in the preceding chapters (Tables 7.5, 8.3 and 8.5).

The practical approach to the patient with post-operative bleeding problems, therefore, is to undertake a skin bleeding time, which if prolonged strongly suggests some platelet abnormality, either quantitative or qualitative, and would suggest the use of platelet transfusions together with cryoprecipitate, usually 6 units of platelets (platelets derived from 3 litres of blood) to be repeated in 6 hours and then 12 hourly intervals for 48 hours and then reassess. This plan would be modified if the clotting screen (Table 10.2) suggested DIC when the measures already outlined in Chapter 9 would be used. If necessary further investigation can be undertaken to detect the precise factors which are lacking and appropriate replacement therapy instituted.

Reference

RATNOFF, O. D. (1980). The psychogenic purpuras: a review of autoerythrocyte sensitization, autosensitization to DNA, 'hysterical' and factitious bleeding and the religious stigmata. *Semin. Hematol.*, **17**, 197

Appendix

SKIN BLEEDING TIME

Thoroughly cleanse and dry the anterior surface of the forearm using chlorhexidine. Wrap the sphygmomanometer cuff around the upper arm and inflate to 40 mmHg. Maintain this pressure throughout the test. Taking care to avoid puncturing surface veins, make three skin punctures of uniform depth with a lancet. Start three stopwatches. Using filter paper, gently remove blood from wound every 30 seconds – take care to avoid actual puncture site. As each wound stops bleeding stop the stopwatch. Average the three times. The normal range is 2–7 minutes.*

* All normal ranges quoted are for our laboratory and must be established individually.

WHOLE BLOOD CLOTTING TIME

Mark three clean 12×75 mm glass test tubes at approximately 1 ml and place in a preheated portable waterbath. Use two syringes for venepuncture discarding the first syringe after collecting 1 ml of blood and then collect in the second syringe (two syringe technique). Add 1 ml of second syringe blood to each tube. Start stopwatch as blood enters syringe and gently tilt the first tube every 30 seconds until clotted, i.e. tube can be taken through a 45° angle. Tilt second and third tubes in succession until clotted. Record clotting times for each tube and average, the normal range is 4–10 minutes. After 1 hour at 37°C, examine retraction. Leave overnight – re-examine after 24 hours for clot lysis and/or increased red cell fallout.

THROMBIN TIME

Reagents

Parke Davis Thrombin Topical.
Reconstitute in saline to 4 U/ml, aliquot and freeze (5 ml lots).
Before use – adjust concentration to give a clotting time equivalent to 15
seconds (suggest 3 parts thrombin and 1 part saline, i.e., 900 μl thrombin and
300 μl saline).

Method

0.2 ml platelet poor plasma (PPP) – leave equivalent of 1 minute to warm.
Then add 0.2 ml thrombin (prewarmed), and measure the clotting time.

Normal range

< 20 seconds using adjusted concentration.
10–13 seconds using 4 U/ml.

Measures

Fibrinogen – level and/or function.
If prolonged: (1)   Estimate fibrinogen
　　　　　　 (2)   Mix 1:1 with normal plasma to see if corrected.
　　　　　　 (3)   Undertake reptilase time.

PROTHROMBIN TIME

Reagents

General Diagnostics Simplastin – reconstitute as directed.

Method

0.1 ml PPP – leave the equivalent of 1 minute to warm. Add 0.2 ml Simplastin
– prewarmed. Measure the clotting time.

Normal range

11–14 seconds.

PARTIAL THROMBOPLASTIN TIME WITH KAOLIN (PTTK)

Reagents for PTTK

Kaolin 50 mg/ml in barbitone buffer.
Barbitone buffer:
   7.3 g NaCl
   2.76 g barbitone – make up to 1 litre with distilled water
   2.06 g sodium barbital. Adjust pH to 7.4
   Make up 500 ml only. Discard if it becomes contaminated
   0.025 mol/l $CaCl_2$
   3.67 g $CaCl_2.2H_2O/l$. distilled water

During the test, store – kaolin at room temperature while performing assays,
   – PPP and platelin packed on ice, and
   – $CaCl_2$ at 37 °C.

Method

   0.05 ml kaolin
   0.05 ml platelin* – allow 1 minute to warm
   Add 0.1 ml PPP (prewarmed)
   Mix quickly then incubate 3 minutes
   Add 0.1 ml $CaCl_2$ and record clotting time

* General diagnostic.

Note: Normal range is 35–45 seconds, so for the first 20 seconds gently agitate mixture in the water bath before commencing regular tilting.

STYPVEN TIME WITH PLATELIN

Reagents

Stypven (Russel Viper Venom) 1/100 000 dilution in saline (i.e. dissolve 0.2 mg vial in 2 ml saline then dilute 1/10 with saline).
Make 1.5 ml aliquots for freezing.

Method

During test have $CaCl_2$ (0.025 mol/l) at 37 °C. PPP, Stypven and platelin on ice.

   0.1 ml Stypven
   0.1 ml platelin – allow approximately 1 minute to warm
   0.1 ml PPP (prewarmed)
   0.1 ml $CaCl_2$ and record clotting time

Normal range

9–11 seconds.

Significance

Acts independently of Factor VIII. Depends on factor X, prothrombin and fibrinogen.

FACTOR XIII

Reagents

0.025 mol/l $CaCl_2$
5 mol/l urea – 30 g urea/100 ml distilled water.

Method

0.5 ml PPP
0.5 ml $CaCl_2$
Leave 30 minutes at 37 °C
Remove clot from tube using orange stick
Place in 3 ml urea
Leave at room temperature (RT) – inspect next day. If factor XIII is absent clot will disappear.

A control urea soluble clot can be produced by clotting EDTA PPP with thrombin.

REPTILASE TIME

Reconstituted reptilase*, if stored at 4 °C, may be used for a period of 28 days.

Method

0.1 ml reptilase – equilibrate 5 minutes at 37 °C
0.3 ml PPP (prewarmed).

Normal range

18–22 seconds

* Abbot Laboratories.

Significance

Thrombin Time	*Reptilase*	*Cause*
Prolonged	Equally prolonged	Hypo/afibrinogenaemia
Prolonged	Prolonged	Dysfibrinogenaemia
Prolonged	Normal	Heparin
Prolonged	Slightly prolonged	FDPs

FIBRINOGEN ASSAY BY CLOT WEIGHT

Method

To a 10 ml tube add 1 ml PPP
$\qquad$ 1 ml 0.025 mol/l $CaCl_2$
$\qquad$ 0.5 ml 4 U/ml thrombin

Mix by inversion and place a glass rod in mixture. Incubate at 37 °C for 15 minutes. Wind fibrin onto glass rod – pressing out excess fluid. Add another 0.5 ml of 4 U/ml thrombin to mixture to check that there is no unclotted fibrinogen left – wait 15 minutes. Place glass rod and fibrin in another 10 ml tube containing distilled water to wash. Leave 5–10 minutes then change water and leave for another 5–10 minutes. Carefully remove fibrin from rod. Blot dry. Dehydrate in 5–10 ml acetone for 10–15 minutes. Dry in hot oven (90–110 °C) for 20 minutes or cooler oven overnight. Weigh clot.

Calculation

$$\text{Fibrinogen} = \frac{\text{Dry weight (mg)}}{\text{Plasma volume (ml)}} \times 100 \, \text{mg}/100 \, \text{ml}$$

EUGLOBULIN LYSIS TIME

Reagents

Borate saline buffer: 9 g NaCl
$\qquad$ 1 g sodium borate
$\qquad$ Make up to 1 litre with dist. H_2O
$\qquad$ Adjust pH to 9.0 with N/10 HCl or N/10 NaOH.

Method

Collect blood into 3.8% trisodium citrate. Place on ice immediately. Spin for 10 minutes at 4000 r/min at 4 °C – blood must be spun within 30 minutes of collection. Pre-cool 9 ml dist. H_2O. Remove PPP and store on ice. Dilute 0.5 ml PPP in 9 ml cold dist. H_2O. Add 0.1 ml 1% acetic acid. Leave on ice for

30 minutes. Spin at 3500 r/min for 3 minutes at room temperature. Tip off supernatant and dry excess liquid from inside tube using a tissue wrapped around an orange stick.

Add 0.5 ml borate buffer to precipitate. Resuspend using a Pasteur pipette – warm to 37 °C. Add 0.5 ml warmed 0.025 mol/l $CaCl_2$. Record clotting time. Continue observation and record time required for complete clot lysis.

ONE STAGE FACTOR VIII/IX ASSAY

Reagents

Factor VIII/IX deficient substrate (DADE).
Standard – factor VIII CSL.* Reconstitute in 1 ml barbitone buffer.
Factor IX – frozen pool obtained by mixing equal volumes of plasma (from five normal people).
Test dilutions 1/10, 1/20, 1/40, using barbitone buffer. Adjust dilutions if any marked variation in concentration.
Platelin.
Calcium – 0.025 mol/l.
Kaolin – 5 mg/ml in barbitone buffer.

Method

In a small clotting tube at 37 °C add:

    50 μl substrate – allow to warm
    50 μl kaolin
    50 μl test dilution
    Incubate 9.5 minutes
    50 μl platelin
    At exactly 10 minutes add 50 μl $CaCl_2$ and record clotting time.

Plot results on log/log graph paper. A straight line should be obtained. Determine the concentration of the test sample knowing that of the factor VIII standard*.

Normal range

    Factor VIII: 62–218%
    Factor IX: 58–144%

Note: Using these dilutions one test or set of tests (i.e. three dilutions) can be set up every 3 minutes.
    Factor IX assay may be done on frozen plasma.
* CSL (Commonwealth Serum Laboratories) Factor VIII standard.

FACTOR XI/XII ASSAY

Reagents

Factor XI/XII deficient substrate (DADE)

Standard – a plasma pool of at least five normal donors. Blood must be non-contacted, i.e. two syringe technique and handled only in plastic or siliconized glassware. Assume standard as 100%.

Test dilutions 1/5, 1/10, 1/20, using barbitone buffer. Adjust dilutions if patients have very low or very high levels.

Platelin

Calcium chloride 0.05 mol/l

Kaolin – 5 mg/ml in barbitone buffer.

Method

In a small clotting tube at 37 °C mix:

$50 \mu l$ deficient substrate
$50 \mu l$ test dilution
$50 \mu l$ platelin

Allow approximately 30 seconds to warm up. Add $50 \mu l$ kaolin and incubate for 5 minutes. Then add $50 \mu l$ CaCl$_2$ record clotting time. Plot results on log/log graph paper and calculate test factor level.

Note: Clotting times for factor XII are very long, so gently agitate tubes in water bath for the first 1 minute before commencing regular tilting. This does not apply to factor XI.

Important Non-contacted plasma must be used, i.e. two syringe technique with no contact with non-siliconized glass.

Normal range

Factor XI: 63–123%
Factor XII: 69–117%

ANTI-FACTOR VIII ANTIBODY DETECTION

Incubate at 37 °C:

(1)   1:1 mix of test PPP with fresh normal PPP. Assay for VIII:C at 0 minute and 2 hours.
(2)   Fresh PPP. Assay for VIII:C at 0 minute and 2 hours.
(3)   Test PPP. Assay for VIII:C at 0 minute.

ANTI-FACTOR IX ANTIBODY DETECTION

Dilute patient's PPP in barbitone buffer. Take PPP neat and dilute 1/2 and 1/5 with barbitone buffer. Mix with an equal volume of fresh normal PPP and assay immediately at usual dilutions, e.g. 1/5, 1/20.

PROTAMINE SULPHATE TEST FOR FIBRIN MONOMERS

Reagents

Citrated PPP
EACA citrated PPP
0.5 ml 3.8% tri Na citrate + 0.04 ml EACA (2.5 g/10 ml)
Collect 4.5 ml blood
1% protamine sulphate
Shelf life 1 month

Fibrin monomers are present in disseminated intravascular coagulation or when a sample is activated by faulty collection, e.g. difficult venepuncture.

Method

Collect blood into two tubes, one containing citrate, the other citrate and epsilon amino caproic acid (EACA). Centrifuge both to obtain PPP. Take 1 ml of citrated PPP and 1 ml of citrated EACA PPP and warm at 37 °C for 2 minutes. Add 0.1 ml protamine sulphate to each tube. Mix gently and leave at 37 °C for 15 minutes. Examine for the presence of flocculation.

Report as negative/mild/moderate/marked. May be cloudy without being positive.

THROMBOPLASTIN GENERATION TEST

Blood

10 ml Citrated patient's blood collected by the two syringe technique using non-contact plastic surface, and centrifuge for PPP. Collect 10 ml whole blood into glass tube.

Control

20 ml Citrated blood collected as above, prepare platelet rich plasma (PRP) and PPP. Collect 10 ml whole blood into a glass tube for serum.

Reagents

Absorbed plasma: incubate 0.9 ml PPP with 0.1 ml Al(OH)$_3$ at 37 °C for exactly 2 minutes. Spin in Sorvall 14 000 r/min for 10 minutes. Dilute 1/5 in barbitone buffer (total volume 1 ml – 0.2 ml absorbed plasma + 0.8 ml buffer).

Serum: stand whole blood at 37 °C for 2–4 hours. Spin and dilute 1/10 with barbitone buffer (total volume 1 ml – 0.1 ml serum + 0.9 ml buffer).

Platelets: * spin down control platelets. Wash twice in normal saline. Resuspend in 1/3 original volume in saline. Spin 3–4 ml PRP. Keep PPP to use as substrate on ice.

Calcium: 0.025 mol/l.

Substrate: control PPP (or fibrinogen).

* If a platelet abnormality is suspected in the patient, a patient platelet suspension should be prepared and substituted for the control platelets.

Method

Prepare six tubes (12 × 75 mm) with 0.1 ml PPP (substrate) at 37 °C. To a glass clotting tube at 37 °C add:

0.2 ml diluted absorbed plasma ⎫
0.2 ml diluted serum ⎬ equilibrate approximately 1 minute
0.2 ml platelets ⎭

Add 0.2 ml CaCl$_2$, start stopwatch and mix.
At 1 minute intervals add 0.1 ml incubating mixture and 0.1 ml CaCl$_2$ simultaneously to substrate tubes and clot. Perform test using:

Absorbed plasma	*Serum*
Control	Control
Patient	Patient
Control	Patient
Patient	Control

Normal result

Times decrease to 8–10 seconds at 3 or 4 minutes.

Interpretation

Absorbed plasma provides factor V and VIII
Serum   IX and X
Both also contain   XI and XII
(*see* Chapter 3)

GLASS ACTIVATION TEST

For contact factors XI, XII.

Blood

Patient 20 ml second syringe (two syringe technique)
Control 10 ml second syringe (two syringe technique)

Reagents

Non-contacted PPP
Activated PPP – non-contacted PPP is rotated with 1 mg/ml glass beads for
   20 minutes at room temperature.

CaCl$_2$ lysed platelet reagent: prepare PRP from 10 ml of patient's blood. Spin
down platelets. Wash three times in normal saline. Resuspend in saline in $\frac{1}{2}$
original volume. Set up platelet count. Freeze/thaw twice using liquid nitrogen
and 37 °C bath. Using platelet count dilute lysed platelets to a final concentration approximately $5 \times 10^9/l$ with 0.1 mol/l CaCl$_2$.

Method

Clot 0.2 ml patient/control non-contacted and activated PPP at 37 °C using
0.05 ml of platelet reagent. Use plastic clotting tubes (or siliconized glass).

Results

Clotting time of non-contacted control plasma 10–25 minutes. Activated
plasma < 350 seconds.

THROMBIN GENERATION TEST

Preparation of standard curve.

Reagents

Prepare fibrinogen (General Diagnostics) to a concentration of 1 mg/ml in
distilled water. Thrombin must be prepared freshly at the following concentrations (dilute using 0.9% NaCl).

Thrombin concentrations (U/ml)	Thrombin (20 U/ml)	Saline
15	0.75 μl	0.25 μl
14	0.7 μl	0.3 μl
12	0.6 μl	0.4 μl
10	0.5 μl	0.5 μl
8	0.4 μl	0.6 μl
U/ml 6	0.3 μl	0.7 μl
4	0.2 μl	0.8 μl
2	0.1 μl	0.9 μl
1	0.05 μl	0.95 μl

Clot by adding 50 μl thrombin dilutions to 200 μl warmed fibrinogen. Plot:

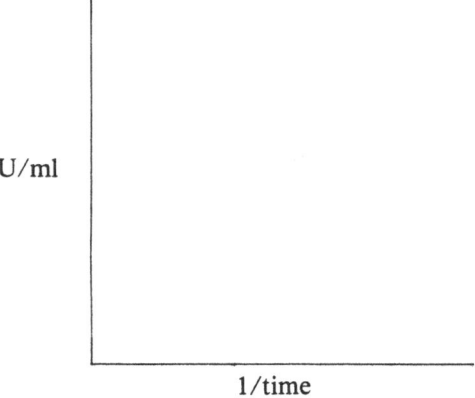

A standard curve must be prepared for each new lot No. of fibrinogen.

Prepare fibrinogen to concentration of 1 mg/ml. Prepare PRP and adjust platelets to $300 \times 10^9/l$ with PPP. Warm $CaCl_2$, NaCl to 37 °C. Prepare 10 tubes containing 0.2 ml fibrinogen at 37 °C.

Method

In a glass tube add: 0.3 ml PRP
                0.3 ml NaCl
                0.3 ml $CaCl_2$.
Start stopwatch. Observe reaction until clot forms (approx. $2\frac{1}{2}$–3 minutes). Quickly remove clot using two orange sticks then sub-sample 50 μl at 1 minute intervals into fibrinogen. (Note a second clot will form about 1 minute after the initial one and must be removed.)

Continue until a peak is reached and times have lengthened again to 30–40 seconds (approx. 12 minutes). Plot thrombin units obtained from standard curve (see Figure 4.4).

THROMBIN GENERATION TEST – VARIATIONS

Stimulation using platelet aggregating agents – ADP and collagen.

Concentrations are those used in platelet aggregation studies, i.e. ADP final concentration 5×10^{-6} mol/l use $100\,\mu l$ collagen final concentration $5\,\mu g/ml$ use $50\,\mu l$.

Method

0.3 ml PRP and aggregating agent. Stir for 5 minutes at 37 °C in the aggregometer. Have ready a glass clotting tube containing the adjusted volume of NaCl. After 5 minutes add PRP mixture to tube. Add 0.3 ml $CaCl_2$. Start stopwatch. Proceed to subsample as for standard thrombin generation test.

DILUTE SIMPLASTIN TEST

Demonstration of 'lupus like' inhibitor.

Reagents

Prepare 1/5, 1/100 and 1/250 dilution of simplastin in barbitone buffer. Add an equal volume of 0.025 mol/l $CaCl_2$ to each, i.e. 1/10, 1/200 and 1/500 dilutions.

Use the above as for a prothrombin time and compare with control. Normal values in our laboratory are: 1/10, 21 ± 3 seconds; 1/200 49 ± 7 seconds; 1/500 66 ± 7 seconds.

Note If patient is on warfarin a 1:1 mix with control PPP should give normal times. Assays can be done on frozen plasma using a 1:1 mix with fresh control.

CHROMAGENIC ANTITHROMBIN III ASSAY

Antithrombin III is a major inhibitor of thrombin, factor Xa, and other coagulation proteases in plasma. Chromagenic Antithrombin III assay utilizes a chromagenic substrate, S-2238, for the specific determination of functional antithrombin III as measured by thrombin inhibition.

Principle

The antithrombin III (AT III or heparin cofactor) activity in plasma is measured in the presence of an excess of heparin. The test plasma is diluted into a buffer containing EDTA and heparin. Thrombin is added in excess, and the mixture is incubated at 37 °C for a certain period of time. An amount of thrombin is inhibited by the complex (AT III. heparin) in proportion to the amount of AT III. After neutralizing the heparin with polybrene, the remaining amount of thrombin catalyses the splitting of p-nitroaniline (pNA) from the tripeptide substrate (S-2238). S-2238 is specific for thrombin. The rate at which pNA is released is measured photometrically at 405 nm.

Reagents

S-2238: 40.85 mg *Ortho* chromagenic substrate with mannitol + 5 mg polybrene (Aldrich). Make up to 15 ml with distilled H_2O.

Heparin buffer
    250 ml 0.2 mol/l Tris (base); MW 121.1 (6.1 g/250 ml)
    20 ml 1.0 mol/l HCl (approx. 11 mol/l conc. Make a 1/11 dilution by taking 2 ml conc. HCl + 20 ml dist. H_2O).
    30 ml 0.25 mol/l K_2 EDTA; MW 404.46 (3.03 g/30 ml).
    0.6 ml 5000 U/ml heparin (3 U/ml final concentration).
    Adjust volume to 1 litre with 0.26 mol/l NaCl; MW 58.44 (11.4 g in 750 ml).
       Adjust pH to 8.4.

Acetic acid: 50%

Thrombin: 10 U/ml, i.e. bovine thrombin reconstituted in isotonic saline (i.e. 1/500 dilution of 5000 U/ml vial). Freeze in 5 ml aliquots.

Control assayed reference plasma (Coagulation ARP Helena Laboratories).

Method

Standard curve dilutions:

    200 μl normal pool + 7.8 ml heparin buffer = 100%...................................(1)
    3 ml of (1) + 1 ml heparin buffer = 75%...(2)
    1 ml of (1) + 1 ml heparin buffer = 50%...(3)
    1 ml of (1) + 3 ml heparin buffer = 25%...(4)

Blank: dilution (1) of the pool, but eliminating the substrate.

Samples are diluted in duplicate using dilution (2) as for pool.

    400 μl of test sample is warmed for 2 minutes at 37 °C (time not critical).
    100 μl of thrombin (10 U/ml), incubate for 2 minutes at 37 °C (critical time).

$200\,\mu l$ S-2238, incubate for 30 seconds (critical time).
$300\,\mu l$ 50% acetic acid.
Measure OD at 405 nm.

Normal range: 80–120%.

Calculations

(1) Draw a standard curve, with activity 0–100% on the x-axis and optical density on the y-axis.
(2) The activity of each sample is read off the graph, and this is then corrected for the dilution, i.e. (2) dilution = activity from graph multiplied by $100/75 = \%$.

To ensure accuracy each run includes one with control assayed reference plasma processed in exactly the same way as test plasma.

LAURELL METHOD FOR DETECTING AND MEASURING FACTOR VIII:RAg

Reagents

Gelbond film (FMC Corporation, Marine Colloids Division, Rockland, USA). Thickness: 0.2 mm, width: 102 mm, length: 16.5 m. Dimensions of film for each Laurell – 102 mm × 82 mm.

NB Before cutting into sections, roll Gelbond opposite way to the way it is rolled; secure with paper clip and leave overnight.

Agarose (Seakam, Electroendosmosis = medium, 0.16–0.19).
(FMC Corporation, Marine Colloids Division, Rockland, USA).

Paper wicks (Miles Laboratories Inc., Research Products, USA). $4'' \times 4''$.

$10\,\mu l$ hole punch

Electrophoresis tank; power pack (preferably with cooling).

Buffers

For electrophoresis tank:
  0.075 mol/l Na barbitone } pH 8.6
  0.015 mol/l barbitone

For gel: Above buffer diluted 1/2 with dist. H_2O

For plasma dilutions:
  barbitone buffered saline, pH 7.4
  0.125 mol/l NaCl
  0.015 mol/l barbitone
  0.010 mol/l Na barbitone.

Stain and destain

Stain – 1.25 g Coomassie Brilliant Blue R (Sigma).
      454 ml 50% methanol
      46 ml glacial acetic acid

Stir for approximately 1 hour (covered) at room temperature then filter, and it is now ready for use.

Destain – ingredients same as for stain but without Coomassie. It can be re-used after destaining – mix with activated charcoal, let charcoal settle then filter.

FVIII antibody

Either use commercially made anti-FVIII or antibody produced by rabbit to purified human FVIII:C. Antiserum from rabbit is adsorbed with von Willebrand plasma until no more visible precipitate is seen.

Method – antiserum heat inactivated 56 °C for 30 minutes, add 1/10 volume of von Willebrand PPP and stand at 4 °C overnight, spin at 10 000 g for 20 min. Repeat until clear.

Standard – normal pooled plasma: plasmas from 20 healthy donors are pooled; snap frozen and stored at − 70 °C in 1 ml aliquots. Aliquot thawed at 37 °C immediately before use.

Preparation of gel

(1) Appropriate size flask containing approximately 10 ml distilled H_2O + stirrer, left to boil on magnetic stirrer with hot plate.

(2) Distilled H_2O discarded; replaced with volume of barbitone buffer (see buffer for gels) + agarose (final concentration of agarose in gel = 0.9% (w/v). After gel has boiled, stirrer removed from flask which is placed in a 56 °C H_2O bath.

(3) When gel has equilibrated to 56 °C, the antibody can be added; mix well.

(4)   Sections of gelbond are secured to level glass plates with three or four drops of water on the hydrophobic side. *NB* Gel must be poured on hydrophilic side. 17 ml of antibody containing gel is then poured onto each section of gelbond. Make sure there is no moisture at the edges of the gelbond or else gel will run over.

(5)   After the gel has set, it is placed in a wet box (airtight container with moistened gauze/filter paper at the bottom) at 4 °C for at least $\frac{1}{2}$ hour (*NB* holes are easier to punch when gel is cold).

(6) $12 \times 10\,\mu l$ holes are punched at one end of each gel so that the leading edge of each hole is 18 mm from the bottom edge.

(7)   Dilutions of normal pooled plasma (NPP) and test samples are made in barbitone buffer, in microtitre trays. For standard curve make 1/8, 1/4, 1/2 dilutions of NPP.

(8)   Place gel in tank with wicks on top and bottom of edges of gel. Run gels at approximately 13 mA/gel (60 volts/tank; 3 gels/tank) toward anode for 18–20 hours.

(9)   Following run, gel is washed in circulating saline (0.9% NaCl) bath at room temperature for at least 4 hours.

(10)   Saline is rinsed off with distilled H_2O. Moistened filter paper is placed over gel. Moisture is removed from gel by placing heavy weight on top of gel sandwiched between paper-towelling. After approximately 15 minutes the gel is dried in front of hair dryer until the filter paper falls away.

(11)   The gel is stained with Coomassie blue for approximately 20 minutes and then destained until peaks are clearly visible.

Determination of results

Height of each peak is measured in mm from leading edge of hole. Standard curve is calculated from height of peak (mm) vs % NPP (1/8 = 12.5%; 1/4 = 25%; 1/2 = 50%) plotted on linear/log graph. Dilutions of test samples are read off and appropriate dilution factors accounted for.

vWf ASSAY USING RISTOCETIN

Reagents

Formalin treated platelets – stored in concentrated form at 4 °C. Remove PRP from 1 pack blood (400 ml blood). Warm equal volumes of PRP and formalin saline separately at 37 °C for approximately 1 hour. Mix and leave at 4 °C for at least 18 hours. Wash three times with Tris-saline containing azide. Store concentrated at 4 °C and dilute to $300 \times 10^9/l$ prior to use.

Formalin saline

2% Formalin	2 ml/100 ml	5 ml/250 ml
0.14 mol/l NaCl, pH 7.4	8.18 g/l	20.5 g/250 ml
0.01 mol/l Tris base	1.21 g/l	0.30 g/250 ml

Washing buffer – as above but without formalin.

Collect blood in 3.8% Na citrate.
Ristocetin initial concentration – 20 mg/ml
Normal pooled plasma – for standard curve (stored at $-70\,°C$)
Patient or test plasma
0.01 mol/l Tris/0.14 mol/l NaCl, pH 7.4 + azide
Payton Aggregometer – chart speed: 2 cm/min.

Method

(1) Dilute concentrated formalinized (form.) platelets to concentration of $300 \times 10^9/l$ with Tris-saline buffer (determine volume needed by roughly calculating how many assays are to be performed).

(2) Set the range between 30 and 80 on the chart paper of aggregometer.

300 μl form. platelets	150 μl. form. platelets
High	**Low**
120 μl buffer	270 μl buffer

Added to aggregometer cuvette with stirrer.

(3) Determination of standard curve – four points are determined by measuring the rate of aggregation, i.e. mm/min.

	Form. platelets	*NPPP*	*Buffer*	*Ristocetin*
100%	300 μl	50 μl	50 μl	20 μl
50%	300 μl	25 μl	75 μl	20 μl
25%	300 μl	25 μl of 1/2 dilution	75 μl	20 μl
12.5%	300 μl	25 μl of 1/4 dilution	75 μl	20 μl

(4) Measure the rate of aggregation and plot against % vWf on log/log graph paper.

(5) Patient/test plasma sample – perform 50% point, i.e. 25 μl PPP. Depending on result do 100% (50 μl PPP) or 25% (25 μl of 1/2 dilution PPP).

COUNTING PLATELETS

Diluting fluid

1% ammonium oxalate. Store in refrigeration and use a fresh aliquot each morning.

Method

Using a 1/100 dilution pipette (i.e. red bead) draw blood to '1' mark, then diluting fluid to 101. Fill chamber. Stand in a moist Petri dish for 20 minutes. minutes.

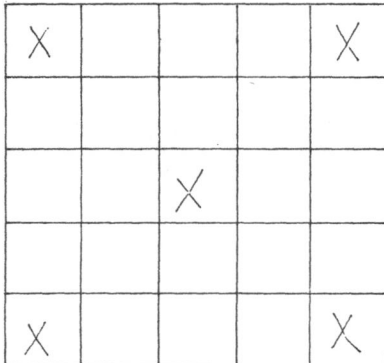

Count cells as shown, adopting same technique as for counting white blood cells. Use phase contrast microscope and × 40 objective. Count both sides of chamber.

Calculations

$$\frac{\text{No. platelets counted} \times \text{dilution}}{0.004 \times \text{no. squares counted}}$$

i.e. if 10 squares counted then:

$$\frac{X \times 100}{0.004 \times 10}$$

i.e. $X \times 2.5 \times 10^9/l$

If platelet count is low ($< 100 \times 10^9/l$) 25 squares are counted on each side. If 25 squares counted then platelets/l $= X \times 10^9/l$.

PLATELET ADHESIONS

Reagents

Add 0.1 ml 2% EDTA (disodium salt) to large clotting tubes. Oven dry and store for use.

Acid washed glass beads (0.5 mm diam. Superbritt):

Soak for 2 days in chromium acid. Rinse.
Soak for 2 days in sodium carbonate solution.
Wash in running tapwater for 2 days.
Wash several times in distilled H_2O.
Dry on filter paper in 37 °C incubator for 2 days.
Store.

Plastic tubing (3 mm diameter)*, length 30 cm. 10.0 ml heparin tube – 150 IU lithium heparin tube.

Method

(1)   Collect 10 ml heparinized blood + EDTA tube and perform test as soon as possible after collection – always < 1 hour.

(2)   Fill the tubing with 2.6 g acid washed beads using a small square of cotton gauze to seal each end. Use a 5 ml syringe as a funnel. Take up approximately 7 ml blood into a 10 ml plastic syringe.

(3)   Fit syringe to constant rate plunger machine. Attach plastic tubing containing the glass beads. Using a rate of 10 ml/min discard the first 1 ml then collect 3 × 1 ml samples into EDTA tubes.

(4)   Perform platelet count on samples 2, 3, and 4 and on patient's whole blood within 20 minutes of passing over glass beads.

* Intramedia polyethylene tubing PE 330 (Clay Adams)

Calculation

$$\text{Platelet retention} = \frac{\text{whole blood platelet count} - \text{average of 2, 3 and 4 samples}}{\text{whole blood platelet count}}$$

Express result as a %. Normal range > 50% adhesion (may be reduced if mHct < 40%). 1 ml commercial sequestrene tubes may be used to collect the samples.

PLATELET AGGREGATES

Reagents

Buffered EDTA formalin		*500 ml*
3 ml 0.077 mol/l EDTA		75 ml
5 ml 4% formalin		125 ml
2 ml 10 × conc. phosphate buffered saline (PBS)	pH. 7.4	50 ml
10 ml distilled H_2O		250 ml

237

Buffered EDTA   *500 ml*

3 ml 0.077 mol/l EDTA   ⎫   75 ml

5 ml 10×conc. PBS   ⎬ pH 7.4   125 ml

12 ml distilled H_2O ⎭   300 ml

10 × conc. phosphate buffered saline

(1)   180 ml NaH_2PO_4. H_2O 234 g/l

(2)   820 ml Na_2HPO_4 213 g/l

(3)   90 g/l NaCl

(1) + (2) is solution A.

(3) is solution B

Mix equal volumes of solutions A and B.

To make 200 ml solution A (1)   5.85 g/25 ml $NaH_2PO_4.H_2O$

                               (2)   17.5 g in 82 ml Na_2HPO_4

Platelet aggregates

Draw 4 ml EDTA buffer into a 10 ml syringe. Label B.

Draw 4 ml formalin/EDTA into a 10 ml syringe. Label F.

Collect blood using a 19 or 21 G butterfly. Use the first 2 ml for platelet count.

Draw 1 ml of blood into syringe, with the tourniquet off. Mix for 15 minutes. Transfer to labelled plastic tubes. Spin 1200 r/min for 15 minutes. Remove PRP using siliconized pipettes.

Perform platelet count using 1/20 dilution of F and B.

Calculate F/B.

Normal range 0.8–1.1

Report platelet count on whole blood with results.

PLATELET FACTOR 3 RELEASE

Prepare eight small clotting tubes* containing 0.1 ml $CaCl_2$ 0.025 mol/l + 0.1 ml Stypven (1 in 10^5 dilution). Place four of these at 37 °C for each assay.

Method

 Prepare PRP to $300 \times 10^9/l$
0.5 ml PRP
0.05 ml kaolin – 50 mg/ml (warmed)
Start stopwatch
Subsample $100 \mu l$ at 1, 5, 10, 20 minute intervals into the Stypven/CaCl$_2$ mixture.

Normal range

 1 min 40–50 s
20 min 18–25 s
Clotting times should fall by > 10 s

*Serology tubes 0.5 cm × 3 cm.

ASSAY FOR DETECTION OF PLATELET ANTIBODIES (PF3 TEST)

Preparation of serum for platelet antibody detection

Blood in glass tube without anticoagulant is incubated at 37 °C for 2 hours then left overnight at 2 °C. Obtain serum by spinning hard (maximum on bench centrifuge). Heat at 56 °C for 30 minutes before testing. Spin hard in either centrifuge or Sorvall to remove any precipitate and test supernatant.

 Normal pooled serum treated in the same way is used as a control.

Method

(1) Collect whole blood from normal person into 3.8% Tri-Nacitrate and mix.

(2) Centrifuge for 20 min at 1200 r/min in bench centrifuge. PRP collected using siliconized pipette, into plastic centrifuge tubes (use graduated test tube).

(3) Count platelets in PRP.

(4) Spin remaining whole blood for 10 minutes at 3500r/minutes to obtain PPP.

(5) Adjust PRP to $400 \times 10^9/l$ with PPP.

(6) Incubate following mixture at 37 °C for 30 minutes (double amounts for duplicate):
    0.4 ml adjusted PRP
    0.05 ml serum (patient or control)
    0.05 ml saline or drug (if suspected drug induced thrombo-cytopenia).

(7)   Add 0.05 ml kaolin (50 mg/ml) to mixture and start stopwatch.

(8)   Sub-sample 0.1 ml of above mixture into 0.1 ml 0.02 mol/l $CaCl_2$ + 0.1 ml 1/100 000 Stypven (preincubated at 37 °C) and start stopwatch. Repeat after 1.5, 3, 5 minutes.

(9)   Record clotting time.

Patient's serum is + ve if clotting time is shortened by 3 or more seconds when compared with clotting time of control serum.

PLATELET AGGREGATION STUDIES

Reagents

Aggregation buffer

Stock solution: 9.147 g Na acetate trihydrate
          14.714 g Na diethyl barbiturate (Na barbitone) in 500 ml CO_2
          free dist. H_2O (boil 30 min).

Working buffer: 12.5 ml stock buffer
          12.5 ml 0.1 N HCl
          225 ml 0.154 mol/l NaCl (i.e. 2.24 g/250 ml)
          Check pH to 7.4.

Aggregating agents

Adenosine-5'-diphosphate (ADP) – concentration used 5×10^{-5} mol/l MW = 427.22 g, therefore use 0.021 g/l ADP (i.e. 2 mg/100 ml, 10 mg/500 ml). Aliquot into approximately 1 ml lots. Freeze. Do not re-freeze after use. Use 40 μl in each aggregation i.e. final concentration is 5×10^{-6} mol/l.

Adrenalin – adrenalin injection BP 1/1000 (1 mg/ml). 1 ml ampoule. Dilute 1/20 with saline. Freeze in 1 ml lots. For each set of aggregations thaw an aliquot and dilute 1/20 in saline (40 μl in 0.95 ml). Use 40 μl of dilute adrenalin, final concentration 1.5×10^{-7} mol/l.

Thrombin – dilute Parke-Davis topical thrombin to a final concentration of 4 U/ml in NaCl. Aliquot into approximately 1 ml lots. Freeze. Do not re-freeze after use. Use 20 μl in each aggregation, i.e. final concentration 0.2 U/ml.

Ristocetin – make a 200 mg/10 ml solution in isotonic saline. Refrigerate in small aliquots of 1 ml. To aggregate use 10 μl (10 mg/ml) 20 μl (20 mg/ml) and 40 μl (20 mg/ml). Return to refrigerator.

Collagen – HORM collagen reagent for platelet aggregations. Dilute 0.2 ml of the collagen with 1.8 ml of the buffer supplied (or isotonic saline). Concentration 100 μg/ml. Freeze in 1 ml lots. For aggregations use 20 μl, i.e. final concentration 5 μg/ml.

Arachidonic acid NB: Air and Light Sensitive – the reagent is supplied in a heavy oil that is insoluble in water. Dissolve 50 mg AA in 0.5 ml absolute alcohol. Then dilute 1/10 with 0.01 mol/l Tris 0.14 mol/l NaCl pH 8.0, i.e. total volume 5 ml. This is an emulsion and must always be mixed before subsampling. Divide stock into 1 ml lots. Cover four of these with foil and freeze. Dilute 1 ml stock with 4 ml buffer. Aliquot approximately 0.5 ml lots with small plastic capped tubes. Cover with large labels to protect from light. Freeze. Thaw one aliquot immediately prior to aggregation. Use 40 μl, final concentration 0.2 mg/ml (6.5×10^{-4} mol/l). Always mix emulsion before subsampling.

To make 0.01 mol/l Tris 0.14 mol/l NaCl buffer use 0.1211 g Tris base and 0.81816-g NaCl. Make up to approx. 80 ml in dist. water, adjust to pH 8.0 with HCl and then make up to 100 ml.

Tris buffer may deteriorate, so always use fresh buffer.

Ionophore A 23187, MW = 523 (Calbiochem–Behring Corp.)
Stock solution 1 mol/l (stored at $-20\,°C$), i.e. 2.615 mg Ionophore/0.5 ml methanol, giving concentration of 10 mmol/l. Then *slowly* add 4.5 ml saline giving 1 mmol/l stock. (If precipitation occurs, sonicate using small probe just below surface of solution which must be in plastic and packed in ice; sonicate four or five times for 30 seconds at 100 watts.)

For each test prepare fresh working solution.
10 μl stock solution + 90 μl saline.
Then slowly add 900 μl saline.
To aggregate use 40 μl working solution. Final concentration of ionophore 10 mmol/l.
If no response use 80 μl.
The ionophore is air and light sensitive.

To aggregate use 0.3 ml PRP + volumes shown in the table over (final volume of 0.4 ml).

Aggregating agent	Stock concentration	Buffer volume	Volume of reagent	Final concentration
ADP	5×10^{-5} mol/l	$60\,\mu l$	$40\,\mu l$	5×10^{-6} mol/l
Adrenalin	1.5×10^{-6} mol/l	$60\,\mu l$	$40\,\mu l$	1.5×10^{-7} mol/l
Thrombin	4 U/ml	$80\,\mu l$	$20\,\mu l$	0.2 U/ml
Ristocetin	10 mg/ml	$80\,\mu l$	$20\,\mu l$	0.5 mg/ml
Ristocetin	20 mg/ml	$80\,\mu l$	$20\,\mu l$	1 mg/ml
Ristocetin	20 mg/ml	$60\,\mu l$	$40\,\mu l$	2 mg/ml
Collagen	100 μg/ml	$80\,\mu l$	$20\,\mu l$	5 μg/ml
Arachidonic acid	6.5×10^{-3} mol/l	$60\,\mu l$	$40\,\mu l$	6.5×10^{-4} mol/l
Ionophore	10 mmol/l	$60\,\mu l$	$40\,\mu l$	1 mmol/l

Method

Preparation

(1) Collect 20 ml blood into 3.8% Tri-Nacitrate. Collect patient and control blood. Spin for PRP (800–900 r/min for 20 minutes). Remove approximately 6 ml PRP. Spin remainder for PPP. Adjust platelets to 300×10^9/l, using PPP.

(2) Turn on aggregometer and recorder. Allow approximately 30 minutes to warm up. Check that temperature is 37 °C.

(3) Remove buffer and reagents from refrigerator/freezer. Use buffer at room temperature. Thaw reagents at room temperature and store on ice.

Notes: Do not store platelets on ice. Always use plastic or siliconized glassware.

Aggregating

Setting a range
Prepare cuvettes as follows:
   Concentrate: 0.3 ml PRP + 100 μl buffer. Using zero knob adjust pen to 90 line on the chart.
   Dilute: 0.3 ml PPP + 100 μl buffer. Using output knob adjust pen to 10 (represents total aggregation).

Repeat the above adjustments until a stable range is established. Mark the exact range on the chart. Once the range is set do not alter zero and output knobs during the aggregation. Recheck when aggregation is complete. Establish a range for each PRP to be aggregated.

The aggregation

To a cuvette add 0.3 ml PRP and the required volume of buffer (*see* Table above). Add a stirrer to the cuvette. Set chart paper running on 2 cm/min.

Allow cuvette to equilibrate in well approximately 1 minute. Add aggregating agent (*see* Table). Label point of addition – volume and reagent added. Run until aggregation is completed, i.e. plateau is reached. If only 1 phase adrenalin (or disaggregation) leave for 5 min. Repeat for each reagent using control and patient.

Calculation of results

(1) *Rate of aggregation* – measure the maximum rate of aggregation by ruling a straight line through the maximum aggregation rate to extent of 1 minute i.e. 2 chart divisions. Express as mm/min.

(2) *Extent of aggregation* – Measure the range of beginning and end of aggregation in mm. Average. Measure extent of aggregation, i.e. the distance from where the reagent is added to the plateau. Express as a % of range, i.e.

$$\frac{\text{Extent} \times 100\%}{\text{Range}}$$

The following Table shows the averaged results of 44 controls (± 2 SD)

	Rate (mm/min)	*Extent* %
ADP	149 ± 50	74 ± 11.6
Thrombin	142 ± 72	53 ± 20
Adrenalin 1st phase	44.2 ± 16.8	25 ± 7.7
2nd phase	70 ± 39	57 ± 14
Arachidonic acid	110 ± 51	84 ± 25
Collagen	139 ± 64	81 ± 23

Extra notes

If there is reduced or absent aggregation for a particular reagent repeat using 0.1 ml control PRP + 0.2 ml patient PRP. If it corrects use a lower proportion of control PRP.

If an arachidonic acid defect is being investigated the studies should be carried out using a control, and blood from a person who has taken aspirin and mixing carried out.

Combinations used:
Patient/Control   PRP/PRP (1:1 volume)
Patient/Aspirin   PRP/PRP (1:1 volume)

SPONTANEOUS AGGREGATION

Refer to section referring to aggregation techniques. Set up aggregation cuvette in usual manner with patient PRP. Allow to equilibrate, and add $40\,\mu l$ buffer, i.e. no aggregating agent. Start recorder. Allow to stir for at least 10 minutes. Observe for aggregation.

Hyperaggregation

Choose two aggregating agents, e.g. ADP, collagen. Perform aggregations at standard concentrations. Repeat aggregations diluting the reagent, 1/5, 1/10, 1/20, 1/30, etc. until no aggregation occurs.
Note: Continue with ADP only until no 2nd phase aggregation occurs.

SEROTONIN RELEASE DUE TO COLLAGEN

Reagents

(1) $0.075\,mol/l$ Na-EDTA, pH 6.7.

(2)   All reagents as used for routine aggregation studies.

(3)   Permablend scintillant 0.3 g Permablend III, 67 ml xylene, 33 ml conc. TritonX-100.

(4)   0.5% Triton, i.e. 0.5 ml TritonX-100 in 100 ml distilled H_2O.

   Note: Triton is very viscous.

(5)   [^{14}C]serotonin (Amersham) – 5-hydroxy-[2-^{14}C]tryptamine creatinine sulphate; $54\,\mu Ci/mmol$, $133\,\mu Ci/mg$, these specifications will vary with batches.
   Use $50\,\mu Ci$ dissolved in 6.25 ml 70% ethanol, i.e. $8\,\mu Ci/ml$ and $0.15\,mmol/l$.

Before you begin

Prepare four 'uptake' tubes, two for patient and two for control – $100\,\mu l$ aggregation buffer and $50\,\mu l$ $0.1\,mol/l$ EDTA, pH 6.7 in each tube.
   Prepare 23 'release' tubes with $50\,\mu l$ $0.1\,mol/l$ EDTA, pH 6.7 (i.e. 1 tube for reagent blank – remaining tubes for number of aggregations performed, equal number for patient and control).
   Use small clotting tubes that can be spun in the Sorvall.

For the patient

Allow 0.3 ml PRP for uptake tube (30 minutes and 60 minutes) and 11 'release tubes'. Similar quantity for a normal control. Approximately 8 ml PRP in each instance.

Method

Prepare PRP – adjust count to $300 \times 10^9/l$. Add approx. $10\,\mu l$ of stock [^{14}C]serotonin for each 2 ml of PRP used. Mix gently and stand at room temperature.

Uptake: 30 minutes after labelling transfer 0.3 ml PRP to an uptake tube. Mix and store on ice till the end of the experiment. Repeat at 60 minutes.

Release: These may be started no sooner than 40 minutes after labelling.

Prepare PRP and aggregometer as for routine aggregations. After 1 minute equilibration add aggregating agent. Stop release after exactly 5 minutes by transferring cuvette contents to a 'release' tube stored on ice (remove stirrer from cuvette).

Aggregating agents

As for routine aggregations include $20\,\mu l$ collagen, allow to mix and aggregate for 5 minutes.

Aggregation blank and total – $40\,\mu l$ aggregation buffer.

Reagent blank – $400\,\mu l$ aggregating buffer.

Take all samples **except total ^{14}C and reagent blank**. Remove stirrer using a magnet and spin in Sorvall 14000 r/min for 10 minutes at 4 °C. Pour off supernatant or mixed sample for ^{14}C total and reagent blank. Add to 5 ml Permablend Scintillant containing 0.5 ml 0.5% Triton. Count on ^{14}C channel for 10 minutes.

Store labelled PRP in small closed vessels. Leave samples for uptake at 37 °C, sub-sample at 30 and 60 minutes. Leave samples for release at room temperature.

Calculations

To calculate net c/min
(1) Subtract reagent blank from uptake samples.
(2) Subtract aggregation blank from release samples.

To calculate % uptake

$$\frac{\text{Net total c/min} - \text{net uptake at 30 min or 60 min} \times 100}{\text{Net total c/min (uptake)}}$$

To calculate % release

$$\frac{\text{Net c/min released (for each aggregation)} \times 100}{\text{Net total c/min (release)}}$$

A normal range should be established for each laboratory. Other aggregating agents can be used in place of collagen (see Table on page 242).

Uptake		Release				
30 min	60 min	ADP	Adrenalin	AA	Thrombin	Collagen
94% ±	93% ± 2	39% ± 11	48% ± 10	43% ± 23	51% ± 17	54% ± 10

PLATELET SURVIVAL

Method

(1) Obtain 1 unit of blood (same blood group and Rh type as patient) from Blood Bank or use patient's blood collected in a triple pack.

(2) Spin blood at *1000 r/min* for *12 minutes* in the IEC centrifuge, Model International PR-6 with pack containing blood in the middle at 24 °C.

(3) Carefully lift triple pack out of centrifuge bucket and place pack containing blood on clamp attached to a retort stand. Undo the two clamps on the tubing leading to the middle empty pack – the PRP will automatically flow into the empty pack. As soon as the red cells start to come through double clamp the tubing again.

(4) Inject approx. 10 ml Anticoagulant Citrate Dextrose (ACD)* (Solution A) into the bag now containing the PRP. Mix.

> *Citric acid anhydrous 7.3 g
> Sodium citrate dihydrate 22.0 g
> Dextrose monohydrate 24.5 g
> Sterile non-pyogenic water 1000 ml

(5) Spin pack at *2000 r/min* with bag containing PRP in the middle for 12 minutes.
Using a 10 ml syringe and a 19 gauge needle draw out ^{51}Cr liquid from bottles – easier to draw out if there is a bubble in the syringe. Recap the needle and release the bubble. Replace the needle with a 25 gauge needle.
Keep empty ^{51}Cr bottle for machine standard.

(6) Gently tip off PPP from middle pack to empty pack – do not tilt so far that bubble upsets platelet button. Clamp.

(7) With 25 gauge needle, inject ^{51}Cr into middle pack. Resuspend platelets in radioactive liquid by kneading the bag with fingers.
When injecting ^{51}Cr draw plunger back and forth or else pressure will cause the syringe to come away from the needle.

(8) Leave the radioactive platelet suspension to sit for approximately 25 minutes.

(9) Transfer non-radioactive PPP (NRA-PPP) into middle pack containing radioactive platelets leaving approx. 20 ml NRA-PPP in third pack. Clamp.

(10) Spin again at 2000 r/min for 12 minutes with the radioactive platelet suspension in the middle.

(11) Place middle pack on stand, pour off radioactive PPP into waste pack (pack containing red blood cells).

(12) Transfer 20 ml NRA-PPP to middle pack. Resuspend platelets in PPP by gently kneading the bag with fingers.

(13) Remove radioactive platelet suspension with 20 ml syringe and 19 gauge needle. After removal, replace needle and cap.

(14) Record the volume of the suspension. Remove a sample for counting (to use as a standard) into an Eppendorf tube.

(15) Inject suspension into patient using a 'butterfly' needle. Record the time.

(16) 18 ml blood samples are taken at 10 minutes and 1 hour after the injection on the first day.

On the following days blood can be taken once or twice a day depending on the circumstances.

Always take 18 ml blood samples, i.e. 2 ml 3.8% sodium citrate + 18 ml blood. The patient is taken for surface scan immediately after injection and once every other day.

Platelet washing procedure

Reagents needed:
Saline
1% ammonium oxalate
2% EDTA in saline. Disodium salt.

Wash platelets in gamma-counting tubes.*

(1) There will be two tubes of blood for each collection. Combine PRPs from two tubes for each collection separately.
Note: 100 μl of the standard should be washed at the same time.

(2) Wash red blood cells with saline (approx. 5 ml saline/tube), spin for PRP again.

(3) Combine PRP from saline wash with appropriate PRP samples.

(4) Record PRP volume and do a platelet count – calculate total platelets.

(5) Spin PRP hard, discard PPP.

*Include standard from this point, i.e. Take 100 μl of standard, wash in approximately 10 ml of washing solution as below. Use 200 μl if suspecting low yield.

(6)   Wash platelet button *once* with 1% ammonium oxalate (approx. 10 ml/tube).

(7)   Spin hard and discard supernatant.

(8)   Resuspend platelets in small volume of 2% EDTA in saline – when suspended make up to 10 ml with 2% EDTA in saline – pipette up and down.

(9)   Spin hard again, discard supernate and wash once more with 2% EDTA in saline.

(10)   Following washings, resuspend platelets in 1–2 ml distilled water.

(11)   Count samples in gamma counter for 10 minutes each.

Calculation

(1)   Calculate total number of platelets in original PRP.

(2)   Call the highest radioactive platelet count 100% (usually day 1, *see* Figure 10.1).

(3)   Work out percentage of platelets in other samples on the basis of (2).

(4)   Subtract the background counts from the other radioactive samples.

(5)   Adjust the counts according to the percentages of the corresponding platelet counts e.g.:

	Platelet count $\times 10^6$	*Gross counts* $-$ *background*	*Adjusted counts*
10 minutes	600 (100%)	10 000	10 000
1 hour	400	5 000	6 650

400×10^6 platelets is 67% of the platelets recovered at 10 minutes. 33% of $5000 = 1650$ must be added on to 5000 (approx. 6650) to make it comparable with the counts, in accordance with the adjustment of the radioactive platelet count to 100%.

(6)   Radioactive count at 10 minutes = 100%. Express the other counts as a percentage of the count at 10 minutes.

(7)   Draw a graph of radioactive counts ^{51}Cr (%) *vs.* time after injection (days).

(8)   Draw a line of best fit through the points and determine the half-life ($t\frac{1}{2}$) – that is, the point at which 50% intersects the line of best fit.

   $t\frac{1}{2}$ in normal range: 4.8–5.4 days. (Figure 10.1)

(9)   Calculate the *yield*

> Need – radioactive count for standard ($-$ background) and
> – rad. count for 10 minute sample ($-$ background)
> – body weight of patient (kg)

Example of calculation to obtain yield:
Standard equals 6500, 10 min $= 6400$, body weight $= 56$ kg.

Total amount of radioactivity (RA) injected
$6500 \times 10 \times 20 = 1\ 300\ 000$

where,

> 10 is the factor to convert the counts in $100\,\mu$l to those in 1 ml. In this case $100\,\mu$l of the standard was washed and counted, and 20 is the volume of the radioactive platelet suspension injected into the patient in ml.

Blood volume
$64 \times$ body weight (kg) $= 64 \times 56 = 3584$

Expected RA/ml blood

$$= \frac{\text{Total amount of RA injected}}{\text{blood volume}}$$

i.e. $\dfrac{1\ 300\ 000}{3584} = 363$

Recorded RA/ml blood

$$\frac{\text{RA count at 10 min}}{\text{Volume of blood taken (ml)}}$$

i.e. $\dfrac{6400}{18} = 356$

Therefore yield

$$= \frac{\text{Recorded RA/ml blood}}{\text{Expected RA/ml blood}}$$

i.e. $\dfrac{356}{363} \times 100 = 98\%$

Report as: Platelet half-life using ^{51}Cr
$T\frac{1}{2} = x$
Normal range 4.8–5.4 days
Yield at 10 min. 98%

References

DACIE, J. V. and LEWIS, S. M. (1975). *Practical Haematology*. 5th edn. (Edinburgh: Churchill Livingstone)

MACFARLANE, D. E., STIBBE, J., KIRBY, E. P., ZUCKER, M. B., GRANT, R. and McPHERSON, J. (1975). A method for assaying von Willebrand factor (ristocetin cofactor). *Thromb. Diath. Haemorr.*, **34**, 306

RICK, M. E. and HOYER, L. W. (1975). Molecular weight of human factor VIII procoagulant activity. *Thromb. Res.*, **7**, 909

WU, K. K. and HOAK, J. C. (1974). A new method for the quantitative detection of platelet aggregates in patients with arterial insufficiency. *Lancet*, **2**, 924

ZIMMERMAN, T. S., ABILDGAARD, C. F. and MEYER, D. (1979). The factor VIII abnormality in severe von Willebrand's disease. *N. Engl. J. Med.*, **301**, 1307

Index

251